THE CARDIAC CYCLE

THE CARDIAC CYCLE

M.I.M. NOBLE

PhD, MD, FRCP,
Senior Investigator, Midhurst Medical Research Institute;
Senior Lecturer in Medicine,
Charing Cross Hospital Medical School;
Consultant Physician,
King Edward VII Hospital, Midhurst and
Charing Cross Hospital, London

BLACKWELL SCIENTIFIC PUBLICATIONS
OXFORD LONDON EDINBURGH MELBOURNE

© 1979 by
Blackwell Scientific Publications
Editorial offices:
Osney Mead, Oxford, OX2 oEL
8 John Street, London, WC1N 2ES
9 Forrest Road, Edinburgh, EH1 2QH
214 Berkeley Street, Carlton
Victoria 3053, Australia

First published 1979

Printed and bound in Great Britain by
William Clowes (Beccles) Limited
Beccles and London

DISTRIBUTORS

USA
Blackwell Mosby Book Distributors
11830 Westline Industrial Drive
St. Louis, Missouri 63141
Canada
Blackwell Mosby Book Distributors
86 Northline Road, Toronto
Ontario, M4B 3E5
Australia
Blackwell Scientific Book
Distributors
214 Berkeley Street, Carlton
Victoria 3053

British Library
Cataloguing in Publication Data
Noble, M I M
    The cardiac cycle.
    1. Heart beat
    I. Title
    612'.17   QP113
    ISBN 0-632-00163-1

CONTENTS

PREFACE

The purpose of this book is to present some ideas, mostly recent, on the events of the cardiac cycle from the pacemaker to the peripheral pulse. When feeling the pulse, we are experiencing something which depends upon a whole train of events which I cover sequentially. The account is not by any means comprehensive and is not intended to be referred to for details of fact. These are covered by fuller texts of which the most recent is *The Mechanics of the Circulation* by Caro, Schroter, Pedley and Seed (1978).

Understanding of any subject does not, in my view, depend so much on the acquisition of more facts as on the development of ideas. One requires working hypotheses in order to design new experiments. We then try to see how well those ideas stand up to critical test. I have done my fair share of such necessary negative work. I hope to redress the balance here by putting up positive ideas for others to try and knock down.

Most of the ideas presented are not my own but are blatantly stolen from many generous friends and colleagues with whom I have been fortunate enough to collaborate. I have had the good luck to work in their widely scattered laboratories and freely acknowledge my debt to them. In Chapter 1, I present new ideas by Gerald Pollack (Seattle) on the mechanism of sinus and atrioventricular nodal function. Chapter 2 derives from a very fruitful recent association with Paul Edman (Lund) through whom I have been able to tap, in addition, the ideas of his young colleagues, Magnus Johannsson and Bjorn Wohlfart. These friends have provided me with the most useful framework I know for understanding force frequency relationships in the heart. Gerald Pollack helped again in Chapter 3 by introducing me to Tatsuo Iwazumi (Seattle). Iwazumi's refreshing views on the mechanism of contraction are brought up to date. In Chapters 4 and 5, I deal with the mechanics of ventricular contraction and its control. The approaches here are taken from the ideas of Lloyd Hefner (Alabama) and from my Dutch colleagues Gijs Elzinga, Gerald Van den Bos and Nico Westerhof (Amsterdam). In Chapter 6, I summarise some accumulated work over the years on steady state effects of changing heart rate and on diastolic pressure-volume relations; in the latter subject I have followed the thinking in Lloyd Hefner's earlier work on pressure-circumference relations.

My interest in the arterial system was first stimulated when I was taught as a student by Donald McDonald whose colleagues at that time were Michael Taylor and Derek Bergel. Donald McDonald (Alabama) has now died but his posthumously published book *Blood Flow in Arteries* remains the standard work on the subject. Donald MacDonald was very kind to me at various stages of my career and introduced me to Lloyd Hefner, who taught me muscle mechanics. Chapter 8 is dominated by the classic work of McDonald and Womersley. The ideas on the arterial system in Chapters 7 and 9 derive from Michael Taylor and from Nico Westerhof and Gerald Van den Bos.

My interest in these topics which led to such fruitful associations stemmed from my original involvement in cardiovascular research in 1962 at the instigation of Abe Guz from whom I have received encouragement ever since. My early experiments with Abe at Charing Cross Hospital Medical School are those of which I am still most proud; they continue to evoke in both of us unique feelings of nostalgia. We had at that time a valuable association with Diana Trenchard, now a close colleague at Midhurst. When I went to U.S.A. in 1966, I was immensely encouraged and helped at the Cardiovascular Research Institute, San Francisco, by Julius Comroe and Julien Hoffman who have also continued to encourage me to the present time.

I should acknowledge my debts to many other colleagues and co-workers. However, when writing a book, which can lead to fatal inaction in the research laboratory, I feel a special sense of obligation to my present co-workers Angela Drake and Demetrius Papadoyannis. The greatest forbearance, however, has been shown by my wife Sheila, who also undertook the mammoth task of typing the manuscript.

CHAPTER 1

THE ELECTRICAL CARDIAC CYCLE

This book principally concerns the mechanical events of the cardiac cycle. However, these events would not cycle at all without being driven by the repetitive electrical signal—the action potential. The distribution of the action potential through the heart is illustrated in Fig. 1.1. These features are well known but there are two which are of particular importance when considering the mechanical consequences, (1) the S-A node has a spontaneous rhythmicity; this provides the basic clock for the other events of the cardiac cycle, (2) the A-V node introduces a delay which allows effective mechanical contraction of atria followed by ventricles. These two features will therefore be discussed in greater detail than the others. The mechanisms are not understood and have recently been the subject of speculation by Pollack. His ideas are presented here.

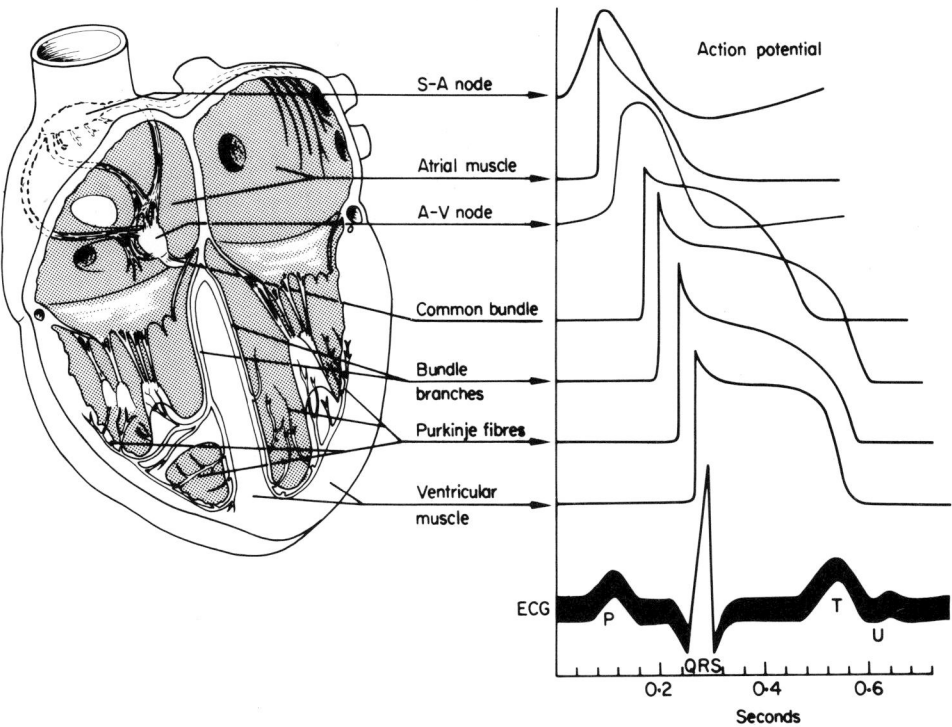

FIG. 1.1. Schematic representation of the sequence of excitation in the heart. The relationship to ECG is also shown (modified redrawing from the CIBA Collection of Medical Illustrations by Frank H. Netter, M.D.).

1

THE MECHANISM OF SINUS NODE RHYTHMICITY

We know that the sinus node pacemaker cells begin in diastole by being well polarised (-50 to -60 mV inside). This potential decreases gradually at first and then more rapidly until complete depolarisation occurs. It is not too difficult to understand why, once one cell or group of cells has done this, the surrounding cells follow (see below). Why does the first group of pacemaker cells spontaneously depolarise and then polarise again?

The potential difference across the cell membrane is maintained actively. The sodium–potassium (Na^+K^+) ATPase of the membrane ensures that the sodium ion concentration is high outside and low inside the cell; the opposite is true for potassium. Calcium (Ca^{++}), like Na^+ is kept at high concentration outside, low inside, probably through a linked mechanism. This active pumping results in the polarisation of the cell. Depolarisation occurs by an inward flow of positive ions, i.e. inward current, positive charges naturally going towards the negative intracellular potential. These ions may be Na^+, Ca^{++} or both. Repolarisation probably occurs by K^+ flowing outwards. In order that these currents can flow, changes must take place in the cell membrane so that ions which previously penetrated slowly because of high resistance (low conductance) can subsequently penetrate the cell quickly, i.e. the membrane conductance for that ion has increased. When we ask the question, 'Why does the sinus node cell spontaneously depolarise?' we are asking, 'What makes the cell membrane of the sinus node cell spontaneously change its conductance?'

Pollack's theory is that the cyclical change in the cell membrane depends on the action of catecholamines on the adenylate cyclase sytem of the membrane. (Fig. 1.2). Activation of this system increases the production of cyclic AMP which then activates protein kinase. Protein kinase catalyses the phosphorylation of membrane

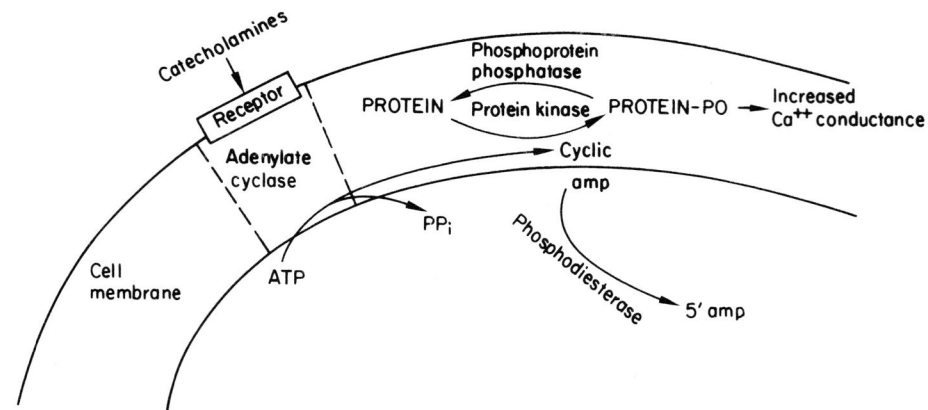

FIG. 1.2.   The mechanism by which catecholamines appear to increase calcium influx into the cell. (Modified from Greengard, 1976.)

proteins, opening calcium channels and allowing calcium ions to enter the cell. It is this inward Ca^{++} current that depolarises the cell membrane. In view of the interest aroused by this suggestion, I include here a fuller account of his ideas from Pollack.

A POSSIBLE MECHANISM OF SPONTANEOUS PACEMAKING

by G. H. POLLACK

Notwithstanding years of study, the mechanism by which the heartbeat is initiated remains uncertain; so uncertain, in fact, that Brooks and Lu (1972) in their excellent review concluded that the mechanism underlying spontaneous pacemaking in the sinus node remains a 'mystery.'

Actually, there appear to be two mysteries. The most obvious, perhaps, is the mechanism by which each of the many cells in the sinus node depolarises and repolarises spontaneously during each heartbeat. The more subtle, but equally intriguing mystery is the manner by which the independent activities of individual cells are coordinated such that the sinus node does not issue forth a barrage of independent, uncoordinated signals to the heart, but an effectively synchronous burst.

Some avenues of approach to the solution of these two mysteries have recently been offered (Pollack 1977). Here, in a more informal way, I would like to recapitulate some of the important pieces of evidence which have led to the formulation of these hypotheses, describe the hypotheses, explore their physiological consequences, and finally touch on their possible implication *vis à vis* the genesis of certain cardiac arrhythmias.

Clues

That catecholamines exert a powerful modulatory influence on pacemaking frequency has been evident for many years. In the mid-fifties, with the advent of microelectrodes, the positive chronotropic action of catecholamines was demonstrated to arise out of an enhancement of the rate of spontaneous depolarisation of the pacemaker cells (Hutter & Trautwein 1956, West *et al.* 1956). It now appears that this modulatory effect on the rate of spontaneous depolarisation is perhaps only one aspect of a more fundamental role; catecholamines may, in fact, be *required* for the generation of spontaneous depolarisation.

Before considering the evidence for this, it is relevant to note that catecholamine stores in the sinus node are not restricted to sympathetic nerve terminals. In dog hearts that had been denervated both surgically and chemically (with 6-hydroxy-dopamine), the sinus node was found to have retained about half the epinephrine present in non-denervated controls (Spurgeon *et al.* 1974). The authors implicated an extraneural storage site, possibly in cells analogous to the catecholamine containing chromaffin cells of the adrenal medulla. Fluorescence histochemical studies (Miyagishima 1975) confirm a rather widespread distribution of catecholamines in the sinus node; the distribution pattern is consistent with localisation within *each* pacemaking cell. Intracellular storage would not be surprising in the light of the 'conspicuously numerous' subsarcolemmal vesicles found in these cells (James *et al.* 1966), vesicles also seen by other investigators (Ruska 1965, Trautwein & Uchizono 1963, Challice 1966, Cheng 1971, Viragh & Porte 1973) and described by some as bearing structural similarity to those in the chromaffin cells of the adrenal medulla that store catecholamines.

That the presence of endogenous catecholamines is *required* for pacemaking has been demonstrated in a series of elegant studies by Tuganowski and colleagues. Tuganowski *et al.* (1973) exposed isolated rabbit sinoatrial node to reserpine, an agent which depletes catecholamine stores. Reserpine (10 μM) reduced the spontaneous rate and brought beating to a halt in 5 to 25 minutes. When catecholamines were added to the bath containing the reserpine, beating resumed within 1 to 3 minutes. In another series of experiments the node was exposed to α-methyl tyrosine (1 mM), a specific inhibitor of catecholamine synthesis. Spontaneous activity ceased in 1 to 4 hours. When catecholamines were added to this bath, beating resumed in 2 to 5 minutes. Although these results implicate a catecholamine requirement in pacemaking, the investigators considered the alternative possibility that the termination of spontaneous activity was not due to catecholamine depletion but to some indirect or non-specific effect of these inhibitors. When the preparations were pretreated with reserpine to deplete catecholamine stores, and washed with fresh Tyrode's solution to restore beating, the time required for α-methyl tyrosine to inhibit beating was reduced 100-fold. This provided powerful evidence that these agents did indeed inhibit beating by depleting endogenous catecholamines.

More recently, the catecholamine requirement has been underscored by the observation that inhibition of adenylate cyclase, the enzyme responsible for catalysing the formation of the 'second messenger' of catecholamines, cAMP, abolished pacing. Exposure of the isolated sinus node to haloperidol or chloropromazine was found to inhibit spontaneous activity (Tuganowski 1977). These effects could be reversed by exposure of the preparation to dibutyryl cyclic AMP, a derivative of cAMP which can diffuse through the plasma membrane. Thus, both catecholamines and cyclic AMP, the first two elements in the beta adrenergic pathway, not only modulate spontaneous activity, but appear to be *required* in some way for pacemaking to occur.

A possible role of endogenous catecholamines

Although the storage site of catecholamines appears to be located *within* the cell, the action of catecholamines on pacemaker (and other) cells is on the *outside* of the membrane (Yamasaki *et al.* 1974, Lefkowitz *et al.* 1973, Reuter 1974). If endogenous catecholamines play an obligatory role in pacemaking, a way must be identified for the catecholamines to leave the cell. Diffusion is the simplest possibility. On the other hand, the numerous exocytic figures seen on the membranes of these pace-making cells (James *et al.* 1966) raises the intriguing possibility that the catechol-amines are stored within the subsarcolemmal vesicles, and discharged from the cell into the extracellular space by exocytosis. The discharge process would then be analogous to that found in neurosecretory tissues.

Could catecholamine discharge and subsequent binding to the outside of the plasma membrane lead to spontaneous pacemaking? This appears possible. Consider first the elements involved in catecholamine discharge. There is little doubt that intracellular Ca^{++} is required, since Ca^{++} influx into the cell is a necessary condition for exocytosis in perhaps all neurosecretory systems studied so far (Douglas 1968, Cochrane *et al.* 1975). Ca^{++} entry also tends to depolarise the cell. Although the complexity of the mechanism by which Ca^{++} entry mediates vesicle discharge presumably transcends mere cellular depolarisation (Dean 1975), there nevertheless appears to be a good correlation between cellular depolarisation and vesicle discharge rate. In the neuromuscular junction, perhaps the best studied secretory system, the rate of discharge varies exponentially with the degree of cellular depolarisation (del Castillo & Katz 1954). Even when the presynaptic cell is fully polarised (about -90 mV), there remains some random, spontaneous discharge of vesicles, the manifestation of which is the miniature end plate potential. As an initial supposition, it seems reasonable to assume that if vesicle discharge did, indeed, occur from sinus node cells, the properties of the discharge system would be similar to those described above. Principally, this means that the rate of cate-cholamine discharge from the cell increases as the cell is depolarised by Ca^{++} entry.

Second, consider the action of the binding of catecholamines to the outside of the cell membrane. Among the most fundamental actions is the increase of calcium flux into the cell (Grossman & Furchgott 1964, Reuter 1965). This appears to occur through the beta-adrenergic pathway, illustrated in Fig. 1.2. Catecholamines stimulate the production of cAMP by activation of adenylate cyclase; this causes phosphorylation of a membrane protein, which results in an increase of calcium conductance (Greengard 1976, Wollenberger 1975).

In view of the fact that an ultimate action of catecholamines is the promotion of Ca^{++} influx, and an action of Ca^{++} influx is the promotion of catecholamine discharge, which in turn increases the availability of catecholamines for further action on the outside of the membrane, one has at hand the elements of a positive feedback, or regenerative, system. Spontaneous depolarisation and repolarisation could then occur by the following scheme (Fig. 1.3a):

(i) Vesicles begin discharging catecholamines spontaneously into the extra-cellular space; the discharge rate is low at first because the cell is relatively polarised (-50 to -60 mV), and intracellular Ca^{++} is relatively low.

(ii) Catecholamines discharged into the extracellular space diffuse away from the discharge site; those molecules which bind to the outside of the cell membrane activate adenylate cyclase, thereby increasing cAMP, bringing about the phosphory-lation of membrane proteins, and transiently opening calcium channels; this allows Ca^{++} to enter and further depolarise the cell.

(iii) The more the cell is depolarised by Ca^{++} entry, the higher the rate of catecholamine discharge; this positive feedback loop results in a depolarisation which has the shape of a rising exponential; ultimately all catecholamines in the releasable pool are discharged.

(iv) With no further catecholamine-mediated adenylate cyclase activity, cAMP returns to baseline levels, and there is no further opening of calcium channels; thus the cell stops depolarising.

(v) As the cell repolarises by Ca^{++} extrusion, the vesicles reform and are replenished with catecholamines; when replenishment is adequate, spontaneous discharge commences and the cycle begins once again.

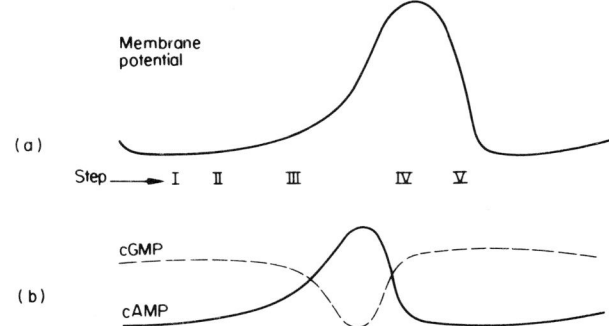

F IG. 1.3.   (a) The time course of the pacemaker potential in primary pacemaking cells. The cycle is broken into five phases, during which the events described in the text may take place. (b) The time course of the concentration of intracellular cyclic AMP expected from the proposed model. Reciprocal fluctuation of cyclic GMP may also occur as it does in another cardiac tissue.

This scheme accounts for the obligatory role of the beta adrenergic pathway in pacemaking. If catecholamines are depleted, or if adenylate cyclase activity is blocked, pacemaking stops; exogenous catecholamines can restore beating by supplementing endogenous stores. Beating can also be stopped by any agent which hyperpolarises the cell (e.g. acetylcholine) to the point where the rate of spontaneous discharge becomes inadequate to initiate the cycle.

An important implication of the proposed scheme is that the concentration of cAMP is expected to oscillate during the pacemaking cycle, as shown in Fig. 1.3b. During steps (i) and (ii) and most of step (iii), the level of cAMP increases, since catecholamine-mediated adenylate cyclase activity increases. When further catechol-amine binding ceases, cAMP production is no longer stimulated. Phosphodiesterase activity then breaks down cAMP and causes a diminution of the pool. Baseline levels of cAMP are reached during step (iv), and with no further adenylate cyclase activity, cAMP remains at this level until the cycle begins again.

Although the concentrations of cyclic AMP during the cardiac cycle have not yet been measured in pacemaker tissue, they have been found to oscillate in frog ventricular tissue (Brooker 1973, Wollenberger *et al.* 1973). In these studies the level of cyclic AMP increased in the early part of the cycle, returned approximately to baseline levels prior to repolarisation and remained there until the beginning of the following cycle, a time course similar to the one in the proposed scheme (Fig. 1.3b).

Maintenance of stable cycling requires that the processes mediating depolarisation be prevented from occurring during the phase of repolarisation; thus Ca^{++} influx must not be allowed to occur beyond step (iii). While this can be achieved in the scheme through phosphodiesterase-mediated diminution of the cyclic AMP level, two additional factors may augment this mechanism and thereby enhance cycling stability.

The first is the acceleration of phosphodiesterase activity during step (iii). The relatively low activity found at low Ca^{++} concentrations increases when the Ca^{++} concentration is elevated above 1 μM to a greatly enhanced activity at 10 μM (Teo & Wang 1973). Because there is good reason (though no conclusive evidence) to believe that intracellular Ca^{++} rises to these concentrations at the peak of the cardiac cycle (Katz 1970, Winegrad 1971), it is possible that a greatly enhanced phosphodiesterase activity in step (iii) may drive cyclic AMP down to baseline levels rapidly.

The second factor may involve cyclic GMP, the other important cyclic nucleotide found in the cardiac cell. In accordance with the so-called 'yin-yang' hypothesis (Goldberg *et al.* 1973) cyclic GMP antagonises the action of cyclic AMP. This probably occurs by dephosphorylation of proteins through activation of phosphoprotein phosphatase (Sandoval & Cuatrecasas 1976). The intracellular concentration of cyclic GMP oscillates during the cardiac cycle of frog ventricle with a time course similar, but in the opposite direction to that of cyclic AMP (Wollenberger *et al.* 1973); this may occur through the conversion of one cyclic nucleotide into the other (Simon 1976). Should cyclic GMP and cyclic AMP fluctuate reciprocally in pacemaker cells as well (Fig. 1.3b) the effect of the cyclic GMP fluctuations would be to enhance phosphorylation at the time in the cycle that the processes mediating Ca^{++} influx required activation (steps (i) to (iii)), and to prevent phosphorylation at the time these processes required inhibition (steps (iv) and (v)). Oscillations of cyclic GMP, if they occurred, would therefore serve to increase cycling stability.

Elements of the pacemaking cycle which are least clear are those occurring in step (v). Repolarisation might occur by a delayed efflux of K^+ as it does in many other cells; a $K^+ - Ca^{++}$ pump would then be required to maintain steady-state concentrations of these ions. A simpler possibility is that repolarisation occurs as a direct consequence of Ca^{++} being pumped out of the cytosol. A Ca^{++}-dependent ATPase is known to exist in the membrane of the catecholamine vesicles of chromaffin cells (Kirschner 1974), and an analogous one might exist in vesicles of the sinus node. If the process of exocytosis involves a continual turnover of vesicle

membrane and plasma membrane (Heuser & Reese 1973), then a Ca^{++}-dependent
ATPase should also exist in the cell membrane; this could mediate Ca^{++} extrusion
from the cell. This area requires further study.

Pharmacologic tests of the proposed scheme

Figure 1.4 shows the elements of the proposed scheme in some detail. Listed
towards the left of the figure are the various classes of agents expected to stimulate

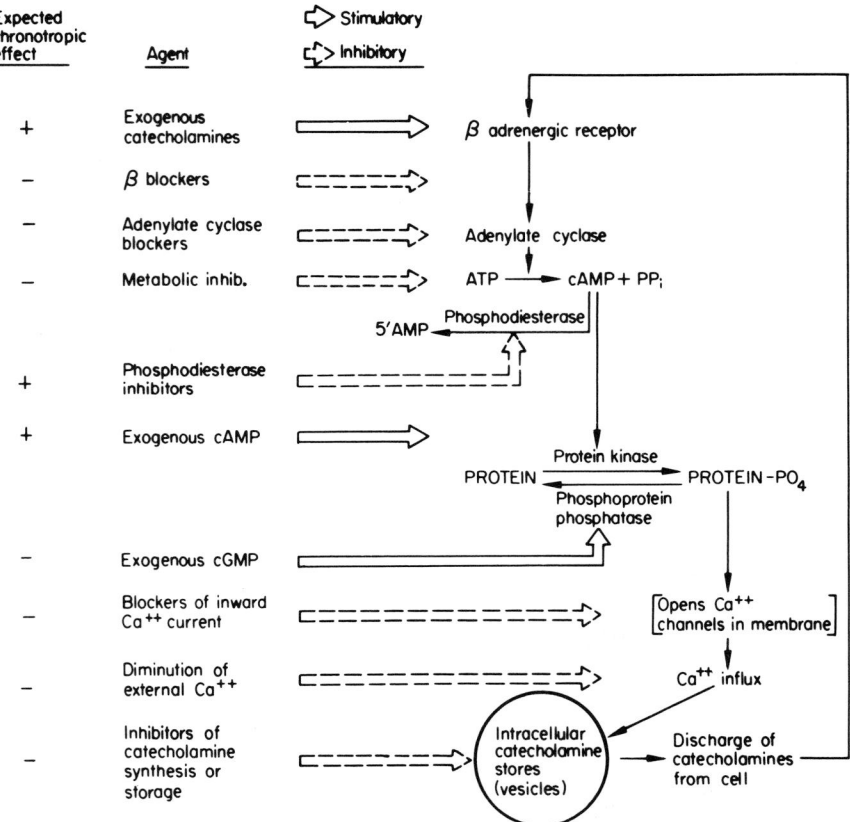

FIG. 1.4. Details of the proposed mechanism of generation of the pacemaker potential.
By inhibiting or accelerating certain processes, the agents listed at the left of the figure should
give rise to increases or decreases of pacing frequency. The expected responses are confirmed
experimentally, as detailed in the text and in the paper by Pollack (1977).

or inhibit certain of the processes along the proposed pathway. The expected effect
on beating frequency of each of these is indicated at the far left. For example,
phosphodiesterase inhibitors (such as caffeine or theophylline) should increase the
amount of cAMP, thereby accelerating spontaneous depolarisation and increasing
beating frequency. Exogenous cyclic GMP, either added directly, or indirectly

through administration of acetylcholine (George *et al.* 1973), should activate phosphoprotein phosphatase, diminishing the degree of protein phosphorylation and Ca^{++} influx, thereby diminishing spontaneous rate.

The actions of some of the agents listed in Fig. 1.4 have been discussed above. A fuller treatment is found elsewhere (Pollack 1977). In general, all agents listed in Fig. 1.4 exert a chronotropic effect which is in the expected direction. While this by no means proves that the hypothesis is valid, it indicates that it is at least a reasonable working hypothesis.

Synchronisation and population dynamics

The second 'mystery' of cardiac pacemaking is the mechanism underlying intercellular synchronisation. Many pacemaker cells comprise the sinus node. Each one begins depolarising at a rate largely independent of the other pacemaking cells, so that there is a spectrum of initial rates of depolarisation ranging from the fastest (primary) to the slower (secondary, latent, or follower) pacemaking cells (Hoffman & Cranefield 1960). But such evidently independent cellular activity does not last throughout the pacemaking cycle; as the primary pacemaker cell undergoes full, regenerative depolarisation, the secondary pacemaking cells are soon made to follow suit, so that a synchronous output emerges from the sinus node to the atrium.

How is the 'turn-on' signal communicated from the primary pacemaking cell to latent pacemaking cells? One possibility is that communication is electrically mediated, i.e. by way of currents flowing between cells. In most cardiac tissues gap junctional channels interconnect contiguous cells, channels which are widely held to represent the sites of current flow between cells (Dewey & Barr 1962, McNutt & Weinstein 1970). Thus depolarisation of one cell establishes a potential gradient between contiguous cells, thereby driving current through the gap junctional channels; this depolarises the contiguous cells sufficiently that they reach threshold, fire, and sustain propagated activity. There is some evidence based upon voltage clamp studies (Noma & Irisawa 1976, Brown, Giles & Noble 1977) and upon measurements of space constant (Bonke 1973) that sinus node cells communicate electrically; however, other considerations indicate that whatever electrical communication might exist is probably far too weak to sustain propagation through the sinus node.

One consideration is based on the very fact that during the phase of spontaneous depolarisation the pacemaking cells depolarise at different rates. Long lasting potential gradients of substantial magnitude develop between neighbouring pacemaker cells during this period (Fig. 1.5), an observation difficult to reconcile with the presumption of tight electrical coupling. Along similar lines of thought, the maximum diastolic potential in sinus node cells is lower than the resting potential in nearby atrial cells, raising once again the question of how such long-lasting gradients could be sustained if the cells were tightly coupled.

Morphologically, the cellular architecture does not lend itself well to electrical

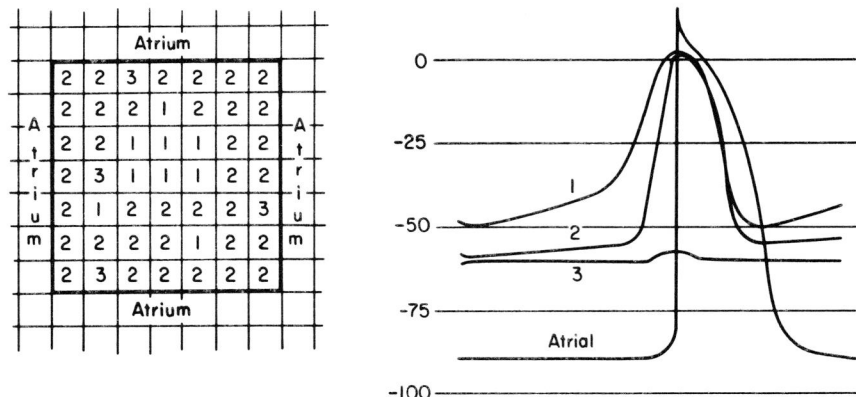

FIG. 1.5. *Left* Schematic representation of the arrangement of pacemaking cells in the sinus node. Primary pacemaking cells (1) are located generally, but not exclusively, near the center of the sinus node. Latent or secondary pacemaking cells (2) are located closer to the periphery of the node. Some cells may show no regenerative activity (3). *Right* Observed waveshapes of depolarization among the various types of cell.

coupling. The gap junctional channels of intercellular communication are rare or absent in the sinus node (James *et al.* 1966, Cheng 1971, Viragh & Porte 1973). This does not rule out the possibility that another type of intercellular communication channel peculiar to the sinus node might one day be identified; however, its properties would have to be remarkable. The required intercellular conductance would have to be much higher than between, say, atrial cells in order that the high intercellular currents required to sustain propagation could flow. Sinus cells are remarkably insensitive to depolarising current, some cells failing to respond to depolarising currents raised to levels sufficient to destroy the cell (Ushiyama & Brooks 1974).

A possibility worth considering is one in which communication occurs mechanically. For example, it has been proposed that propagation through the A-V node occurs by a stretch-induced depolarization mechanism (see below): proximal cells are excited, depolarise, contract, and thereby stretch more distally placed cells. Stretch depolarises these latter cells, causing them to contract and stretch cells which are still more distally placed, and so on (Pollack 1974). Could such a mechanism apply in the sinus node?

The required contractile machinery is present in sinus node cells, though the myofilament packing density is relatively lower than in 'working' myocardium (James *et al.* 1966). Contractile activity of the sinus node has been observed and measured (Irisawa & Noma 1976). Since the primary pacemaking cells depolarise first, presumably they also contract first. Neighbouring latent pacemaker cells, as yet unactivated, should offer little resistance to stretch; if stretch could abruptly accelerate their slow spontaneous rate of depolarisation, propagation could be sustained. In such a way an excitation signal from a primary pacemaking cell could propagate through the sinus node and synchronise the action of the constituent pacemaking cells.

Pacemaking cells do appear to be sensitive to stretch. For example, in mammalian sinus node stretch increases the frequency of discharge (Deck 1964); this effect is mediated by an increase in the rate of spontaneous depolarisation. This action can be sufficiently strong to induce spontaneous depolarisation in those cells within the sinus node in which activity had been absent prior to stretch (Brooks & Lu 1972). In cells of many species throughout the animal kingdom, particularly in the more primitive phyla, the distension caused by filling of the cardiac chambers is often the physiologic 'trigger' of pacing; i.e. unless sufficiently stretched some pacemakers will not pace.

Returning to the proposed mechanism of spontaneous pacemaking, we can identify a possible mechanism by which stretch might accelerate depolarisation. Consider, again, the analogy to other vesicle discharge systems. At the myoneural junction, where the effect of stretch is best documented, stretch increases the presynaptic vesicle discharge rate (Hutter & Trautwein 1956). The action is instantaneous (Ypey 1975), and the sensitivity to stretch is exquisite: stretch of 10–15%, depending upon the frequency of stimulation, increases the probability of vesicle discharge by five to ten times (Ijpeij *et al.* 1974).

If an analogous situation existed in pacemaking cells, the means by which stretch induces depolarisation would be evident. Stretch of a latent pacemaking cell would provoke a more intense discharge of catecholamines, thereby providing the means by which its rate of depolarisation could be accelerated. Through such a mechanism the action of the latent cells could be synchronised to the action of the more primary cells.

One powerful feature of such a communication mechanism is its inherent safeness. As the number of depolarised cells increases, a progressively larger fraction of the cells stretches the remaining diminishing fraction; consequently the 'gain' increases progressively. Once a critical fraction of the cells is contracting, stretch of the remaining cells should be sufficiently vigorous for their full activation to be inevitable. Synchronisation is thereby achieved by an effectively regenerative mechanism. Yet the safeness inherent in the redundancy of multiple independent pacemaking cells is retained. If the communication occurs this way, nature will have created an elegant mechanism.

The stretch mechanism explains the paradox of independent cellular behaviour during the early phase of the cycle, but highly coordinated behaviour later in the cycle. During the early phase, the cells are sufficiently polarised that contraction would not be expected to occur; consequently, synchronisation is effectively turned off, and the cells behave independently. Later in the cycle, as cells depolarise further and the communication mechanism turns on, the independent behaviour of individual cells gives way to synchronised behaviour.

The mechanism also accounts for the fact that the speed of propagation through the sinus node is about two orders of magnitude lower than through cardiac tissues where intercellular propagation is electrically mediated (Sano & Yamagishi 1965). Propagation by stretch is limited in speed by the time required to activate the myofilaments and by the maximum velocity with which the cells can contract, factors which are not relevant in electrically mediated propagation.

Arrhythmias

Sinus arrhythmias, according to the proposed hypothesis, can be caused either through some action on the mechanism of spontaneous cellular depolarisation, or through some action on the mechanism of intercellular synchronisation. Sinus tachycardia, often the result of excessive sympathetic drive, is readily explained in terms of increased supply of catecholamines. Sinus bradycardia, usually the result of excessive vagal tone, is explained in terms of the inhibitory effect of acetylcholine, as described above.

The cyclic variation of heart rate during the repiratory cycle—an increase during inspiration and a decrease during expiration—is generally attributed to cyclic variations of vagal tone. An alternative possibility stems from the direct effect of stretch. The sinus node is probably stretched during inspiration as a result of the reduced intrathoracic pressure, and consequently should depolarise more rapidly and discharge at a relatively elevated frequency.

'Sick sinus syndrome,' otherwise known as sinus block, is possibly the manifestation of diminished efficacy of communication. It is a condition in which not every depolarisation generated by primary pacemaking cells propagates sufficiently to reach the atrium. According to the hypothesis, the efficacy of communication depends upon the vigour of contraction, the susceptibility to stretch, and the level of catecholamines in the latent pacemaking cells. Sick sinus syndrome often occurs in the elderly, where contractile strength may be reduced, where increased connective tissue deposition is likely to limit cellular stretch, and where diminished enzymatic activity could reduce the rate of catecholamine synthesis.

The conditions leading to sinus block should be pharmacologically evocable by agents which impair contractility, inhibit catecholamine synthesis, or block catecholamine discharge. The effects of some of these agents have already been explored. Impaired communication results from the application of acteylcholine, vagal stimulation, Mn^{++}, electrical overdrive, hypothermia, propranolol and reserpine, (Brooks & Lu 1972, Bouman *et al.* 1968, Sano & Yamagishi 1965, Lu *et al.* 1965). Conversely synchronisation is improved by stretch (Brooks & Lu 1972), an agent which should increase both contractility and the rate of vesicle discharge.

Could stretch be a useful clinical tool to alleviate sick sinus syndrome?

PROPAGATION OF ELECTRICAL IMPULSES IN THE HEART

The electrical impulse is generated in the S-A node by an as yet undetermined mechanism for which Pollack has made a postulate (above). This is as yet unproved and designed to stimulate further research. Now we turn to the question—how it is that the electrical impulse may move throughout each cell (intracellular conduction) and from one cell to the next (intercellular conduction).

Intracellular conduction of impulses

If a nerve or muscle cell is stimulated and a depolarisation induced at any point, that depolarisation will be conducted throughout the whole cell. The mechanism in heart muscle is similar to that in nerve in which, in the region of the depolarisation, the transmembrane potential is reversed (Fig. 1.6). Since the fluid medium on either

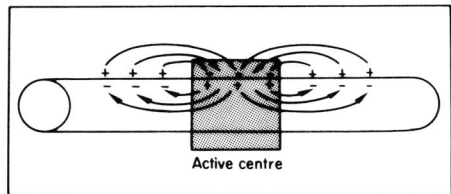

Active centre

FIG. 1.6. Movement of charged particles around the active centre of a cell.

side of the membrane is a conductor, an electrical gradient will be created between the adjacent oppositely charged regions of the membrane which will tend to cause the charged particles to move. Hence on the outer surface of the fibre, positive ions will be attracted into the negative region. This means that the transmembrane potential of the regions from which these now come will be reduced until these neighbouring segments of the membrane also reach their firing potential. Hence the depolarisation will be propagated in both directions from the point of stimulation.

Similarly, if we visualise a three dimensional structure it is obvious that the depolarisation will be propagated in all directions forming concentric spheres of depolarisation about the point of stimulation.

Movement of an impulse is always unidirectional, however, since once it is moving in one direction, the region from which it has just come will be refractory and thus relatively unexcitable.

In addition, the refractory area, which is still partly depolarised, will be a less plentiful source of ions for the local currents. Most of the ions which move into the

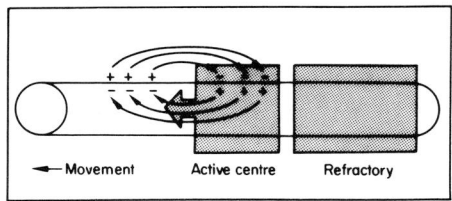

◄—Movement   Active centre   Refractory

FIG. 1.7. Constraint on the movement of charged particles around the active centre due to the presence of a refractory zone. As a result the active centre continues to move in the same direction.

depolarised area will therefore have to come from in front of the action potential. The electrical field caused by the action potential will thus be 'concentrated' in front of the depolarised area and this assists its propagation in that direction (Fig. 1.7).

In this way the depolarisation spreads across the whole surface area of the membrane, whatever its shape. When two active centres meet, for example travelling in different directions around the circumference of a spherical cell, the depolarisation

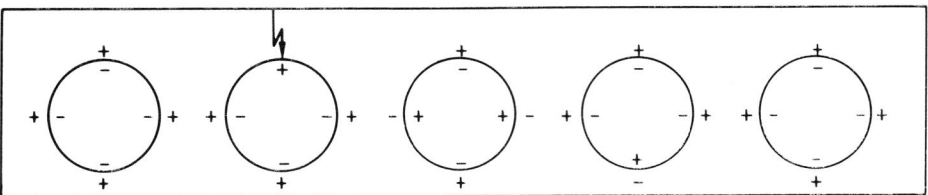

FIG. 1.8.   Two active centres traversing the surface of the cell in opposite directions will annihilate one another as they meet because they are now surrounded by refractory membrane.

cannot progress any further since it is surrounded by refractory membrane (Fig. 1.8). The impulse thus decays unless it is possible for it to be transmitted to another neighbouring cell.

Intercellular conduction of impulses

Under most circumstances it would be most disadvantageous for impulses to move from one cell to another since this would mean that a depolarisation in any nerve would be propagated throughout the nervous system, and similarly a depolarisation in any muscle cell would be propagated throughout the whole muscle mass and into neighbouring nerves or muscles. Thus a stimulus anywhere would lead to an uncontrollable epileptic convulsion. However, there are many situations where intercellular conduction is essential, such as between a nerve cell and the muscle cell which it innervates or between one nerve cell and the next in a line of communication. In these particular situations a chemical intercellular messenger is used, e.g. acetylcholine or noradrenaline.

In the heart the individual myocardial cells are not separately innervated and hence must be stimulated by conduction from their neighbours. The intercellular transmission of impulses in the heart occurs because the cells are joined to each other by special structures called intercalated discs (Fig. 1.9). These junctions allow the cells to be structurally separate but provide pathways of very low resistance between the cells so that ions may pass freely. Thus the action potential may be propagated from one cell through the discs to its neighbours. Since electrical impulses can therefore travel freely throughout the myocardial muscle mass, the heart is often described as being a 'functional syncytium'.

Although such cell to cell conduction occurs extensively in the heart, the presence of the anatomical conduction system enables many points in the myocardium to be

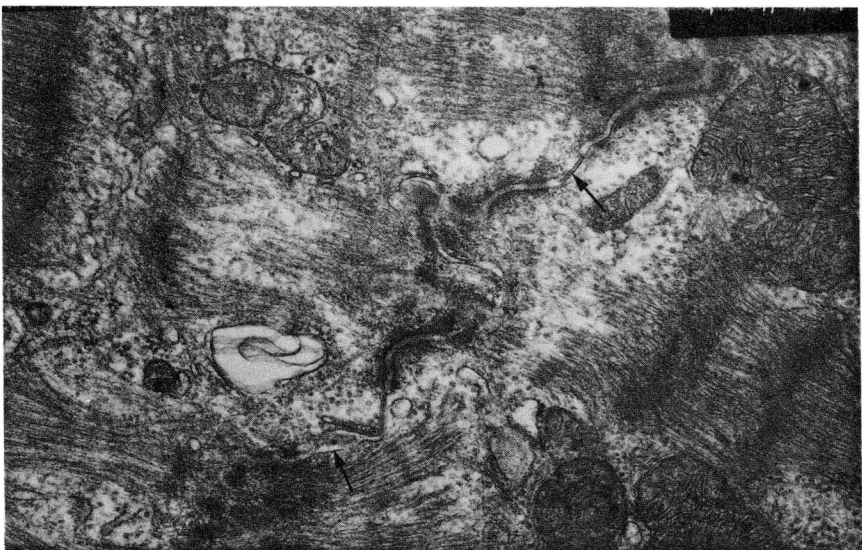

FIG. 1.9. Electronmicrograph showing intercalated disc ensuring good electrical communication between cells, particularly at specialised junctions (arrowed).

stimulated within a very short interval. In addition, the conduction system synchronises these various points in the myocardium to the 'master timer' such that the relevant time delays are introduced (Fig. 1.1).

Thus we can see how the impulse is propagated and the correct timing achieved. The most crucial timing is the atrio-ventricular sequence which requires the main delay provided by the A-V node. Propagation through the A-V node is a special case which will be considered in a later section.

Microelectrodes inserted into cells of the conduction system other than the A-V node show that they undergo a sequence of changes which result in regular depolarisations. The events in the membrane accompanying these action potentials will be discussed later. It can be shown that the resting membrane potential is unstable in cells of the conducting system (some specialised atrial cells, Purkinje fibres) and decays progressively until it reaches its firing potential. Following each depolarisation it returns to its resting potential but once again this is unstable and decays and the cycle thus repeats itself (Fig. 1.10).

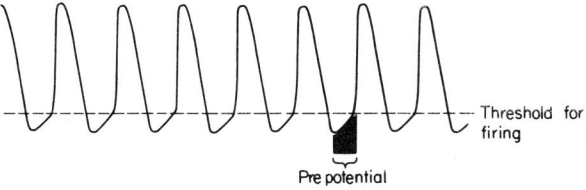

Threshold for firing

Pre potential

FIG. 1.10. Cell in the conducting system with unstable diastolic potential (pre-potential) and firing potential (threshold level for rapid complete depolarisation).

The phase between the resting and firing potentials is termed the pre-potential. The slope of the pre-potential in these cells defines their intrinsic rate of spontaneous firing, since the steeper the slope, the sooner the firing potential is reached. The origin of this slope is not known for certain. It is affected by many factors such as changes in temperature and the prevailing levels of catecholamines. This tendency of many cells in the conduction system to depolarise spontaneously before the onset of the action potential means that there are a multitude of potential pacemakers in the heart in addition to the sinus node. These take over the role of actual pacemaker should the sinus node fail.

How then is it possible to synchronise the heart to just one pacemaker, and which one will it be? The solution to this problem becomes apparent when one appreciates that cells in the conducting system outside the S-A and A-V nodes may be depolarised by an electrical stimulus coming from any direction. Thus if two pacemaker cells with unequal rates are connected to one another, the one with the faster rate will cause the slower one to depolarise at the same rate (Fig. 1.11). The S-A node, which is the pacemaker with the fastest intrinsic rate of depolarisation and repolarisation will control the heart unless for any reason another group of cells starts to depolarise at a faster rate.

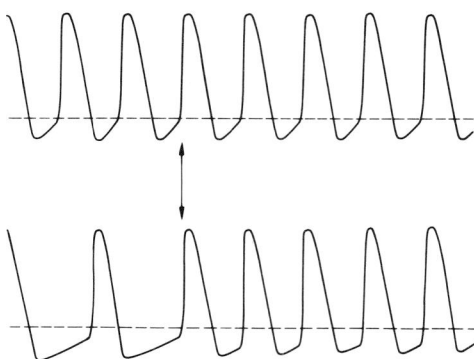

FIG. 1.11.   Upper conducting cell has faster intrinsic rate than lower. When connected at arrows, the slower cell is triggered and takes on the rate of the faster. Their differing pre-potential slopes remain unchanged but the effective firing potential in the lower trace is reduced.

A-V nodal transmission

The mechanism of propagation of the impulse in the conducting system described above, i.e. local current flow from depolarised to non-polarised cells is unlikely to apply to the A-V node in which conduction is very much slower than in atrial cells, Purkinje cells or working ventricular cells. The sites generally thought to be responsible for current pathways between working myocardial cells and between Purkinje cells are notably rare and possibly absent among cells deep in the A-V node, i.e. between 'N' cells. The scarcity of these low resistance gap junctions is suggestive of an impediment to intercellular current flow. Quantitative considerations based on the rate of passage of fluorescein dye between N cells indicate that they may not be sufficiently well coupled to permit impulse propagation through the A-V node by intercellular current flow alone (Pollack 1976). Another consideration is that, in contrast to working myocardial or Purkinje cells, the low rate of rise and magnitude of the depolarisation in N cells would further limit the availability of current to depolarise a contiguous quiescent N cell. Finally, in the face of low cell to cell current flow, the current required for threshold depolarisation in N cells is reported to be at least an order of magnitude higher than in most other cardiac tissues.

In those cardiac tissues where propagation is clearly by intercellular current flow (see above), a tenfold increase of intercellular resistance or current required for depolarisation would inhibit propagation. In the A-V node, where these impediments appear to sum to a higher order of magnitude, it is difficult to view propagation by local currents as the certain mechanism.

Another relevant observation is the consistently lower resting membrane potential recorded in nodal cells compared with surrounding myocardial cells. If substantial electrical communication pathways existed between nodal and surrounding cells, the nodal cells would act necessarily as a source of continuous current flow into these surrounding cells. A growing ionic imbalance would result unless some hypothetical restorative mechanism were assumed. On the other hand, if nodal cells were electrically insulated, as electron microscope evidence suggests, no such mechanism need be postulated.

In order to overcome these difficulties, Pollack has put forward another hypothesis which is given below.

HYPOTHETICAL ELECTROMECHANICAL MECHANISM FOR A-V NODAL TRANSMISSION

by G. H. POLLACK

The postulated mechanism of nodal transmission is based on the assumption that upon being stretched, nodal (N) cells depolarise somewhat like stretch receptors. The essential features of this hypothesis are as follows:

(1) Electrical excitation waves in the atria traverse the atrial septum and excite the proximal margins of the A-V node (the so-called atrinodal region).

(2) The signal traverses the node electromechanically as shown in Fig. 1.12, i.e. tension development in atrionodal tissues stretches the nodal cells just distal to the excited areas. This stretch in turn brings about cellular depolarisation which, if adequate, results in active contraction, shortening and consequent stretch of the more distally placed N cells. In this manner, an electromechanical stretch-depolarisation-contraction wave (S-D-C) propagates through the A-V node.

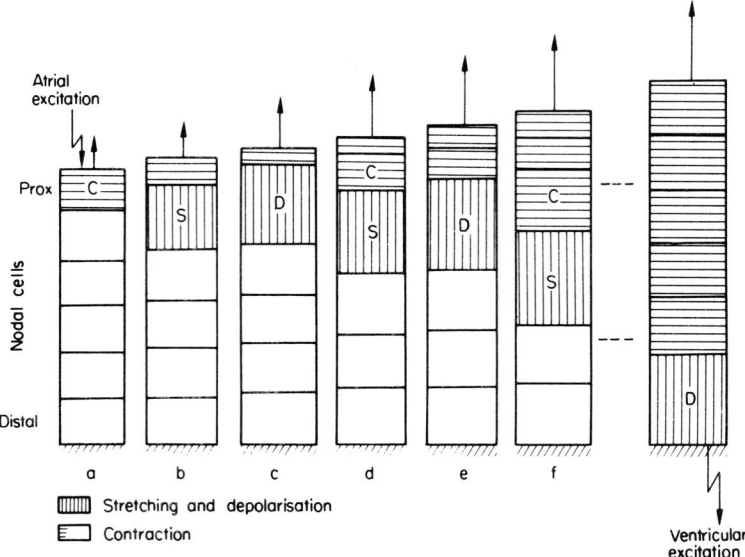

FIG. 1.12. Diagram illustrating the sequence of stretch-depolarisation-contraction of nodal cells (highly schematic). In (a), the most proximal cell is excited electrically and begins (b) to shorten. The adjacent cell is stretched to the point (c) where it achieves sufficient depolarisation and (d) contracts, stretching the next cell. The process continues (e, f . . .) until a distal cell of the node—which communicates electrically with the His bundle—is depolarised. Increasing atrial tension (arrows) keeps the node taut during transmission.

(3) The final event in this sequence is the stretching and attendant depolarisation of cells which communicate electrically with cells of the His bundle.

(4) The depolarisation of N cells does not occur in an all-or-none fashion; its magnitude and time course depend upon the magnitude and time course of applied stretch, in a manner similar to that of mechanoreceptors.

Evidence for an electromechanical mechanism

The proposed electromechanical mechanism for A-V nodal transmission requires that (1) cellular stretch results in cellular depolarisation; (2) sufficient depolarisation brings about tension development and consequent cellular shortening; (3) the stretch-depolarisation characteristics are similar to those of stretch receptors; and (4) the cellular architecture of the A-V node is appropriate to support an S-D-C wave.

Stretch induced depolarisation

Evidence for this in SA nodal cells was given in the discussion of pacemaking (above). Stretch also causes depolarisation in working myocardium. Kaufman and Theophile (1967) have reported diastolic depolarisation and initiation of spontaneous activity with stretch in papillary muscle and atrial trabeculae. Lab (1969) found decreased resting potential in ventricular fibres of rat hearts during the distension induced by acute aortic clamping. Numerous clinical reports describe the initiation of ventricular ectopic beats (presumably by depolarisation) with increased distending pressure. It is not unreasonable to predict that stretch induced depolarisation, apparently an ubiquitous phenomenon in other cardiac tissues, also applies in some degree to fibres of the A-V node.

Contraction

The second requirement of contraction following depolarisation is not too difficult to accept provided A-V nodal cells have contractile machinery. Moreover, as will be discussed in greater detail in Chapter 2, tension development depends on the magnitude and duration of depolarisation which controls calcium ion influx.

A-V nodal cells do have myofilaments. There are fewer myofibrils per cell but according to James and Sherf (1968), the myofilament density per myofibril approaches that of working ventricular cells (as opposed to weakly contractile Purkinje fibres which have only few myofilaments per myofibril), i.e. they resemble miniature working myocardial cells in appearance. Nodal motion can be observed directly in the rabbit interatrial septum—A-V node preparation. This motion appears to be more than in parts of the interventricular septum. Markers on the A-V node reveal a contractile wave progressing distally along it.

Receptor-like behaviour

The most obvious characteristic of mechanoreceptors like the muscle spindle, stretch receptor and Pacinian corpuscle is the absence of an 'all-or-none' depolarisation. Electrical responses in mechanoreceptors are graded in accordance with the intensity of the mechanical stimulus. If nodal cells behaved like mechanoreceptors, cellular depolarisation ought not to be fixed in magnitude. Considerable variation ought to be found among different nodal cells of the same preparation as there is little reason to expect that each cell will be stretched equally. Moreover, within a given cell, if the stretch intensity is altered by some agent, variation of the magnitude of depolarisation ought also to be evident.

Such variations are found. The records of Janse et al. (1971) (Fig. 3 of their paper) indicate a gradation of depolarisation magnitude among different cells in which the extremes differed by two to one. Depolarisation magnitude varies depending on whether stimulation is from the right atrium, interatrial septum, His bundle or whether the right atrium and His bundle are stimulated simultaneously. There are also variations with the rate and rhythm of the heart.

The refractory period of conducting cells after repolarisation is very brief whereas in mechanoreceptors it is three to five times the interval of depolarisation. Meredith et al. (1968) found that in Purkinje fibres, as in other cells which exhibit all-or-none properties, the refractory period ended when the action potential ended whereas in A-V nodal cells it persisted four times the duration of depolarisation; this is exactly the same situation which is found in mechanoreceptors! This refractoriness also appears to apply to mechanical stimuli as well as the electrical stimuli used by Meredith *et al.* Mendez and Moe (1966) present records indicating a relative refractory period for N cells completed at about three times the duration of depolarisation.

A stretch occurring when a mechanoreceptor is still depolarised from a previous stretch will bring about a secondary depolarisation. In Fig. 1.13 are presented records of Janse *et al.* (1971) showing that such secondary depolarisations occur in nodal cells. They occur at any time through the course of the first depolarisation. This behaviour is characteristic of mechanoreceptors but not of 'all-or-none' cells found in other areas of the heart.

Other features, perhaps less exclusive than the three mentioned above, are shared by mechanoreceptors and nodal cells. These properties shared by N cells and mechanoreceptors contrast markedly with the well-known recorded properties of atrial, ventricular, and Purkinje fibres which are indicated briefly in other sections of this chapter and are detailed in any standard text.

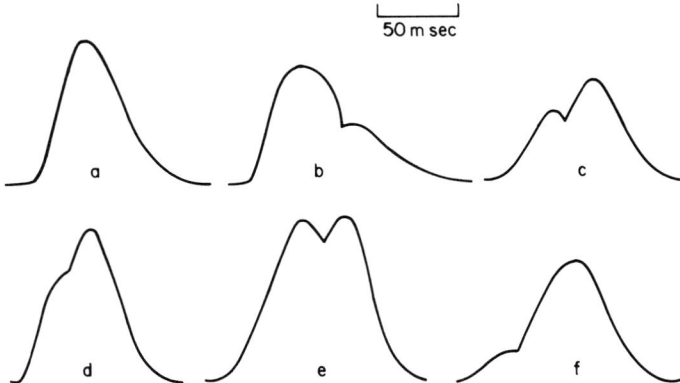

FIG. 1.13. Intracellular potentials in nodal cells illustrating summation. All records are redrawn from Janse *et al.* (1971). The one in (a) is a typical N cell potential observed when excitation is initiated in the right atrium. The ones in (b)–(f) are records typical of those seen when the atrial excitation is followed by another closely coupled atrial excitation. A secondary depolarisation summating with the first is generally observed. Note that the secondary depolarisation can begin at any time during the course of the primary depolarisation. The characteristics of the potentials shown here are similar to those reported by Hoffman and Cranefield (1960) and Mendez and Moe (1966). N cells do not appear to be all-or-none.

Architecture

The fourth requirement for this hypothesis is that nodal architecture be compatible with the proposed stretch-depolarisation-contraction mechanism. Two contrasting cellular arrangements may be envisaged as depicted in Fig. 1.14a, a highly cross-linked, basketweave arrangement or 1.14b, strings of cells in series which are free of any such lateral contraint. The first arrangement 1.14a is best suited for the proposed type of transmission and there is ample evidence that the cells of the A-V node are tightly interwoven in this way. Transmembrane potentials recorded from N cells indicate that depolarisation is usually not preceded by a pre-potential of any consequence such as that found in S-A nodal cells. Instead, a well-defined upstroke of depolarisation is generally preceded by a period of latency. The existence of latency in distal cells during the time in which activity is approaching from the proximal

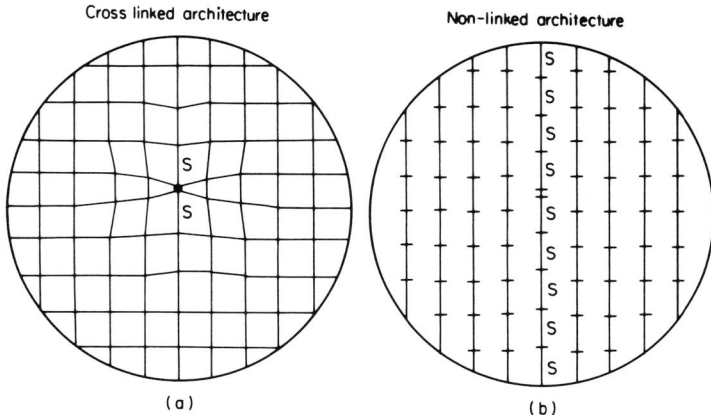

Cross linked architecture   Non-linked architecture

(a)   (b)

FIG. 1.14. Models of two contrasting cellular arrangements, a highly cross-tethered, basket-weave type (a) versus one in which strings of cells are free of any such lateral constraint (b). As a model of the highly tethered architecture, consider a rubber sheet placed under tension from all sides with grid lines painted on. If two points on the sheet are pinched together (representing a contracting cell), will the resultant lengthening (representing stretch of contiguous cells) be localised or distributed ? One can try this simple experiment and verify, as shown in (a), that the resultant stretch of such a sheet is largely localised and maximised in the area immediately surrounding the pinch (labelled 's'). At the opposite extreme, suppose parallel slits were cut along the pinching axis, throughout the sheet, as shown in (b). Long, parallel, untethered rubber bands, or strings of cells would now be represented. If two neighbouring points on one rubber band are now pinched together, the resultant stretch will be uniformly distributed over the remainder of that band, as shown; in no single area (or cell) would the stretch be of appreciable magnitude. Transmission would therefore be least effective in such a non-tethered architecture, and most likely to fail. Since A-V nodal architecture most closely resembles that in (a), rather than (b), it appears to be well suited to the proposed S-D-C mechanism.

cells indicates that the process of transmission must be a highly localised one, an observation consistent with the tightly interwoven nodal architecture and the proposed mechanism.

The manner in which stretch induced depolarisation and depolarisation induced contraction results in the characteristic delay of A-V nodal transmission is illustrated schematically in Fig. 1.15. Depression of either mechanism causes an increased delay and, if sufficiently severe, complete A-V block.

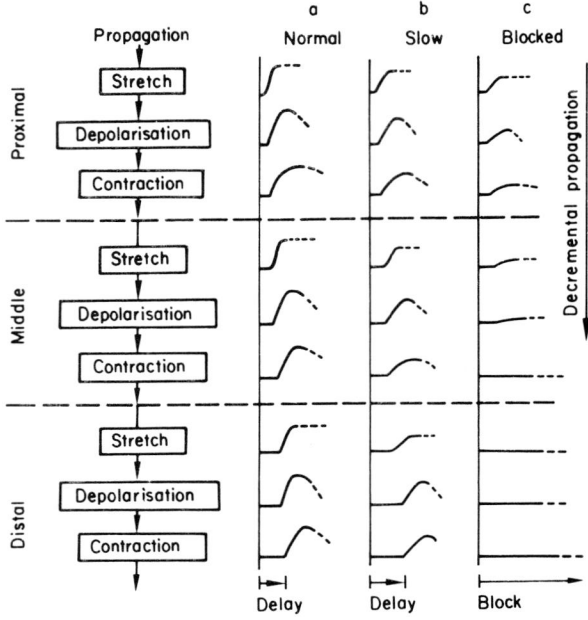

FIG. 1.15. Factors associated with impaired transmission through the A-V node. Stretch-depolarisation-contraction sequences are shown for representative cells in proximal, middle and distal areas of the A-V node. During normal propagation (a), stretch, depolarisation and contraction have maximal rate of rise and magnitude, and the electromechanical wave is perpetuated without decrement. If stretch-induced depolarisation or depolarisation-induced contraction is impaired, the situation in (b) obtains. Reduced rate of stretch gives rise to smaller depolarisation, hence reduced contractile vigour. The cycle is perpetuated through the node, resulting in longer transit time. If impairment is sufficiently high (e.g., for a highly premature beat) the wave cannot be sustained, and attenuation, or decremental propagation, occurs. If the decrement is sufficiently large, as in (c), the His bundle will fail to be excited and a ventricular beat will be dropped. Very rapid wave attenuation will occur distal to the point where depolarisation is less than the threshold required to bring about minimal contraction. In reality, small 'abortive' depolarisations may still occur beyond this point as a result of some stretch by atrial or proximal nodal cells.

THE CARDIAC ACTION POTENTIAL

When the impulse has been propagated to any part of the working ventricular myocardium, an action potential with a form shown in Fig. 1.16 is recorded. As with other excitable tissues, current thinking concerning the mechanism of depolarisation and repolarisation stems from the theory put forward by Hodgkin and Huxley for the case of squid axons. The voltage across the cell membrane was controlled and the ionic current measured. The total ionic current was measured as a function of voltage and time and separated into sodium and non-sodium components by measuring the current in the presence and absence of external sodium ions. The conductance of the cell membrane for each ion is obtained by dividing these currents by the electrochemical potential gradient. Both sodium and potassium

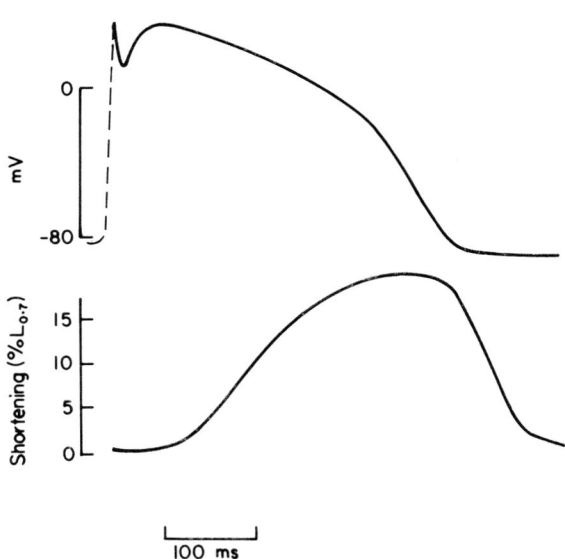

FIG. 1.16. Record of an action potential (above) recorded by intracellular microelectrode, together with shortening of muscle (below). Cat papillary muscle. Tracing kindly provided by Max Lab.

conductances increase on depolarisation but the sodium increase is very much faster than the increase in potassium conductance. Therefore, initially the major effect is a rapid increase in sodium current which is inward and causes further depolarisation. It is thought to be responsible for the initial fast rapid upstroke of the action potential. Subsequently, potassium conductance becomes predominant, causing outward flow of positive charge and repolarisation.

These phenomena in cardiac muscle have mostly been studied in Purkinje fibres. The behaviour of sodium conductance has considerable similarities to that in squid axon and is responsible for the fast rapid upstroke depolarisation of the action potential. However, the behaviour of potassium current in Purkinje fibres differs considerably from nerve. Moreover the action potential shows a long plateau quite different from the brief spikes in nerve. Considerable modification of the equations postulated to account for the changes in membrane conductances were therefore required to predict the cardiac action potential.

Subsequently, it was realised that depolarisation during the cardiac action potential consisted of two components—an initial fast component is a sodium spike similar to that of squid axon and a slow component which produces both slow depolarisation and the plateau of the action potential. This slow component depends upon a slow inward current due predominantly if not exclusively to inward flow of calcium ions. In the voltage range where the slow component threshold is thought to lie, potassium conductance appears to decrease so that outward flow of potassium ions and repolarisation are delayed. Thus, the action potential duration is prolonged compared to nerve. Repolarisation by potassium current appears to be dependent on the duration of the inward calcium current which is under the influence of a number of controlling factors (Chapter 2).

Detailed consideration of the electrophysiology of the cardiac cell will not be carried out here; it is available in specialised texts. However, in view of the particular ideas about the heart which this book attempts to highlight, two points which emerge from the foregoing brief description will be emphasised.

(1) There appears to be no fast component sodium current spike in S-A nodal and A-V nodal cells, making them unique and quite different from other cardiac cells. As will be seen from the ideas already put forward by Pollack above, this property may well be an essential component in the mechanism of action of these cells. In the case of the S-A nodal cells, this property accords well with the fact that they initiate, not conduct, excitation of the heart. It also accords well with Pollack's idea that spontaneous pacemaking results from a slow depolarisation due to increased calcium ion conductance. This pacemaking mechanism has been emphasised here because it constitutes the basic clock which controls the frequency of all the other oscillations during the cardiac cycle to be considered in the rest of the book.

(2) The plateau phase of the action potential of working myocardium and the associated inward flow of calcium ions constitutes the major route for entry of calcium ions into the cell. These calcium ions may then participate in the events of 'the calcium cardiac cycle' (Chapter 2). It therefore constitutes a major factor in the control of the contraction of the heart. More detailed consideration of this control will be taken up in the next chapter.

REFERENCES

BONKE F.I.M. (1973) Electronic spread in the sinoatrial node of the rabbit heart. *Pflügers Arch.*, **339**, 17–23.

BOUMAN L.N., GERLINGS E.D., BIERSTEKER P.A. & BONKE F.I.M. (1968) Pacemaker shift in the sino-atrial node during vagal stimulation. *Pflügers Arch.*, **302**, 255–267.

BROOKER G. (1973) Oscillation of cyclic adenosine monophosphate concentration during the myocardial contraction cycle. *Science*, **182**, 933–934.

BROOKS C.M. & LU H-H. (1972) *The Sinoatrial Pacemaker of the Heart.* Thomas, Springfield, Ill.

BROWN H.F., GILES W. & NOBLE S.J. (1977) Membrane currents underlying activity in frog sinus venosus. *J. Physiol.*, **271**, 783–816.

CHALLICE C.E. (1966) Studies on the microstructure of the heart. *J. Royal Microscopical Soc.*, **85**, 1–21.

CHENG Y-P. (1971) The ultrastructure of the rat sino-atrial node. *Anatomica Niponica*, **46**, 339–358.

COCHRANE D.E., DOUGLAS W.W., MOURI T. & NAKAZATO Y. (1975) Calcium and stimulus-secretion coupling in the adrenal medulla: Contrasting stimulating effects of the ionophores X-537A and A23187 on catecholamine output. *J. Physiol.*, **252**, 363–378.

DEAN P.M. (1975) Exocytosis modelling: An electrostatic function for calcium in stimulus-secretion coupling. *J. Theor. Biol.*, **54**, 289–308.

DECK K.A. (1964) Dehnungseffekte am spontanschlagenden, isolierten Sinusknoten. *Pflügers Arch.*, **280**, 120–130.

DECK K.A. & TRAUTWEIN W. (1964) Ionic currents in cardiac excitation. *Arch. Ges. Physiol.*, **280**, 63–80.

DEFELICE L.J. & CHALLICE C.E. (1969) Anatomical and ultrastructural study of the electrophysiological atrioventricular node of the rabbit. *Circulation Res.*, **24**, 457.

DEL CASTILLO J. & KATZ B. (1954) Changes in end-plate activity produced by pre-synaptic polarisation. *J. Physiol*, **124**, 586–604.

DEWEY M.M. & BARR L. (1962) Intercellular connection between smooth muscle cells: the nexus. *Science*, **137**, 670–672.

DOUGLAS W.W. (1968) Stimulus-secretion coupling: The concept and clues from chromaffin and other cells. *Br. J. Pharmac.*, **34**, 451–474.

GEORGE W.J., WILKERSON R.D. & KADOWITZ P.J. (1973) Influence of acetylcholine on contractile force and cyclic nucleotide levels in the isolated perfused rat heart. *J. Pharmacol. Exp. Ther.*, **184**, 228–235.

GIBBONS W.R. & FOZZARD H.A. (1971) Voltage dependence of contraction in sheep cardiac Purkinje fibres. *Circulation Res.*, **28**, 446.

GOLDBERG N.D., HADDOX M.K., HARTLE D.K. & HADDEN J.W. (1973) In *Proceedings of the fifth International Congress of Pharmacology*. R.A. Maxwell and G.H. Achson, Eds. Karger, Basel, p. 146.

GREENGARD P. (1976) Possible role for cyclic nucleotides and phosphorylated membrane proteins in postsynaptic actions of neurotransmitters. *Nature*, **260**, 101–108.

GROSSMAN A. & FURCHGOTT R.F. (1964) The effects of various drugs on calcium exchange in the isolated guinea-pig auricle. *J. Pharmacol. Exp. Ther.*, **145**, 162–172.

HEUSER J.E. & REESE T.S. (1973) Evidence for recycling of synaptic vesicle membrane during transmitter release at the frog neuromuscular junction. *J. Cell Biol.*, **57**, 315–344.

HODGKIN A.L. & HUXLEY A.F. (1952) A quantitative description of membrane current and its application to conduction and excitation in nerve. *J. Physiol.*, **117**, 500–544.

HOFFMAN B.F. & CRANEFIELD P.F. (1960) *Electrophysiology of the Heart*. McGraw Hill, New York.

HUTTER O.F. & TRAUTWEIN W. (1956) Vagal and sympathetic effects on pacemaker fibres in sinus venosus of heart. *J. Gen. Physiol.*, **39**, 715–733.

IJPEIJ D., KERKHOF P.L.M. & BOBBERT A.C. (1974) Muscle length and neuromuscular transmission in the frog. *Pflügers Arch.*, **347**, 309–322.

IRISAWA H. & NOMA A. (1976) Contracture and hyperpolarisation of the rabbit sinoatrial node cells in Na-depleted solution. *Jap. J. Physiol.*, **26**, 133–144.

JAMES T.N. & NADEAU R.A. (1963) Sinus bradycardia during injections directly into the sinus node artery. *Amer. J. Physiol.*, **204**, 9.

JAMES T.N. & SHERF L. (1968) Ultrastructure of the human atrioventricular node. *Circulation*, **37**, 1049.

JAMES T.N., SHERF L., FINE G. & MORALES A.R. (1966) Comparative ultrastructure of the sinus node in man and dog. *Circulation*, **34**, 139–163.

JANSE M.J. (1969) Influence of the direction of the atrial wave front on A-V nodal transmission in isolated hearts of rabbits. *Circulation Res.*, **25**, 439.

JANSE M.J., VAN CAPELLE F.J.L., FREUD G.E. & DURRER D. (1971) Circus movement within the A-V node as a basis for supraventricular tachycardia as shown by multiple microelectrode recording in the isolated heart. *Circulation Res.*, **28**, 403.

KATZ A.M. (1970) Contractile proteins of the heart. *Physiological Rev.*, **50**, 63–158.

KAUFMAN R. & THEOPHILE U. (1967) Automatic fordernde Dehnungseffekte an Purkinje-Fäden, Papillarmuskeln und Vorhoftrabekeln von Rhesus-Affen. *Pflügers Arch.*, **297**, 174.

KIM S. & BABA N. (1971) Atrioventricular node and Purkinje fibres of the guinea pig heart. *Am. J. Anat.*, **132**, 339.

KIRSHNER N. (1974) Function and organisation of chromaffin vesicle. *Life Sci.*, **14**, 1153–1167.

LAB M.J. (1969) The effect on the left ventricular action potential of clamping the aorta. *J. Physiol*, **202**, 73.

LEFKOWITZ R.J., O'HARA D.S. & WARSHAW J. (1973) Binding of catecholamines to receptors in cultured myocardial cells. *Nature New Biol.*, **244**, 79–80.

LOWE R.D. & LAVERY H.A. (1971) Atrial ectopic beats in response to atrial oscillations in the dog. *Cardiovascular Res.*, **5**, 90.

LU H-H. (1965) Factors controlling pacemaker action in cells of the sinoatrial node. *Circulation Res.*, **17**, 460–471.

MENDEZ C. & MOE G.K. (1966) Some characteristics of transmembrane potentials of A-V nodal cells during propagation of premature beats. *Circulation Res.*, **19**, 993.

MEREDITH J., MENDEZ C., MUELLER W.J. & MOE G.K. (1968) Electrical excitability of atrioventricular nodal cells. *Circulation Res.*, **23**, 69.

MIYAGISHIMA Y. (1975) Studies on catecholamine (CA) of the heart—fluorescence histochemical method. *Jap. Circ. J.*, **39**, 361–375.

McNUTT N.S. & WEINSTEIN R.S. (1970) The ultrastructure of the nexus. A correlated thin-section and freeze-cleave study. *Cell Biol.*, **47**, 666–688.

NOBLE D. (1966) Applications of Hodgkin-Huxley equations to excitable tissues. *Physiol Rev.*, **46**, 1–50.

NOMA A. & IRISAWA H. (1976) Membrane currents in the rabbit sinoatrial node cell as studied by the double microelectrode method. *Pflügers Arch.*, **364**, 45–52.

PAES DE CARVALHO A, HOFFMAN B. & DE PAULA CARVALHO M. (1969) Two components of the cardiac action potential. *J. Gen. Physiol.*, **54**, 607–635.

POLLACK G.H. (1974) A-V nodal transmission: A proposed electromechanical mechanism. *J. Electrocardiol.*, **7**, 245–258.

POLLACK G.H. (1976) Intercellular coupling in the atrioventricular node and other tissues of the rabbit heart. *J. Physiol.*, **255**, 275–298.

POLLACK G.H. (1977) Cardiac Pacemaking: An obligatory role of catecholamines? *Science*, **196**, 731–738.

REUTER H. (1965) Über die wirkung von adrenalin auf den cellulären Ca-umsatz des meerschweinchenvorhofs. *Naunyn-Schmeidebergs Arch. Pharmakol. Exp. Path.*, **251**, 401–412.

REUTER H. (1967) The dependence of slow inward current in Purkinje fibres on the extracellular calcium concentration. *J. Physiol.*, **192**, 479.

REUTER H. (1968) Slow inactivation of currents in Purkinje fibres. *J. Physiol.*, **197**, 233.

REUTER H. (1974) Localization of beta adrenergic receptors, and effects of noradrenaline and cyclic nucleotides on action potentials, ionic currents and tension in mammalian cardiac muscle. *J. Physiol.*, **242**, 429–451.

RUSKA H. (1965) In *International Symposium on Electrophysiology of the Heart*. B. Taccardi and G. Marchetti, Eds. Pergamon, New York.

SANDOVAL I.V. & CUATRECASAS P. (1976) Opposing effects of cyclic AMP and cyclic GMP on protein phosphorylation in tubulin preparations. *Nature*, **262**, 511–514.

SANO T. & YAMAGISHI S. (1965) Spread of excitation from the sinus node. *Circulation Res.*, **16**, 423–430.

SIMON M. (1976) Conversion of guanosine 3′,5′-monophosphate to adenosine 3′,5′-monophosphate in frog myocardial tissue. *Biochem. Biophys. Res. Commun.*, **68**, 1219–1225.

SPURGEON H.A., PRIOLA D.V., MONTOYA P., WEISS G.K. & ALTER W.A. Ill. (1974) Catecholamines associated with conductile and contractile myocardium of normal and denervated dog hearts. *J. Pharmacol. Exp. Ther.*, **190**, 466–471.

TEO T.S. & WANG J.H. (1973) Mechanisms of activation of a cyclic adenosine 3′5′-monophosphate phosphodiesterase from bovine heart by calcium ions. Identification of the protein activator as a Ca^{++} binding protein. *J. Biol. Chem.*, **248**, 5950–5955.

TRAUTWEIN W. & UCHIZONO K. (1963) Electron microscopic and electrophysiologic study of the pacemaker in the sino-atrial node of the rabbit heart. *Z. Zellforsch.*, **61**, 96–109.

TUGANOWSKI W., KRAUSE M. & KORCZAK K. (1973) The effect of dibutyryl 3′,5′ cyclic AMP on the cardiac pacemaker, arrested with reserpine and alpha-methyl-tyrosine. *Naunyn-Schmiederberg's Arch. Pharmacol.*, **280**, 63–70.

TUGANOWSKI W. (1977) The influence of adenylate cyclase inhibitors on the spontaneous activity of the cardiac pacemaker. *Arch. int. Pharmacodyn.*, **225**, 275–286.

USHIYAMA J. & BROOKS C.M. (1974) Intercellular stimulation and recording of the cardiac pacemaker. *J. Electrocardiol.*, **7** (2), 119–126.

VAN CAPELLE F.J.L., JANSE M.J., VARGHESE P., FREUD G.E., MATER C. & DURRER D. (1972) Spread of excitation in the atrioventricular node of isolated rabbit hearts studied by multiple microelectrode recording. *Circulation Res.*, **31**, 602.

VIRAGH Sz. & PORTE A. (1973) On the impulse conducting system of the monkey heart (macaca mulatta). II. The atrio-ventricular node and bundle. *Z. Zellforsch.*, **145**, 363–388.

WEST T.C. & LANDA J. (1956) Transmembrane potentials and contractility in the pregnant rat uterus. *Am. J. Physiol.*, **187**, 333–337.

WEIDMANN S. (1955) The effect of the cardiac membrane potential on the rapid availability of the sodium-carrying system *J. Physiol.*, **127**, 213–224.

WINEGRAD S. (1971) Studies of cardiac muscle with a high permeability to calcium produced by treatment with ethylenediaminetetraacetic acid. *J. Gen. Physiol.*, **58**, 71–93.

WOLLENBERGER A. (1975) The role of cyclic AMP in the adrenergic control of the heart. In *Contraction and Relaxation in the Myocardium*. W.G. Nayler, Ed. Academic Press, New York.

WOLLENBERGER A., BABSKII G.B., KRAUSE E.G., GENZ S., BLOHN D. & BOGDANOVA E.V. (1973) Cyclic changes in levels of cyclic AMP and cyclic GMP in frog myocardium during the cardiac cycle. *Biochem. Biophys. Res. Commun.*, **55**, 446–452.

YAMAGISHI S. & SANO T. (1967) Effect of temperature on pacemaker activity of rabbit sinus node. *Am. J. Physiol.*, **212**, 829–834.

YAMASAKI Y., FUJIWARA M. & TODA N. (1974) Effects of catecholamines injected into sinoatrial nodal cells on their electrical activity. *Japan. J. Pharmacol.*, **24**, 383–391.

YPEY D.L. (1975) Feedback of isotonic muscle contraction on neuromuscular impulse transmission in the frog. *Pflügers Arch.*, **355**, 291–306.

CHAPTER 2
THE CALCIUM CARDIAC CYCLE

After considering the initiation of the depolarisation pulse by the S-A node and the spread of the action potential to the rest of the heart, it is necessary to have a working hypothesis for the mechanism by which the action potential causes a contraction. This process is referred to as excitation–contraction coupling. There is universal agreement that this process is achieved by the release of calcium ions (Ca^{++}) into the cytoplasm of the cell interior and that the calcium ions react with the contractile proteins to produce contraction.

The simplest demonstrations of this are:

(1) The cell membrane can be stripped from muscle cells, including cardiac muscle cells. Thus the structure responsible for propagation of the action potential and isolating the cell interior from the extracellular fluid is removed. Under these circumstances, the calcium ion concentration of the fluid bathing the preparation must be kept extremely low in order to keep it relaxed—below 10^{-7} molar. As the calcium ion concentration increases, the preparation develops tension (Fig. 2.1) and reaches full tension at concentrations above 10^{-5} molar. At these concentrations, the contractile system is fully saturated and no more tension can be produced.

(2) In heart muscle, if the calcium ions are removed from the extracellular fluid, the

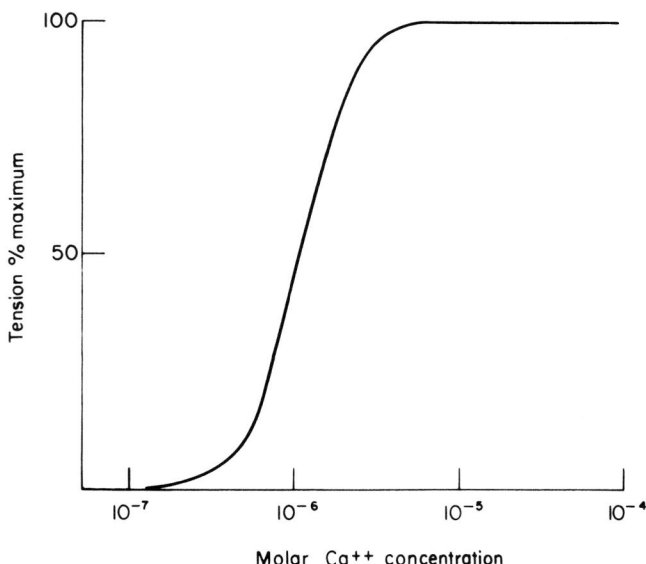

FIG. 2.1. Relationship between tension development and calcium ion concentration in a skinned cardiac cell. Redrawn from Fabiato and Fabiato (1975a).

muscle becomes non-contractile. This is because calcium ions are 'washed out' of the cell and are no longer available for their function of excitation–contraction coupling. (3) Aequorin, a bioluminescent protein which emits light in the presence of calcium ions, can be injected intracellularly into a muscle cell. The light signal obtained from this indicator follows the action potential and precedes the development of tension. This is shown for a skeletal muscle fibre and an atrial trabecula in Fig. 2.2.

It is not clear exactly where the calcium release takes place in the cell and how

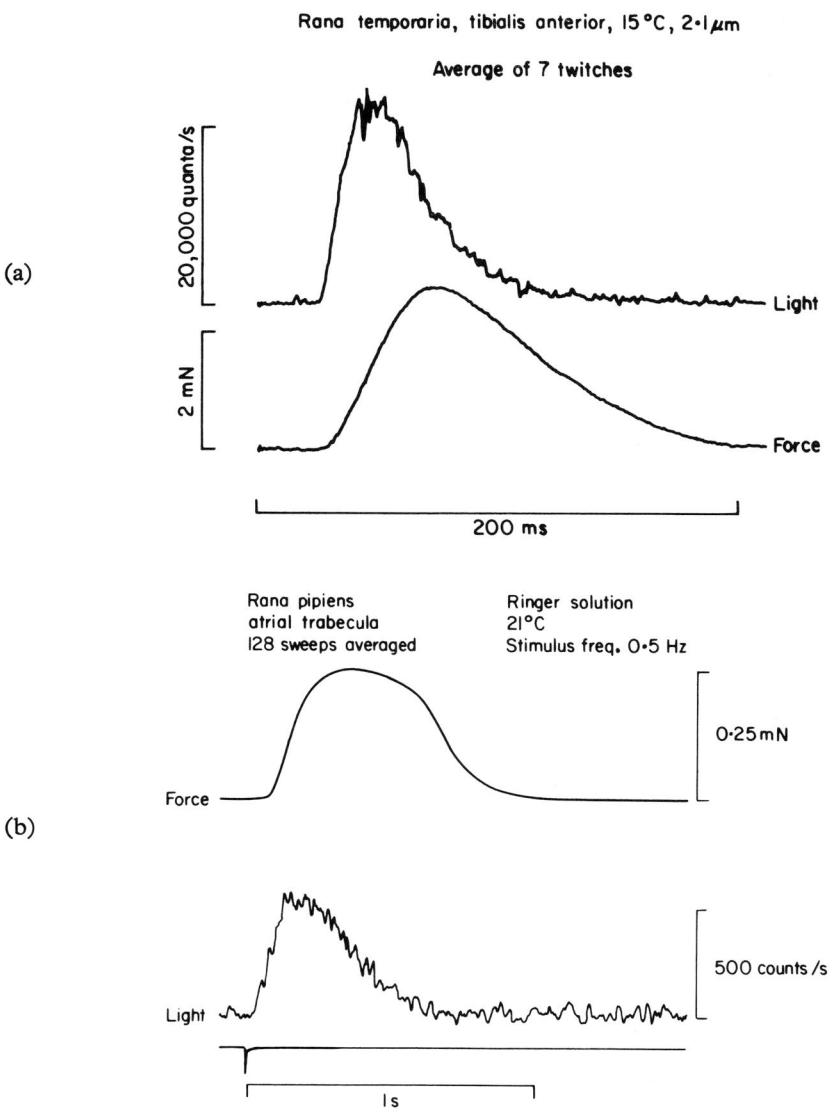

F IG. 2.2. (a) Time relation between free calcium ion release (aequorin signal) (above) and tension (below) in a skeletal muscle fibre. (b) Tension (above) and light from aequorin (below) in frog atrial trabecular muscle twitch. Average of 128 contractions at a stimulus frequency of 0·5 Hz at 21°C. Tracings kindly provided by John Blinks.

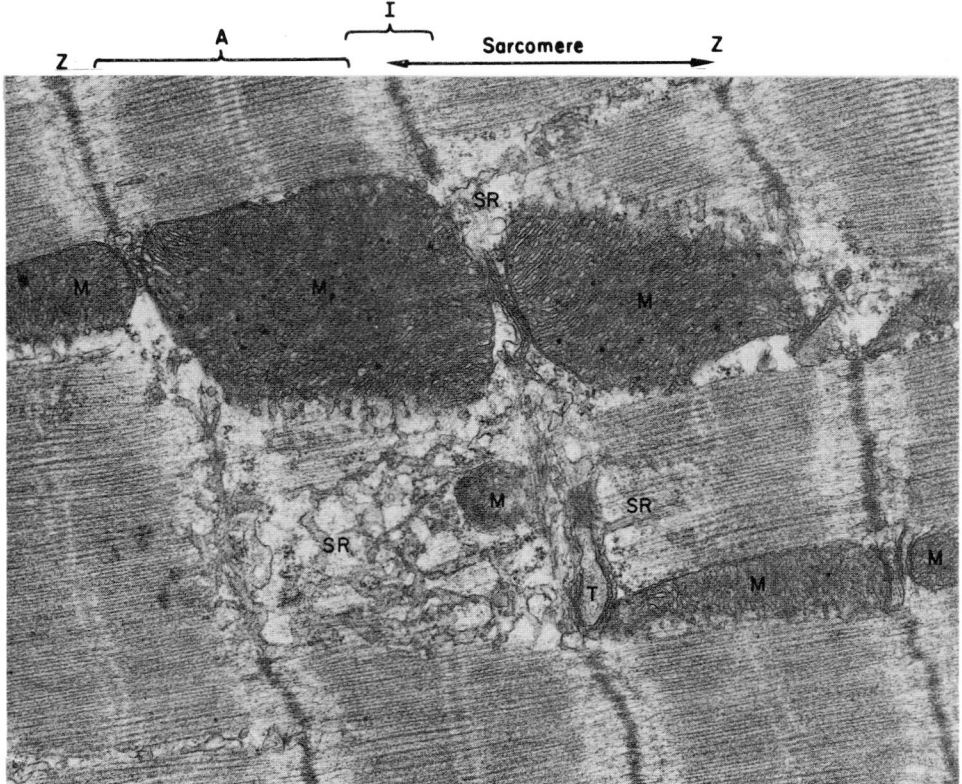

FIG. 2.3. Electronmicrograph of cardiac muscle showing sarcoplasmic reticulum (SR). Also shown are mitochondria (M), *T*-tubules (T), *A* and *I* bands and *Z* disc.

the release is triggered by the action potential. This question is inseparable from the consideration of the function of the sarcoplasmic reticulum. This complex network of tubules is wrapped around the contractile proteins (Fig. 2.3). If myocardium is homogenated, the sarcoplasmic reticulum can be separated out from other cellular constituents and forms vesicles in fluid suspension which actively *accumulate* calcium ions (consuming ATP). This ability to sequester calcium ions is responsible for relaxation, which occurs when the sarcoplasmic reticulum removes calcium ions from the contractile proteins. Agents which inhibit calcium uptake★ by sarcoplasmic reticulum (e.g. caffeine, strontium ions) also cause slower relaxation. Agents which accelerate ion uptake by sarcoplasmic reticulum (e.g. catecholamines) also cause faster relaxation.

When considering calcium ion release, one therefore has to ask whether this same structure releases its calcium ions again when triggered by an action potential. The alternative sources of calcium ions are (1) mitochondria which actively accumulate and are rich in calcium, (2) the lateral sacs or cisternae. These are connected to the rest of the sarcoplasmic reticulum and are thought to be part of that system.

★ By 'uptake' I mean both 'binding' and 'true uptake', i.e. sequestration.

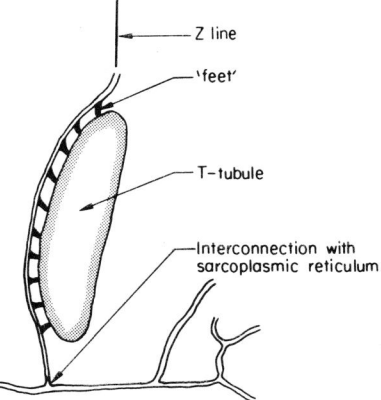

Z line

'feet'

T–tubule

Interconnection with
sarcoplasmic reticulum

FIG. 2.4.   Diagram of proposed interconnection between *T*-tubule and sarcoplasmic reticulum.

They lie in close approximation to the cell membrane or to the *T*-tubules—invaginations of the cell membrane which occur at the position of the *Z* discs of the sarcomeres. Specialised structures associated with these cisternae have been described as 'feet' which form very close connections with the cell membrane (Fig. 2.4). (3) A store of calcium ions just outside the cell membrane where the concentration may be higher than in the general extracellular fluid because of the presence of a layer of mucopolysaccharide. (4) Calcium from the general extracellular fluid.

Of these alternatives, the mitochondria seem unlikely candidates because it is difficult to think of a way in which they would be triggered by the action potential. In the case of the two extracellular sources (3 and 4 above), entry into the cell would occur during the plateau phase of the action potential (Chapter 1) which is the only time in the cardiac cycle when the cell membrane is highly permeable to calcium ions. Reuter has measured the magnitude of this calcium 'current' and calculated that only part of the total amount of calcium necessary to produce the recorded tensions could come into the cell in this way. Thus a large part of the calcium released must come from the cisternae or the sarcoplasmic reticulum or both.

This can also be shown by applying a prolonged depolarisation to the cell artificially. There is an initial twitch similar to a normal twitch but, during continued depolarisation, relaxation is not complete and a level of tension is maintained—so called 'tonic tension'. The initial twitch is due to the normal release of internal Ca^{++} triggered by the depolarisation; the continued tonic tension is due to the effect of the depolarisation *per se* and for arguments sake, will be assumed to be due to direct flow of Ca^{++} from outside the cell membrane to the contractile proteins. This tonic tension is much less than the twitch peak tension* showing that the amount of Ca^{++}

* Results depend on technique. If Tritthart *et al.*'s claim is correct that much of the tonic tension found by others is artefact, then the contrast between tonic tension and twitch peak tension is very great indeed (10% in their Fig. 3b).

coming in during depolarisation is insufficient to produce the full amount of tension in a normal beat.

Calcium ion release from sarcoplasmic reticulum

This subject has been comprehensively reviewed by Fabiato and Fabiato. The two principal ways in which the phenomenon can be investigated are (1) to study isolated sarcoplasmic reticulum as described above or (2) to use the 'skinned' muscle cell without cell membrane and study calcium release by measuring tension production. Unfortunately, both these methods lump the main part of the sarcoplasmic reticular network and the cisternae together and do not allow one to investigate whether they have different, possibly complementary functions.

Nevertheless it can be concluded that the following factors influence this 'lumped' sarcoplasmic reticulum to release Ca^{++}:

(1) Depolarisation. The hypothesis is that the depolarisation of the cell membrane by the action potential spreads directly to the sarcoplasmic reticulum and causes calcium ion release. This is usually demonstrated in these preparations by using an increase in concentration of anions. It appears to be the dominant mechanism in skeletal muscle. Although present in cardiac muscle preparations, it is difficult to demonstrate because of the dominance of the second mechanism.

(2) Ca^{++} induced Ca^{++} release. A strange paradox is that although the sarcoplasmic reticulum is certainly responsible for relaxation by extracting Ca^{++} from the contractile system, it is also triggered to release all its Ca^{++} again by the addition of Ca^{++}. This mechanism is much more easily demonstrated in cardiac than in skeletal muscle. Cardiac sarcoplasmic reticulum is triggered by concentrations of Ca^{++} between 3 and 5×10^{-8} molar according to Fabiato and Fabiato.

In cardiac muscle therefore, one can postulate that because of the long plateau of the action potential, associated as it is with a considerable inward flux of Ca^{++}, enough Ca^{++} enters the cell at this time to release the Ca^{++} stored in the cisternae and sarcoplasmic reticulum. However, it is equally possible, according to available evidence, that the cisternae (with their intimate structural connections to the cell membrane) are depolarised and that this induces release of calcium ions which is either sufficient for contraction or which releases more Ca^{++} from the rest of the sarcoplasmic reticulum. This view is favoured by the fact that in intact muscles a twitch is produced by an artificially curtailed action potential with no plateau. This finding has been interpreted as showing that internal stored Ca^{++} is released as a consequence of the fast Na^+ inward current of the initial part of the action potential (Chapter 1) and that the Ca^{++} which enters during the plateau goes into replenishment of the internal Ca^{++} store (see below).

There is still a conceptual difficulty in accepting a situation in which the same structure (sarcoplasmic reticulum) both releases the calcium to activate contraction and then immediately goes into reverse and takes the calcium up again to cause relaxation. For this to be the case, the system must have some intrinsic oscillatory tendency like that of pacemaker cells (Chapter 1). It is not unreasonable to suppose that this cyclical process in the membrane of the sarcoplasmic reticulum is similar to that in the membrane of sinus node cells as postulated by Pollack. Both have the same catecholamine—adenyl cyclase—cyclic AMP system. (Ca^{++} uptake is accelerated by catecholamines and cyclic AMP, which cause accelerated relaxation.) One could then postulate that the Ca^{++} uptake process is analogous to the depolarisation process of the sinus pacemaker cell. This sequestered Ca^{++} might be bound to the membrane in an unreleasable form and take time to be taken up into the lumen of the sarcoplasmic reticular tubules. Conceivably, it is only in this latter form that the Ca^{++} can be released, requiring different conditions which are set up by the action potential (discussed above). Release is followed by uptake again as a result of the intrinsic oscillatory properties of the sarcoplasmic reticulum.

Compartmentalisation of the calcium ion uptake/release system

The description of the uptake and release system given above omits an enormous amount of available information which shows that the system is very much more complicated. However, I think that it is more important to focus on the evidence that can be gleaned from intact cardiac muscle preparations and whole hearts. This evidence already shows conclusively that the Ca^{++} uptake and release system is functionally compartmentalised. The structural correlates of these compartments must remain speculative.

There are various ways in which the calcium ions entering the cell during a depolarisation can be increased. The reader need not concern himself with the details of the techniques used. The important fact is that the extra calcium ions entering have little effect on that contraction. However, the following contraction with a normal or even attenuated action potential is potentiated. Thus there is a delay between calcium ions entering the cell during the action potential and that extra calcium being released. The calcium is entering some compartment of the calcium handling system separate from the 'release' compartment and only subsequently enters that release compartment. A large number of studies of this type of phenomenon have appeared and are still appearing. They all make use of the fact that cardiac muscle is normally not fully activated especially at short lengths (see Chapter 5). This means that the isometric tension developed by the muscle (usually papillary muscles) is a measure of the amount of calcium ions released and reaching the contractile proteins. The relationship between the isometric tension and quantity of Ca^{++} is not linear (Fig 2.1) but the use of tension development is adequate for the present purpose.

Post-extrasystolic potentiation

This is the best example of the operation of the principle outlined above. Extrasystoles occur in normal individuals and are a frequent problem in heart disease.

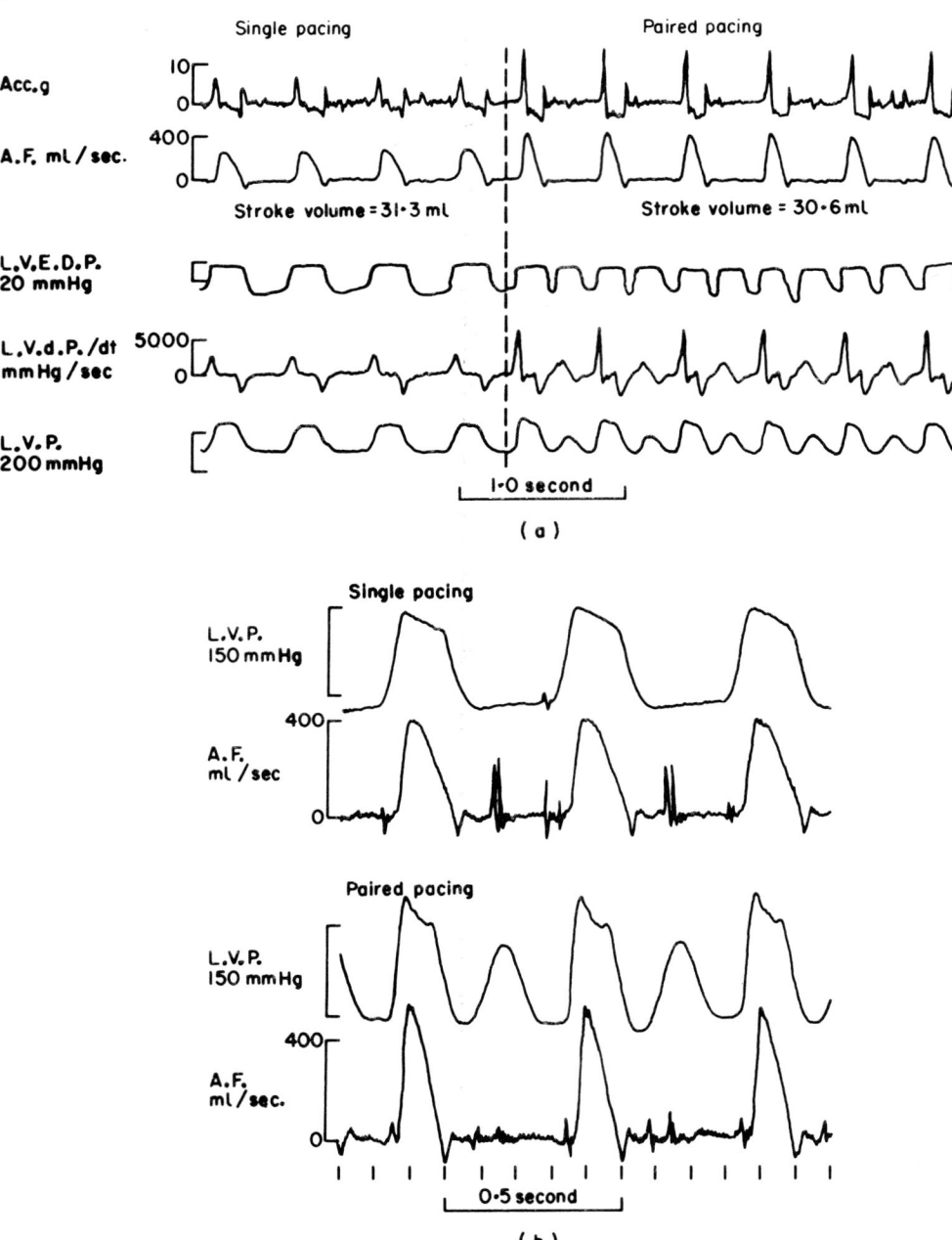

FIG. 2.5. Effect of paired pulse stimulation of the right atrium to produce sustained post-extrasystolic potentiation in a dog with chronic cardiac denervation. (a) Left: single pulse stimulation. Right: paired pulse stimulation at the same basic heart rate but with ectopic beats between each ejecting beat. LVEDP of the ejecting beats is the same. (b) Left ventricular pressure (LVP) and aortic flow (AF) during the same experiment recorded on a high frequency response photographic recorder for clearer display of the primary signals. Potentiation is indicated by the greater rate of rise of pressure (LV dP/dt) and of flow, i.e. acceleration (Acc). EDP = end-diastolic pressure. Redrawn from Noble *et al.*, *Cardiovascular Res.*, **6**, 467 (1972).

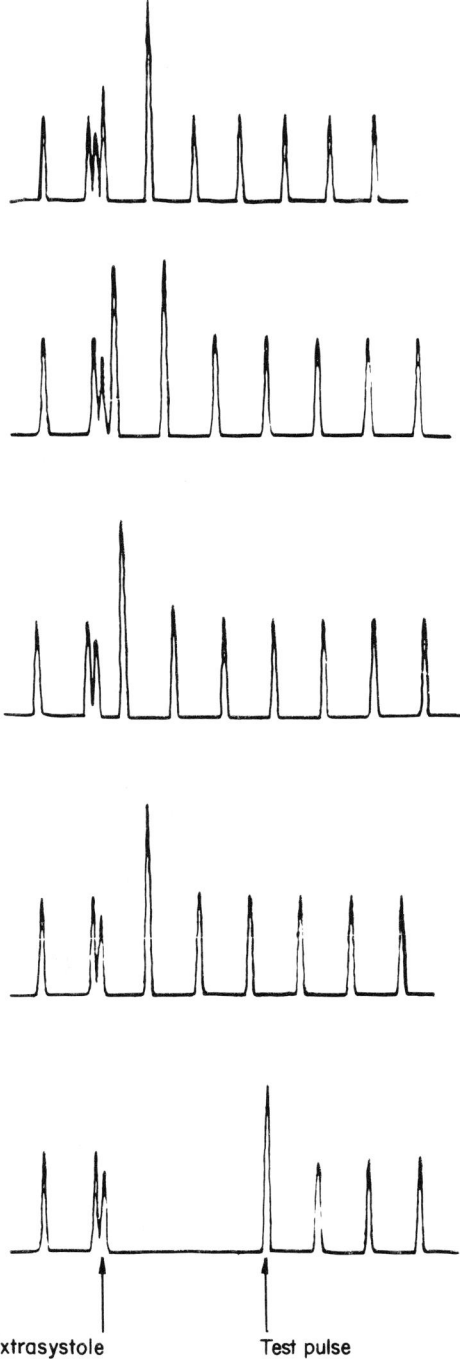

Extrasystole   Test pulse

FIG. 2.6.   Effect of a premature contraction (extrasystole, EC) on the subsequent contraction (1). The interval between EC and a test pulse (test pulse interval, TPI) was varied. The interval between control contraction and EC was fixed at 0·25 sec. The test pulse is always potentiated and is greatest at a TPI of 0·8 sec, i.e. optimum contractile response after EC occurs at a TPI of 0·8 sec. Data kindly provided by Björn Wohlfart.

It is thus a very common experience that the beat following the extrasystole is much stronger than a normal beat in the steady state. This is true even if the extrasystole is not followed by a compensatory pause.

In Fig. 2.5 an intact dog heart has been paced electrically so that the beat after the extrasystole occurs without a compensatory pause (from the same end-diastolic pressure). It can be seen to be a much stronger beat. This can be shown formally in a papillary muscle preparation (Fig. 2.6). Everything about the post-extrasystolic beat can be made normal, i.e. normal time interval before contraction, normal action

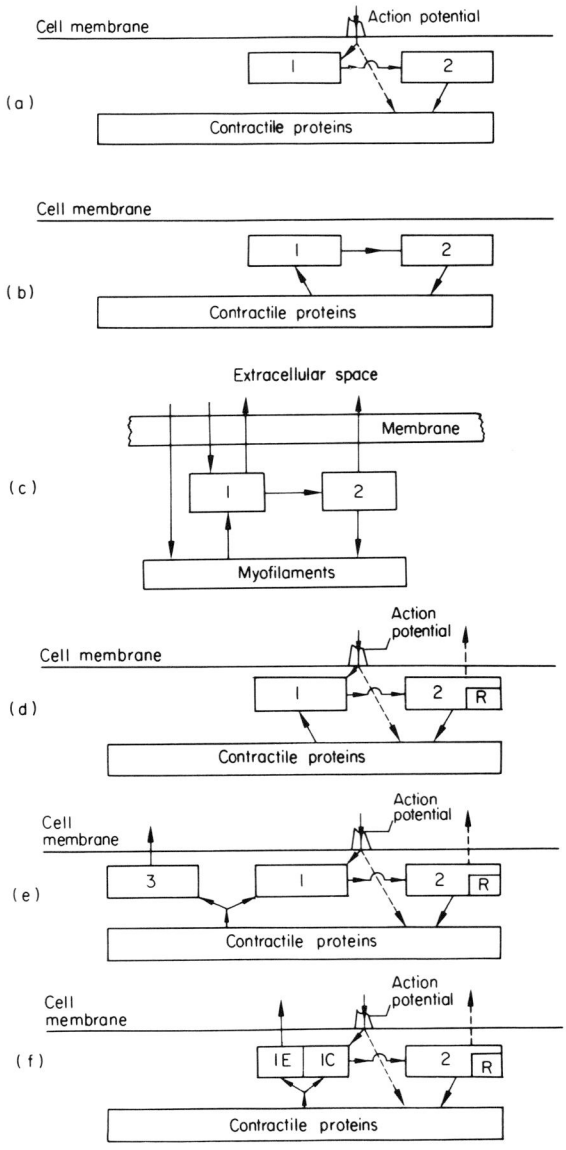

FIG. 2.7.   Development of models of the recirculation of calcium ions.

potential, etc. However it is always potentiated, indicating more Ca^{++} delivered from the release compartment.

The only cause of this potentiation is the occurrence of the premature beat. The action potential of the premature beat may or may not be prolonged but even such prolongation as may occur is insufficient to account for the extra Ca^{++} entry.* For some reason as yet unknown, more calcium enters during the action potential of the premature beat. The situation can now be summarised in Fig. 2.7a where I have depicted two boxes representing two compartments. Compartment 1 receives the calcium ion entry during the action potential and passes it to compartment 2 from which it is released by the following action potential.

The optimal contractile response and rested state contraction

It is now necessary to consider the route taken by the calcium which is taken up during relaxation. This can be examined by pacing a papillary muscle regularly and then introducing a test pulse. (Of the various good studies of the subject, I choose to follow the analysis of Edman and Johannsson.) If the test pulse occurs early after the last beat in the steady series, a small contraction results (Fig. 2.8a). This means that the calcium removed from the contractile proteins by the uptake system in the previous relaxation is not all in the release compartment (compartment 2 in Fig. 2.7a). It must be in some other compartment. If the test pulse occurs later, a larger contraction occurs (Fig. 2.8b), i.e. with the passage of time, Ca^{++} has moved from the uptake compartment to the release compartment. With longer and longer test pulse intervals, the test pulse reaches a maximum strength and then declines (Fig. 2.8c, 2.9a).

Thus there is an optimum time between beats when the maximum amount of Ca^{++} has reached the release compartment from the uptake compartment. This is called the optimal contractile response by Edman and Johannsson. In rabbit papillary muscle this occurs at 0·8 sec but there are differences between species and preparations. The important point at the moment is that we have to postulate two compartments for the Ca^{++} taken up during relaxation (Fig. 2.7b). The second (release) compartment is identical to compartment 2 of Fig. 2.7a. Is the uptake compartment identical to compartment 1 in Fig. 2.7a?

An affirmative answer to this question would simplify the situation since up to this point in the argument, one would still have only two functional compartments. There is some evidence to support the idea, e.g. if one introduces various test pulse intervals as in Fig. 2.8 after a premature extrasystole (Fig. 2.6) one obtains an optimal contractile response at the same test pulse interval as following a steady series of beats (Fig. 2.8). Therefore, since the time required for Ca^{++} taken up

---

* Prolongation may occur in isolated papillary muscle; in intact heart shortening appears to be the rule. There is extra Ca^{++}, as judged by optimal contractile response (below) over and above that produced by doubling the steady state frequency.

during relaxation in the steady state to reach the release compartment is the same as the time required for extra Ca^{++} entering during an extrasystole to get to that compartment, I will continue with the simpler postulate that the uptake compartment is the same as compartment 1 in Fig. 2.7a.

However, we now have to account for the fact that with longer intervals than the optimal test pulse interval, the strength of contraction decays (Fig. 2.9b). This presumably means that with the passage of time, Ca^{++} leaks out of compartment 2. Therefore, there must be some pathway for slow loss of Ca^{++} from compartment 2.

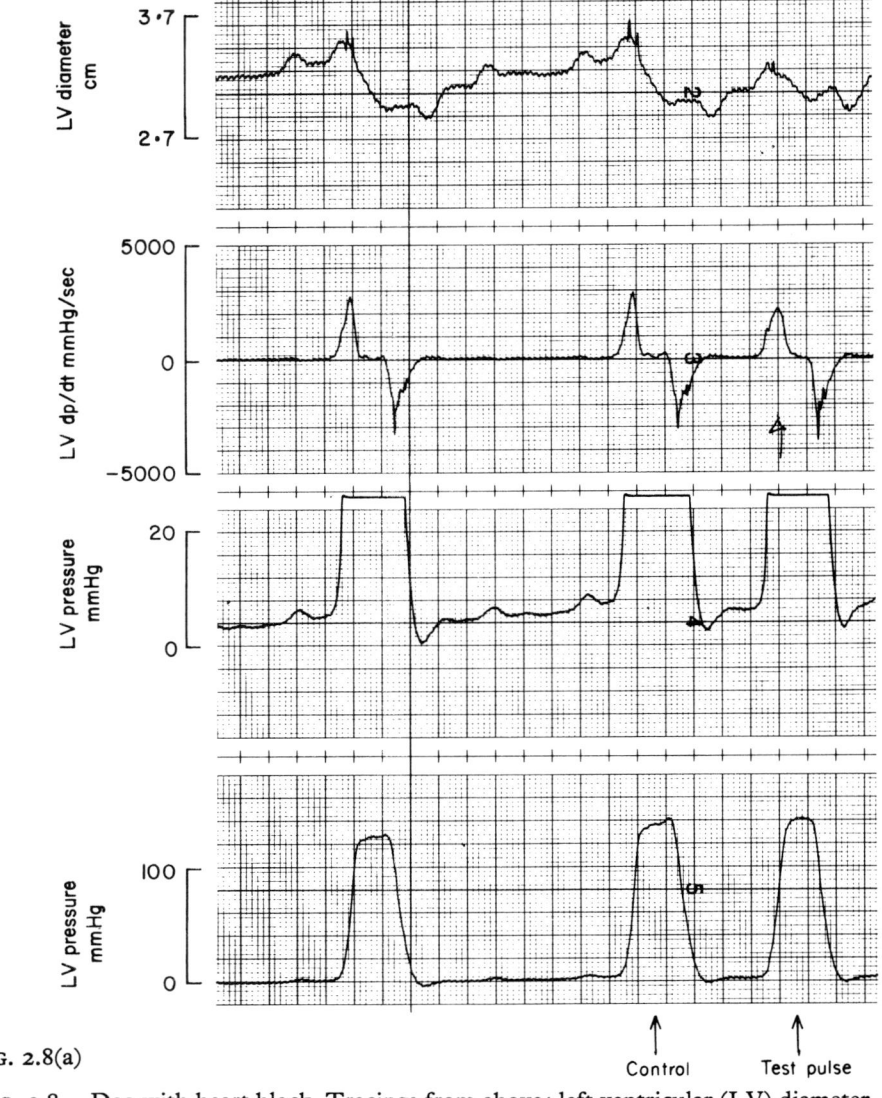

FIG. 2.8(a)

Control   Test pulse

FIG. 2.8. Dog with heart block. Tracings from above: left ventricular (LV) diameter (ultrasonic crystals), maximum rate of rise of LV pressure (LV *dP/dt*), LV end-diastolic pressure and LV pressure. Steady state stimulation rate 1/sec. (a) test pulse interval = 0·5 sec. (b) test pulse interval = 0·8 sec. (c) test pulse interval = 1·5 sec. See (b), (c) on pp. 39 and 40.

However, even this is an oversimplification because if one lets cardiac muscle rest for a long time, it will still produce a contraction when stimulated, i.e. the curve in Fig. 2.9b does not decay away to zero with extremely long intervals. This contractile response after a long rest is called rested state contraction. To deal with this problem one has to assume part of compartment 2 is 'leak-tight'. This subcompartment is however affected by changes in the extracellular Ca^{++} and Na^+ concentrations, i.e. it is the initial filling level of compartment 2.

To recapitulate the situation so far I present Fig. 2.7c which is the model of Edman and Johannsson and Fig. 2.7d which is similar but includes a subcompart-

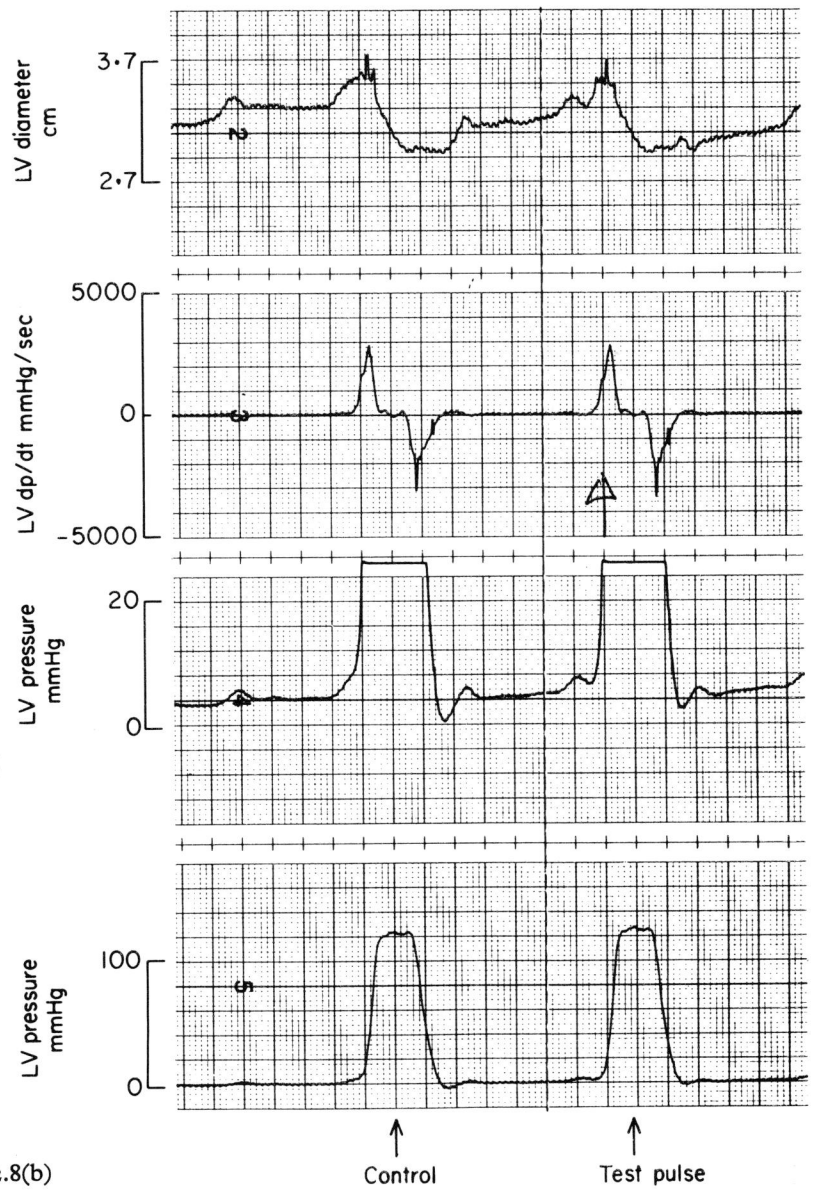

FIG. 2.8(b)

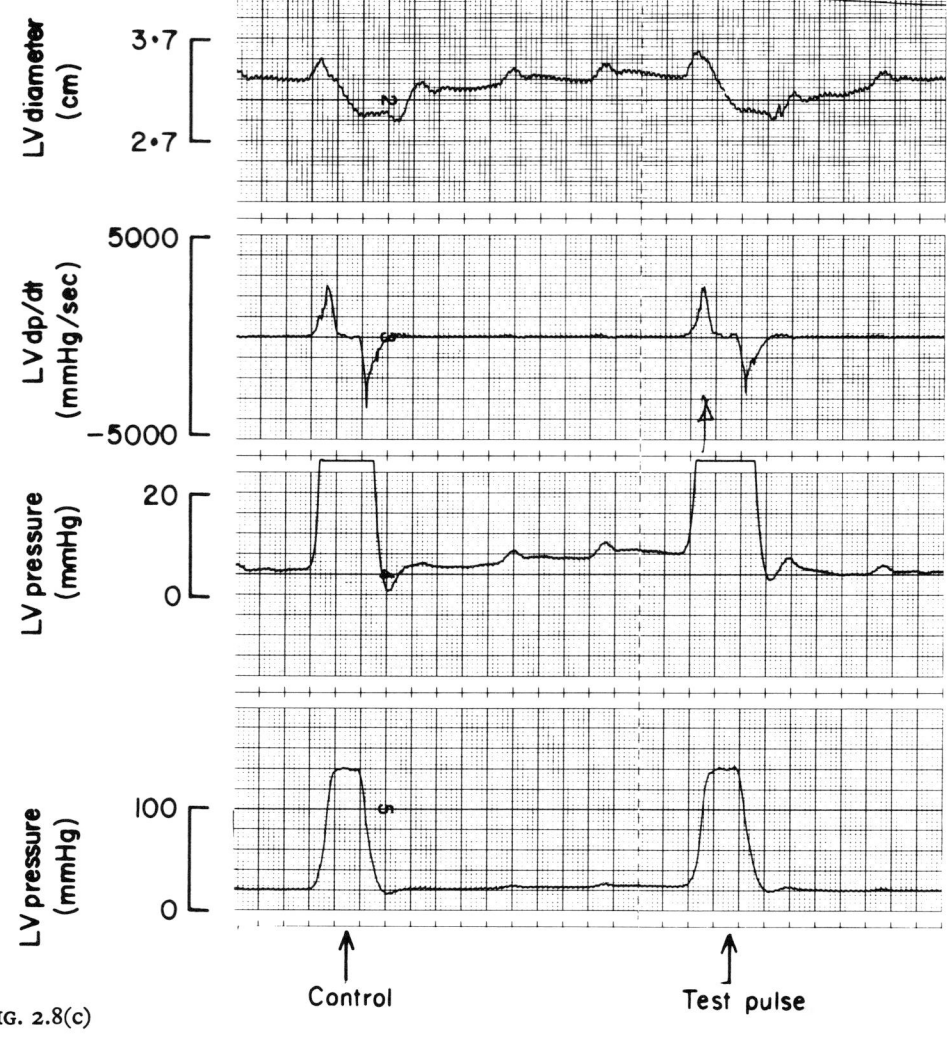

FIG. 2.8(c)

ment of Edman and Johannsson's compartment II, labelled R (residual or resistant or 'rested state Ca^{++}'). For the moment I leave out the exit arrow from compartment I since this has not been discussed above; consideration of this must now be taken up.

Calcium ion loss from the cell

The only loss of calcium ions from the cell described so far is that from compartment 2 which accounts for the decay in contractile state with long intervals (Fig. 2.9b). However this loss is very slow (over ten seconds) and therefore for practical purposes at normal heart rates of 1/second or more, it can be ignored. It is therefore clear from Fig. 2.7d that the system is unstable. Ca^{++} enters the cell with every action potential but there is no exit of Ca^{++}. This would mean that intracellular Ca^{++} accumulates indefinitely.

We know that this is not the case. With steady pacing at a fixed rate the isometric tension is constant so that the amount of calcium leaving and entering the cell must be equal in the steady state. Reuter has described a system whereby internal Ca^{++} is exchanged for external Na^+ during diastole; there may be other calcium extrusion systems.

The rapid calcium ion exit system depends on the presence of contractions and relaxations. If one has a potentiated state, it decays slowly in the absence of contractions as in Fig. 2.9b but decays rapidly within about six beats in the presence of cardiac cycles (Fig. 2.10). This can be explained by saying that part of the calcium taken up during relaxation is extruded. This means one needs a second uptake compartment (compartment 3 in Fig. 2.7e) which performs this function. The alternative is to divide compartment 1 into two subcompartments (Fig. 2.7f)

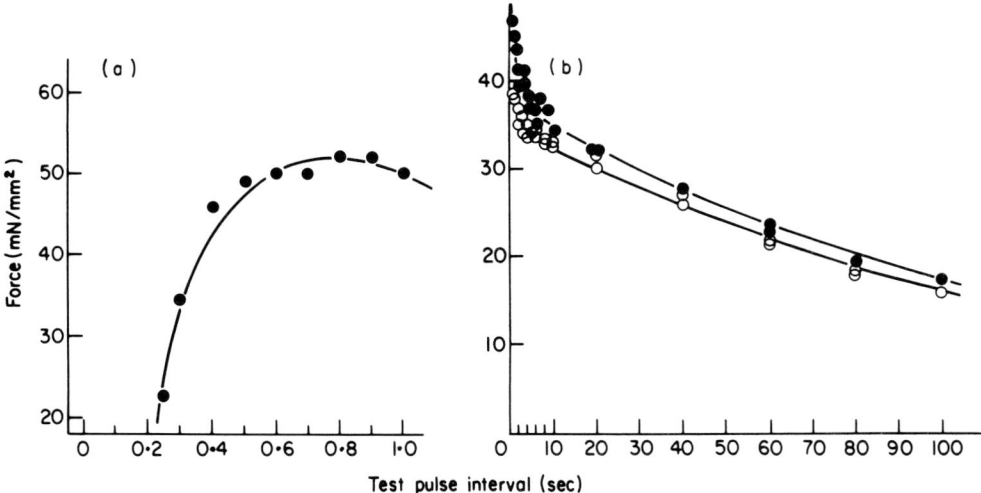

FIG. 2.9. Rabbit papillary muscle. (a) Relationship of contractile force to test pulse interval. (b) Forces obtained when test pulse intervals longer than the optimum are used. From Edman and Johannsson (1976).

labelled C and E (C for Ca^{++} circulating subcompartment and E for Ca^{++} extrusion subcompartment). A separate compartment 3 has an advantage if one wants to postulate that it is a separate structure, e.g. mitochondria.

An important property of compartment 3 or subcompartment 1E is that the amount of Ca^{++} extruded increases to equal any increase of Ca^{++} entering the cell during action potentials. This is necessary in order to satisfy steady state conditions. It will be seen in the next section that such increases in steady state Ca^{++} entry and exit do occur and are associated with an increase in the total amount of Ca^{++} recirculating within the cell. The regulation of Ca^{++} extrusion could be assumed at this stage to be a relatively simple dependence on the amount of Ca^{++} in compartment 3.

It is tempting to speculate on the anatomical sites of these compartments.

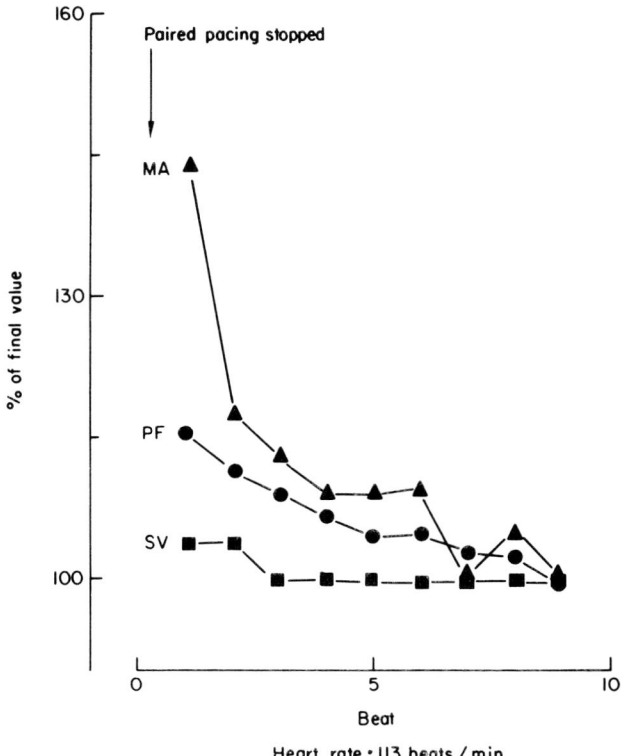

FIG. 2.10.   Beat by beat decay of post extrasystolic potentiation in a conscious dog after stopping paired pulse stimulation. MA = maximum acceleration of blood from the left ventricle. PF = peak outflow velocity. SV = stroke volume.

Morad and Goldman, and Kaufman for instance suggest that the release compartments are in the cisternae and lateral sacs and the uptake compartment is the 'longitudinal' sarcoplasmic reticulum. However, it is strange in that case that incoming Ca^{++} during the action potential goes to the more distant longitudinal sarcoplasmic reticulum and is then passed back to the superficially placed cisternae after 0·8 sec. There is no direct evidence for this suggestion and no evidence against postulating the reverse. I prefer to think that maybe the uptake compartment is due to binding of Ca^{++} to the sarcoplasmic reticulum membrane and that time is required for this bound calcium to be truly taken up into the tubules. It is possible that the latter process must take place before the Ca^{++} can be released again. The Ca^{++} in the sarcoplasmic reticulum lumen is the release compartment (2). It is not unreasonable to suppose that part of the Ca^{++} entering during the action potential is bound to the sarcoplasmic reticulum membrane (i.e. compartment 1). However, whatever the mechanisms, there seems no reason to doubt that the functional compartments exist somewhere and this is all one needs to explain the force frequency relationship (below), i.e. the effect of an increase in heart rate.

Force-frequency relationship and Bowditch 'staircase' or 'treppe'

The Bowditch 'staircase' is illustrated in Fig. 2.11. A rabbit papillary muscle was stimulated at 1/sec in the control period, *a*. The stimulation frequency was then increased to 4/sec during the next period, *b*. One sees a progressive build up of tension until a steady state is reached. It has been common in the intact heart literature to interpret the Bowditch effect as an increase in contractility caused by an increase in heart rate. However in intact dogs in good condition, there is hardly any difference in contractility in the steady state when heart rate is increased. In the isolated muscle literature it is well known that the steady state force-frequency relationship is highly variable. The usual finding is a marked increase in steady state force development with increasing stimulation frequency as is the case in Fig. 2.11. When the force-frequency relationship has been compared in the same heart *in vitro* and *in vivo*, it has been found that whereas force plotted against frequency has a positive slope *in vitro*, it is flat when determined *in vivo*. Can these apparent inconsistencies be clarified by use of the analysis presented in the preceding sections?

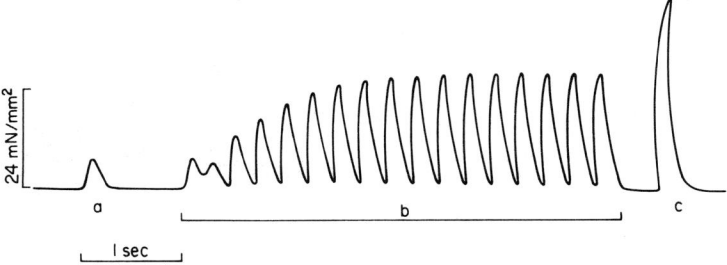

FIG. 2.11. (a) low frequency, (b) high frequency. Note increase in force development. *c* is an optimal contractile response pertaining to frequency *b*. From Edman and Johannsson (1976).

After a period of pacing at 4/sec, *b* in Fig. 2.11, a test pulse interval was introduced at *c* of 0.6 sec. This beat, *c*, was much stronger than the steady state beats in period *b*. This shows that the amount of calcium circulating in the cell is greater than the amount released in any one steady state beat. This is because the steady state interval is too short for all the calcium to pass from compartment 1 to compartment 2 which takes 600–800 msec in this preparation (Fig. 2.9a). One only detects the full amount of calcium present when one stops and puts in a stimulus at the optimum interval.

The effect of increasing the stimulation rate in the steady state is seen in Fig. 2.12a where the relationship of force to test pulse interval is depicted at four rates. This figure shows that the optimal contractile response occurs at the same time at each steady state frequency. It also shows that with increasing steady state frequency the optimal contractile response also increases, i.e. the total amount of circulating Ca^{++} increases as revealed by the force generated after waiting the optimum interval. If the steady state interval is shorter than the optimum, less force than this

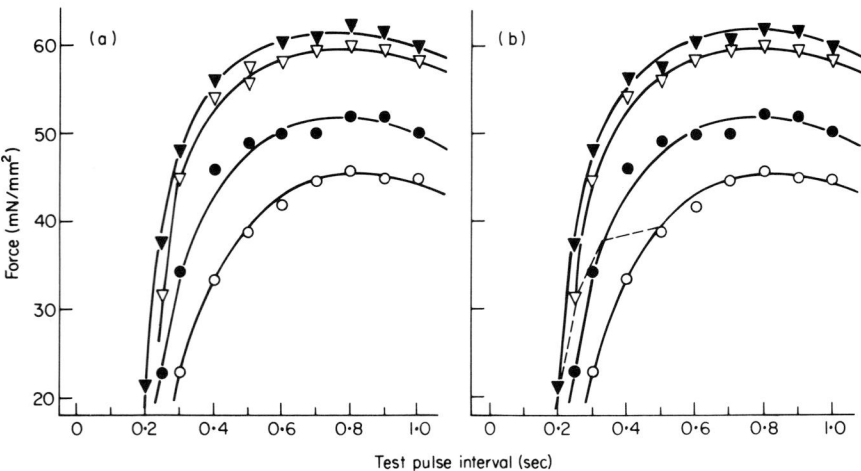

FIG. 2.12.   (a) Test pulse interval curves following stimulation at four priming intervals of
2 (○), 3 (●), 4 (▽) and 5 (▼) stimuli/sec. (b) dashed line joins values at steady state
(priming) frequency. From Edman and Johannsson (1976).

will be produced in steady state contractions. These forces for the four rates shown
in Fig. 2.12a are joined together by the dashed line in Fig. 2.12b. In Fig. 2.13, the
steady state forces are plotted against rate using the filled circles and it can be seen
that the values rise to a plateau between 3 and 4/sec and then fall. On the other
hand, the optimal contractile response, indicating the amount of Ca^{++} circulating,
continues to increase even when steady state force begins to fall. In this preparation
(rabbit papillary muscle) the muscle is still not full of Ca^{++} at 5/sec since the

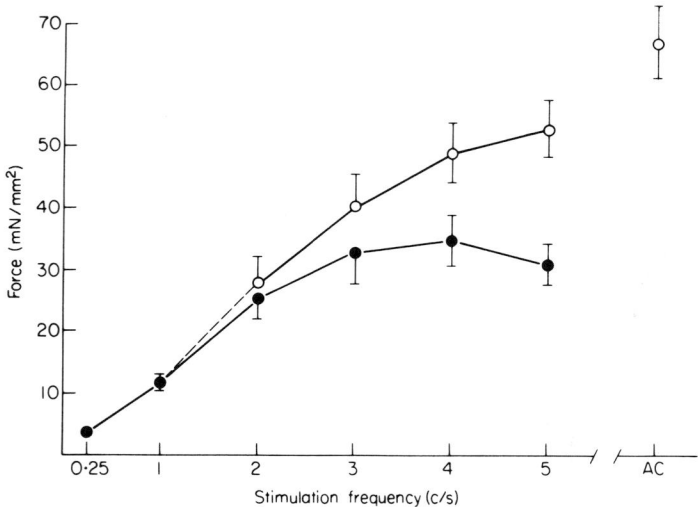

FIG. 2.13.   ● : Amplitude of steady state twitch responses. ○ : Optimum contractile
response at different frequencies and, top right at 20/sec a.c. stimulation. From Edman and
Johannsson (1976).

optimal contractile response after pushing more Ca^{++} in with a.c. stimulation is even higher than that at 5/sec (open circle on right).

Clearly the shape of the steady state force-frequency relationship (solid circles in Fig. 2.13) and the position of the plateau will be highly variable depending on the shapes and positions of the test pulse interval curves (Fig. 2.12). These in turn depend on the physiological condition of the Ca^{++} uptake and release compartments leading to variation between the *in vivo* and *in vitro* conditions. In the intact, conscious dog, the plateau of the steady state force-frequency curve occurs in the physiological range of 1·5–2·5 cycles per sec (90 to 150 beats/min) instead of between 3 and 4 cycles/sec in the rabbit papillary muscle. However, the test pulse interval curves and optimal contractile response increasing with frequency are still present in the intact dog. There is no fundamental difference in mechanisms as can

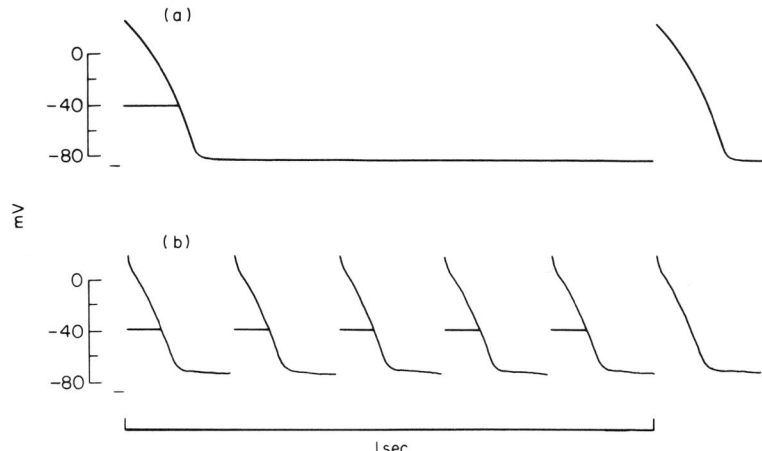

FIG. 2.14. Oscilloscope traces illustrating action potentials at 1/sec (upper) and 5/sec (lower). The time during which the cell membrane is depolarised beyond the −40 mV level during a 1 sec interval is indicated by horizontal bars. From Edman and Johannsson (1976).

be confirmed by observing the transient changes following a sudden increase in heart rate (initial weaker beat followed by Bowditch staircase) and decrease in heart rate (initial strong beat followed by a decay).

Why is the optimal contractile response increased by increased heart rate? Edman and Johannsson correlated this with the fact that because there are more action potentials in a given time (Fig. 2.14) the fraction of time during which the membrane is depolarised is increased, i.e. the time for calcium influx is increased and therefore the calcium influx will be higher. When the optimum contractile response is correlated with the fraction of time for membrane depolarisation, an excellent linear relation is obtained (Fig. 2.15). However, the fraction of time for membrane depolarisation was measured in the steady state as an index of calcium influx, i.e. at a time when this is equal to calcium efflux. Since both calcium ion influx and efflux increase with increased heart rate, one might wonder why there is a correlation between these fluxes and the optimal contractile response reflecting total circulating Ca^{++}.

The answer lies in the fact that there is a time lag for extra Ca^{++} entering compartment 1 (with the action potential) to reach compartment 3 (Fig. 2.7e), raise the level of Ca^{++} there and stimulate Ca^{++} extrusion. The relationship shown in Fig. 2.15 does not hold true for transient non-steady state conditions. The sequence of events accompanying an increase in heart rate is illustrated in Fig. 2.16. At the time of a step increase in frequency (arrow), there is an increase in Ca^{++} influx (continuous line) followed after a transit time by an equal increase in efflux (dashed line). The difference is obtained by subtracting efflux from influx. The change in

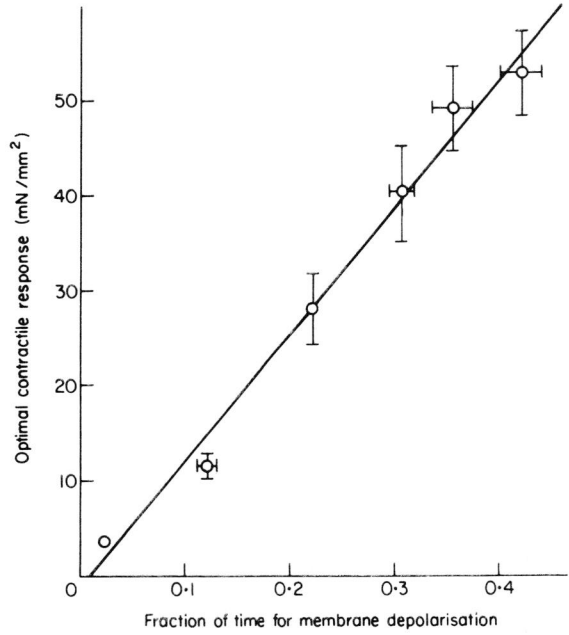

FIG. 2.15. Relationship between optimum contractile response and the fraction of time during which the cell membrane is depolarised beyond −40 mV at stimulation frequencies between 0.25–5/sec. From Edman and Johannsson (1976).

total circulating Ca^{++} is obtained by integrating the area under the curve of difference between influx and efflux. When an increase in influx occurs, there is an increase in circulating Ca^{++} only because of the time lag between the increases in influx and efflux. When the influx increase is greater because of a greater increase in heart rate, the increase in total Ca^{++} is also greater. In the right hand panel the influx was doubled, the total Ca^{++} is doubled, i.e. the total Ca^{++} is proportional to the influx increase. The reason why optimal contractile response is proportional to the fraction of time for membrane depolarisation, considered here as an index of influx, is thus clarified.

However, this is still an oversimplification because there is also less time between

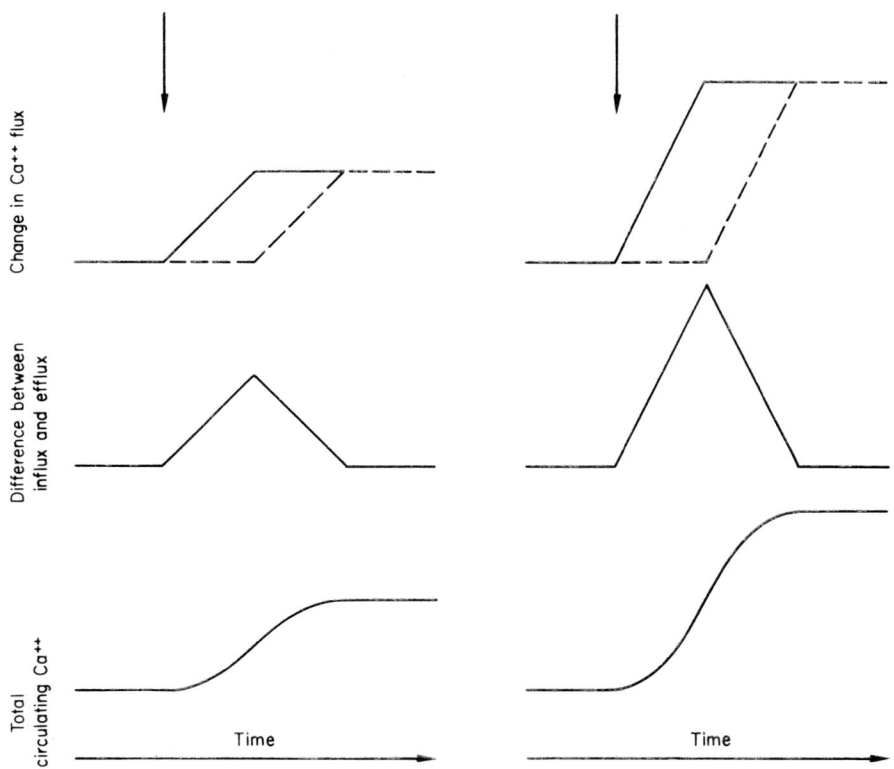

FIG. 2.16. Scheme for events following an increase in calcium ion influx. Continuous line = influx, dashed line = efflux.

action potentials (Fig. 2.14) and therefore less time for Ca^{++} efflux between action potentials. This will lead to all the consequences of decreased Ca^{++} efflux discussed below and depicted in Fig. 2.17; these will add to the effects of increased Ca^{++} influx transiently. Both effects must therefore be reduced by negative feedback mechanisms in order for them to equalise in the steady state condition.

Inotropic effects

An important feature of cardiac function is that the strength of the beat can be varied considerably by external influences. Increases in beat strength are usually called increases in contractility or positive inotropic effects. These are now thought to be mediated by increases of Ca^{++} concentration following activation. In following some of these effects, use can be made of the same scheme as was used for increase in heart rate (Fig. 2.16).

A relatively simple and effective positive inotropic effect is that of increased external Ca^{++} concentration. In the steady state, the twitch tension is a function of external Ca^{++}. In Fig. 2.16 the arrow indicates the time of a step increase in external Ca^{++}. This results in more Ca^{++} entering the cell with each action

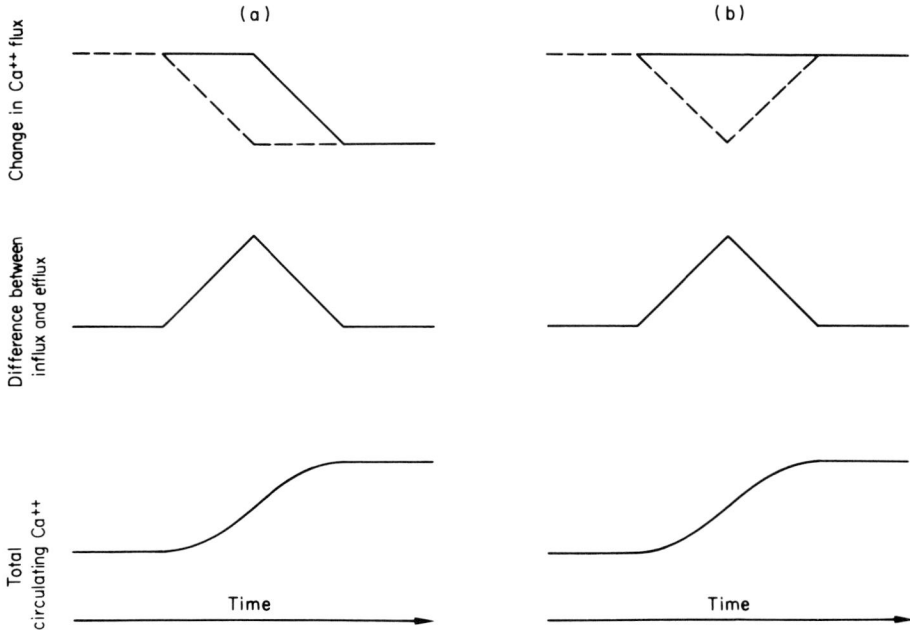

FIG. 2.17.   Scheme for events following a decrease in calcium ion efflux.

potential because of the increased concentration gradient across the membrane. The increased influx is indicated by the continuous line. Efflux (dashed line) will increase by the same amount to produce steady state requirements. As with increased heart rate, the total circulating Ca^{++} increases because of the transient difference between influx and efflux and is equal to the integral of this difference.

Most probably the increased efflux is caused by the increase in total circulating Ca^{++}. This would be expected with the diastolic exchange of internal Ca^{++} for external Na^{++}. It is also indicated by the fact that contractility is more closely related to the Ca/Na concentration ratio than to Ca^{++} concentration alone. It seems reasonable to suppose that the positive inotropic effect of decreased external Na^{+} concentration is partly due to decreased efflux by the Ca^{++}/Na^{+} exchange mechanism, rather than just competition between Na^{+} and Ca^{++} for the slow inward channels of the action potential plateau, allowing decreased external Na^{+} to cause increased Ca^{++} inflow, and a sequence of events as depicted in Fig. 2.16.

The suggested sequence of events with this intervention is shown in Fig. 2.17a. At the arrow, Ca^{++} efflux (dashed line) is reduced by a step decrease in external Na^{+} concentration. Influx (continuous line) will decrease by the same amount to produce steady state requirements. The total circulating Ca^{++} increases because of the transient difference between influx and efflux and is equal to the integral of this difference. An interesting consequence of these considerations is that there has to be a negative feedback mechanism whereby an increase in total circulating Ca^{++}

causes a decrease in influx. Alternatively, the increase in total circulating Ca^{++} must force the efflux rate back to the control level (Fig. 2.17b). Without one or other of these control mechanisms, the system for control of contractility would be unstable.

The first mechanism, i.e. that circulating Ca^{++} affects Ca^{++} inflow inversely is suggested by the fact that when the internal circulating Ca^{++} is depleted by a series of beats with artificially shortened action potentials, there is a large difference in the tensions resulting from action potentials with and without plateaus, i.e. the depletion of circulating Ca^{++} leads to a much greater Ca^{++} inflow during the action potential plateau.

If we return for a moment parenthetically to the effect of Ca^{++} increase extra-cellularly—this will tend to decrease Ca^{++} efflux by the Ca^{++}/Na^{+} exchange system and tend to accentuate the build up of internal Ca^{++} greatly and in an unstable fashion unless that increased internal Ca^{++} has an inhibitory effect on Ca^{++} influx. Thus, increased external Ca^{++} and increased heart rate are both likely to involve a combination of the sequence of events in Figs. 2.16 and 2.17 (Fig. 2.18) and steady state conditions in these and perhaps all inotropic phenomena depend on the presence of negative feedback control of both Ca^{++} influx and Ca^{++} efflux.

The simplest hypothesis to account for a decrease in Ca^{++} inflow (Fig. 2.17a)

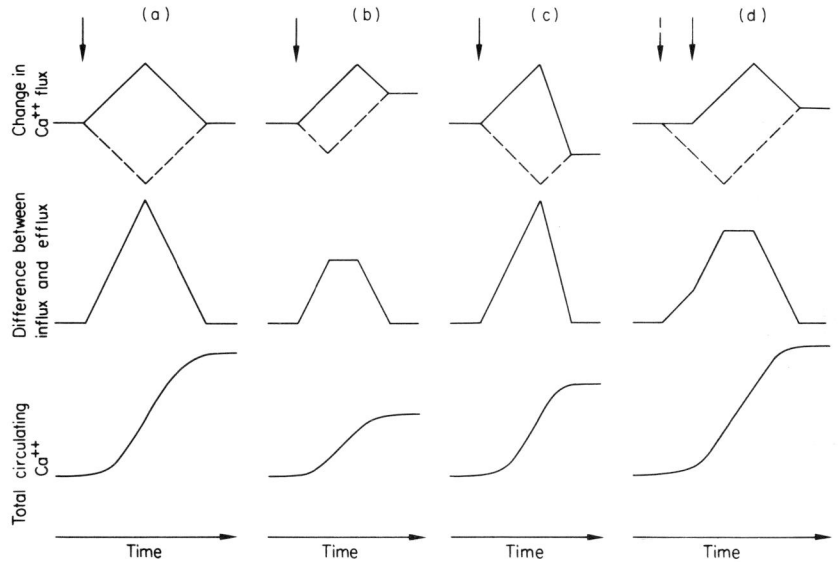

FIG. 2.18.   Various hypothetical schemes leading to a positive inotropic response.

seems to be that Ca^{++} inflow during the action potential is inhibited by an increase of Ca^{++} in compartment 1 (Fig. 2.7). However in this case the timing is wrong. At the time of the action potential in a steady state at the optimum interval, the Ca^{++} (mainly) is in compartment 2. This might indicate compartment 2 Ca^{++} as the most likely inhibitor of Ca^{++} influx. This is further suggested by the effect of pre-mature extrasystoles. A premature beat comes just after a normal contraction when compartment 2 is 'empty', i.e. low in Ca^{++}. As a result there would be no inhibitory effect of compartment 2 Ca^{++} on Ca^{++} inflow which would therefore be greatly augmented. Thus the positive inotropic effect of extrasystoles (as judged by optimal contractile response) is much greater than a doubling of steady state frequency.

Most other positive inotropic interventions have more than one action. For instance, catecholamines, the principal agents for increase of contractility in life, have an acceleratory action on Ca^{++} sequestration by the sarcoplasmic reticulum causing earlier and more rapid relaxation. It is possible that this causes preferential uptake of Ca^{++} by compartment 1 at the expense of compartment 3, i.e. a greater fraction of Ca^{++} taken up is recirculated (hitherto this fraction has been assumed to be constant). The drop in Ca^{++} in compartment 3 would lead to reduced efflux and

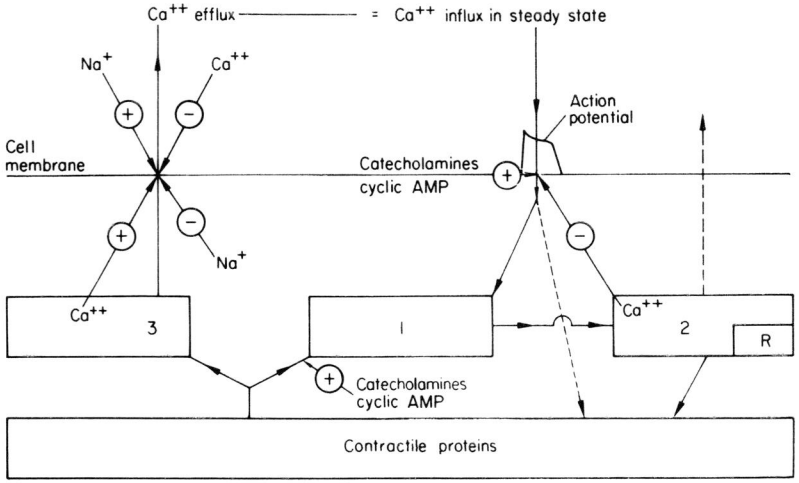

FIG. 2.19. Working hypothesis for control of contractility. —⊕→ accelerating influence on calcium ion flow. —⊖→ decelerating influence.

a sequence of events as illustrated in Fig. 2.17. Otherwise it is necessary to postulate an effect of catecholamines to increase Ca^{++} influx during the action potential and a sequence of events as illustrated in Fig. 2.16.

The other favourite agents, digitalis and caffeine are even more complicated. There are several rival hypotheses to account for the positive inotropic effect of digitalis which are outside the scope of this work, as are the mechanisms of action of many other drugs. The increase in intracellular Na^+ concentration (and possibly a decrease in the Na^+ concentration of a restricted extracellular space between cells) leads to decreased efflux by the Ca^{++}/Na^+ exchange from compartment 3 and a sequence of events as illustrated in Fig. 2.17. Caffeine has a direct action to release Ca^{++} from sarcoplasmic reticulum and also inhibits the uptake of Ca^{++} by sarcoplasmic reticulum. It therefore produces larger, more prolonged contractions in low concentrations and contracture in high concentrations.

It is now thought by many that the effect of increased muscle length is also due to increased activation by Ca^{++} (Chapter 5). This conclusion is partly based on the fact that skinned cells are little affected by changes in muscle length, indicating possibly that it is not stretch of the sarcoplasmic reticulum that mediates the effect of length but stretch of the cell membrane. It would be interesting to check this point by indirect methods in intact cells, e.g. does an increase in length affect the optimum interval between beats? Stretch of the cell membrane could influence its properties in such a way as to produce increased Ca^{++} inflow* during the action potential, or decreased outflow by the Ca^{++}/Na$^+$ exchange, or both. What is the relative effect of increased length on twitch tension and tonic tension during prolonged artificial depolarisation?

I suggest as a working hypothesis for the Ca^{++} cardiac cycle and control of contractile tension the functional model depicted in Fig. 2.19.

REFERENCES

ALLEN D.G., JEWELL B.R. & WOOD E.H. (1976) Studies of the contractility of mammalian myocardium at low rates of stimulation. *J. Physiol.*, **254**, 1–17.

BAILEY L.E., ONG S.D. & QUEEN G.M. (1972) Calcium movement during contraction in the cat heart. *J. Molec. Cell. Cardiol.*, **4**, 121–138.

BASS B.C. (1975) Restitution of the action potential in cat papillary muscle in relation to stimulation frequency. *J. Physiol.*, **254**, 565–581.

BASS O. (1976) The decay of the potentiated state in sheep and calf ventricular myocardial fibres. *Circulation Res.*, **39**, 396–399.

BEELER G.W. Jr. & REUTER H. (1970) Relation between membrane potential, membrane currents and activation of contraction in ventricular myocardial fibres. *J. Physiol.*, **207**, 211–229.

BOWDITCH H.P. (1871) Uber die Eigenthumlichkeiten der Reizbarkeit, welche die Muskelfasern des Herzens zeigen. *Ber. Verhandl. Saechs. Akad. Wiss. Leipzig*, 652–689.

EBASHI S., ENDO M. & OHTSUKI I. (1969) Control of muscle contraction. *Q. Rev. Biophys.*, **2**, 351–384.

EDMAN K.A.P. & JOHANNSSON M. (1976) The contractile state of rabbit papillary muscle in relation to stimulation frequency. *J. Physiol.*, **254**, 565–581.

FABIATO A. & FABIATO F. (1975a). Contractions induced by a calcium-triggered release of calcium from the sarcoplasmic reticulum of single skinned cardiac cells. *J. Physiol.*, **249**, 469–495.

FABIATO A. & FABIATO F. (1975b). Relaxing and inotropic effects of cyclic AMP on skinned cardiac cells. *Nature*, **253**, 556–558.

FABIATO A. & FABIATO F. (1977). Calcium release from the sarcoplasmic reticulum. *Circulation Res.*, **40**, 119–129.

FORD L.E. & PODOLSKY R.J. (1970) Regenerative calcium release within muscle cells. *Science*, **167**, 58–59.

FORD L.E. & PODOLSKY R.J. (1972) Intracellular calcium movements in skinned muscle fibres. *J. Physiol.*, **223**, 21–33.

GIBBONS W.R. & FOZZARD H.A. (1975) Slow inward current and contraction of sheep cardiac Purkinje fibres. *J. Gen. Physiol.*, **65**, 367–384.

* This seems to be what happens in barnacle muscle cells where there is a greater depolarisation for a given current stimulation at longer fibre lengths. Calcium ion release dependence on length has been documented in this preparation with aequorin.

GORDON A.M. & RIDGEWAY E.B. (1976) Length-dependent electro-mechanical coupling in single muscle fibres. *J. Gen. Physiol.*, **68**, 653–669.

HARIGAYA S. & SCHWARTZ A. (1969) Rate of calcium binding and uptake in normal animal and failing human cardiac muscle. *Circulation Res.*, **25**, 781–794.

HOFFMAN B.F., BINDLER E. & SUCKLING E.E. (1956) Postextrasystolic potentiation of contraction in cardiac muscle. *Am. J. Physiol.*, **185**, 95.

HUXLEY A.F. (1971) The Croonian Lecture 1967: The activation of striated muscle and its mechanical response. *Proc. Roy. Soc., Lond.*, **178**, 1–27.

KALIN M.L., KAVALER F. & FISHER V.J. (1976) Frequency-force relationships of mammalian ventricular muscle *in vivo* and *in vitro*. *Am. J. Physiol.*, **230**, 631–636.

KAUFMAN R., BAYER R., FURNISS T., KRAUSE H. & TRITTHART H. (1974) Calcium-movement controlling cardiac contractility. II. Analog computation of cardiac excitation-contraction coupling on the basis of calcium kinetics in a multi-compartment model. *J. Molec. Cell. Cardiol.*, **6**, 543–559.

KOCH-WESER J. (1966) Potentiation of myocardial contractility by continual premature extra-systoles. *Circulation Res.*, **18**, 330–343.

KOCH-WESER J. & BLINKS J.R. (1963) The influence of the interval between beats on myocardial contractility. *Pharmacol. Rev.*, **15**, 601.

LANGER G.A. (1968) Ion fluxes in cardiac excitation contraction and their relation to myocardial contractility. *Physiol. Rev.*, **48**, 708–757.

LANGER G.A. (1973) Heart: Excitation-contraction coupling. *Ann. Rev. Physiol.*, **35**, 55–86.

LEWARTOWSKI B. & CZARNECKA M. (1970) Relation between the shape of the cellular action potentials and the strength of contraction of the heart muscle. *Acta Physiol., Pol.*, **1**, 1–14.

MORAD M. & GOLDMAN Y. (1973) Excitation-contraction coupling in heart muscle: membrane control of development of tension. *Progress Biophys. molec. Biol.*, **27**, 257–308.

MORAD M. & TRAUTWEIN W. (1968) The effect of the duration of the action potential on contraction in the mammalian heart tissue. *Pflügers Arch.*, **299**, 66–82.

NAKAJIMA Y. & ENDO M. (1973) Release of calcium induced by depolarisation of the sarcoplasmic reticulum membrane. *Nature New Biol.*, **246**, 216–218.

NEW W. & TRAUTWEIN W. (1972) Ionic nature of slow inward current and its relation to contraction. *Pflügers Arch.*, **334**, 24–38.

NIEDERGERKE R. (1956) The 'staircase' phenomenon and the action of calcium on the heart. *J. Physiol.*, **134**, 569–583.

NIEDERGERKE R., PAGE S. & TALBOT M.S. (1969). Calcium fluxes in frog heart ventricles. *Pflügers Arch.*, **306**, 357–360.

REPKE D.I. & KATZ A.M. (1972) Calcium-binding and calcium uptake by cardiac microsomes: a kinetic analysis. *J. Molec. Cell. Cardiol.*, **4**, 401–416.

REUTER H. (1974). Exchange of calcium ions in the mammalian myocardium. Mechanisms and physiological significance. *Circulation Res.*, **34**, 599–605.

SANDOW A. (1965) Excitation-contraction coupling in skeletal muscle. *Pharmacol. Rev.*, **17**, 265–320.

TRAUTWEIN W. (1973) Membrane currents in cardiac muscle. *Physiol. Rev.*, **53**, 793–835.

TRITTHART H., KAUFMAN R., VOLKMER H-P, BAYER R. & KRAUSE H. (1973) Ca-movement controlling myocardial contractility. *Pflügers Arch.*, **338**, 207–231.

WOOD E.H., HEPPNER R.L. & WEIDMANN S. (1969) Inotropic effects of electric currents. I. Positive and negative effects of constant electric currents or current pulses applied during cardiac action potentials. II. Hypothesis: Calcium movements, excitation-contraction coupling and inotropic effects. *Circulation Res.*, **24**, 409–445.

WOODWORTH R.S. (1902) Maximal contraction, 'staircase' contraction, refractory period and compensatory pause of the heart. *Am. J. Physiol.*, **8**, 213.

CHAPTER 3

THE MECHANISM OF CONTRACTION

INTRODUCTION

In the previous chapter, I presented some ideas about how changes in the strength of cardiac contraction might be achieved by varying the amount of Ca^{++} ion circulating in the cell. Since a number of authors have presented similar kinds of model, the basic idea can be considered not too controversial. However, attempts to show changes in Ca^{++} uptake, e.g. by radioactive Ca^{++} tracer methods have failed to produce convincing results. This can be put forward as disproof of the theory. I think that in the case of the Ca^{++} cardiac cycle theory, this is not the case because of the inadequacy of the method. In postulating molecular mechanisms at sub-cellular level, one is often beyond the resolution of current methods of investigation of intact cells or tissue.

When considering the question of how contraction occurs by interaction of thin actin filaments and thick myosin filaments with active cross projections, this problem also applies, but research workers have been too inclined to explain any results from such methods in terms of the cross-bridge theory of contraction. I think it is rather unlikely that molecules would grip the thin filaments, pull them along, detach, grip and pull again at high frequency. Unfortunately, results which give strong evidence against that theory have been ignored, or rather fanciful extra hypotheses put forward to explain them away. One obvious example is the fact that in skeletal muscle, when overlap between thick and thin filaments is reduced in actively contracting fibres, the force increases even though fewer cross-bridges can interact and less force would be predicted (Deleze 1961, Edman, Elzinga & Noble 1978). Another is the fact that ATP causes the cross-bridge and thin filament to dissociate (Eisenberg & Kielly 1973). Another is the finding of Oplatka that contractions can occur in the absence of thick filaments. More detailed consideration of the pros and cons of cross-bridge theory and Iwazumi's theory (below) is given in an article by Noble and Pollack (1977).

As we are particularly interested here in cardiac muscle, I must draw attention to the problem of double overlap of thin filaments which commonly occurs in the working range of heart muscle. How does a cross-bridge sort out the need to pull only the thin filament of its own side and make sure it does not pull the thin filament from the opposite side in the wrong direction? One of the great attractions of Iwazumi's theory is that thin filaments are always pulled in the 'right' direction as a natural consequence of the principle of force generation. The consequences of double overlap will be discussed in greater detail by Iwazumi.

In discussing the question of the mechanism of contraction, one of the difficulties is that while cross-bridge theory is familiar and there are many articles describing it, Iwazumi's alternative ideas have never been seriously considered. For this reason I take this opportunity to concentrate on them. The characteristics of a theory are often determined by the first question one asks. In the case of cross-bridge theory, the question was, 'How can force and movement be generated between the two sets of filaments?' I think this has tended to lead us to forget that the filament array is not a semi-rigid skeleton. Iwazumi, on the other hand, asks a more fundamental question first, namely, 'How is the orderly array of the filamentous structure maintained in the face of high mechanical forces?' The obvious pulling function of the cross-bridge theory is immediately rejected because it causes collapse of the structural order.

A THEORY OF SARCOMERE DYNAMICS

by TATSUO IWAZUMI

1. Introduction

How does muscle contract? What is the molecular mechanism? How can we explain and predict the complex behaviour of muscle on a unified and self consistent basis? These are questions that have been asked by scientists for so long. Yet, no satisfactory or convincing answers have emerged despite tremendous efforts that have gone into research on muscle contraction. A great number of theories have been proposed, refuted and forgotten since the turn of this century. In the past two decades cross-bridge theory (Huxley 1969, Huxley & Simmons 1971) has enjoyed widest acceptance among muscle researchers, but the situation is far from settled. No theory of science has been found to be perfect, and cross-bridge theory is no exception. We must still strive for a unified and self consistent theory that explains every aspect of muscle in order to fully understand its mechanism of contraction. To this end we need to develop alternative theories toward perfection.

The purpose of this chapter is to introduce the reader to a relatively new theory of muscle contraction (Iwazumi 1970) and to discuss some selected topics to demonstrate how this theory predicts and explains various phenomena.

2. Conceptual background of theory

Without resort to any scientific measurement we know that muscle generates a contractile force upon activation. In addition, with the help of modern instruments, we now have positive evidence that muscle expends a small amount of energy at rest and varying amounts during contraction, and that certain ultrastructural features are invariant among all functionally intact striated muscles. The cellular subunit of striated muscle, the sarcomere, has highly distinct features. The major constituents are two different kinds of filaments: the thick filament, consisting mostly of myosin to form the *A*-band; and the thin filament, consisting mostly of actin and occupying the *I*-band as illustrated in Fig. 3.1. Two *Z*-lines delineate the sarcomere, and the distance between them is defined as sarcomere length. Optical and electron micrographs indicate that the thick and thin filament interdigitate and slide past each other upon contraction (Huxley & Niedergerke 1954, Huxley & Hanson 1954).

Because of the fact that an isolated single fibril (membrane free, and many sarcomeres connected in series) can contract normally in an appropriate medium, there is no doubt that a contractile force is developed between the thick and thin filaments. Experimental evidence supporting the sliding filament mechanism derives solely from electron microscopy. However, it is not yet certain whether the length of these two kinds of filaments remains invariant with sarcomere length changes.

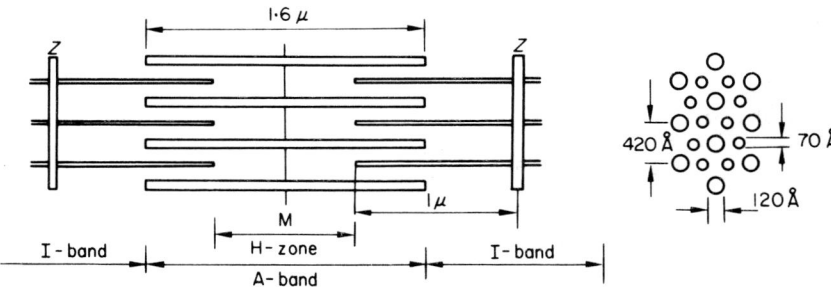

FIG. 3.1. A schematic sarcomere to show the spatial relationship and sizes of the thick and thin filament. The dimensions are approximate values found in typical skeletal and cardiac muscle.

A conspicuous feature of the sarcomere is that the *A*-band remains at the centre of the sarcomere at any sarcomere length which is less than the sum of the thick filament and twice the thin filament lengths, i.e. any length that allows some overlap of thick and thin filaments. This central positioning of the *A*-band has been observed universally in all normal sarcomere of striated muscles. The *A*-band may not be at the centre, however, if the sarcomere length has been extended beyond the overlap limit; such over-extension invariably results in impaired contractile force and significantly increased variation of sarcomere lengths. Other ultrastructural features revealed in transverse sections are the thick filament, arranged in hexagonal array, and the thin filaments, about equidistant from neighbouring thick filaments (the thin filament of cardiac and skeletal muscle is usually located at the trigonal point of three thick filaments, but this is not true in most other types of muscles).

The fundamental question from which this theory evolved is as follows. *If a force is generated between the thick and thin filaments, what are the requirements for the high degree of structural orders of the sarcomere?* For the *A*-band to remain at the centre of the sarcomere the laws of physics demand that the potential energy associated with the force on the A-band be minimum at the centre. This is called the longitudinal stability condition. Furthermore, the equidistant position of a thin filament from the adjacent thick filaments requires that another potential energy be minimum. This is called the lateral stability condition. These two independent stability conditions can be mathematically formulated independent of the physical mechanism of force generation in muscle. In other words, any mechanism must satisfy the longitudinal and lateral stability conditions in order for the muscle ultrastructure to retain its structural orders and remain functionally intact during the large deformations that take place during contraction.

In principle, many mechanisms of force generation could satisfy the longitudinal

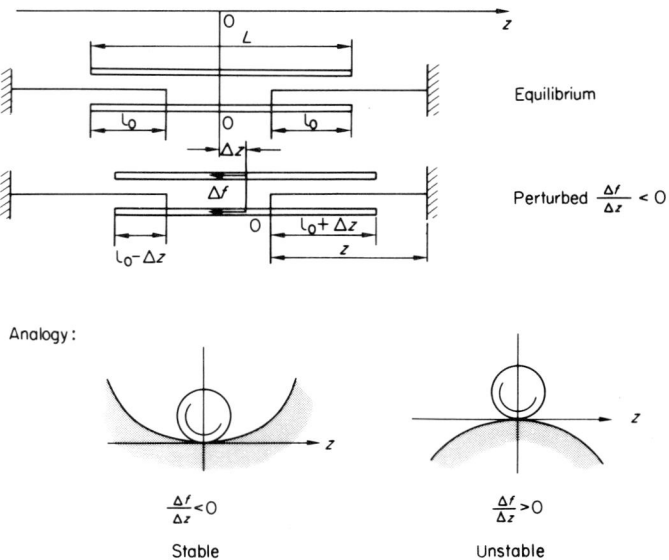

FIG. 3.2. Longitudinal stability condition of the thick filament. In order for the thick filament to be stable at the centre, as seen in all striated muscle, the restoring force Δf must always point towards the centre.

and lateral stability conditions. As we shall see later, there are many additional constraints that must be imposed because muscle is a biological system that derives its energy from chemical reactions. Let us consider what limitation the longitudinal stability condition imposes upon possible force generation mechanisms. A simple method to derive the longitudinal stability condition is shown in Fig. 3.2. In order that the thick filaments tend to remain at the centre of the sarcomere, the direction of the restoring force, Δf, must always point to the centre; hence, $\Delta f/\Delta z$ must be negative. In other words, a greater contractile force must be generated at the side with less overlap. Because of the symmetry of the structure and the continuously variable overlap length from zero to maximum, we must conclude that the contractile mechanism is required to generate greater force with decreasing overlap length.

Note that this argument is valid independent of filament length. In order to assure that the thick filaments never drift away during steady contractions that can be realised in a skinned fibre preparation with ATP and Ca^{++} activation, the above requirement must hold true both statically and dynamically.

In the following sections is a theory which assumes that force is generated by the action of an electrostatic field on a dielectric body. This mechanism not only satisfies both longitudinal and lateral stability conditions but also is compatible with other biochemical, energetic, and ultrastructural requirements.

3. Electrostatic fields and force

Hypothesis 1. The principle of force generation in muscle is the electrostatic force that acts on a dielectric body.

The principle may conveniently be represented by a capacitor model as shown in Fig. 3.3. The energy source is a battery which delivers positive and negative

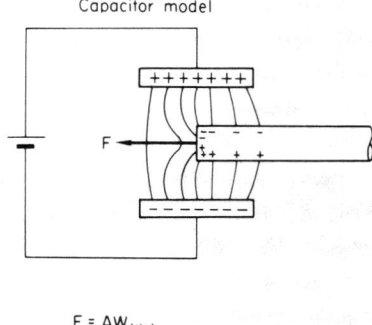

Capacitor model

$$F = AW_{(tip)}$$

F: Axial force acting on the thin filament

A: Cross sectional area of the thin filament

$W_{(tip)}$: Energy density at the tip of the thin filament

FIG. 3.3. Capacitor model of a contractile force generation. The dielectric cylinder between two capacitor plates induces surface charges which results in a net axial force by Coulomb's law. The field energy is supplied by a battery.

charges to the capacitor plates and establishes an electrostatic field. When a dielectric cylinder is introduced into the field, induced charges appear on the cylinder surface, thus resulting in an axial force. In this capacitor model the cylinder is a passive element representing the thin filament, and the capacitor and battery together constitute an active element representing a part of the thick filament. However, one should not hastily assume the existence of metallic parallel plates on the thick filament, as the capacitor model is used only to illustrate the principle.

The polarity and amount of the induced charges depend on the dielectric properties of the thin filament. The dielectric properties of polymerized macro-molecules in an aqueous solution are very complex and beyond the scope of this chapter. The interested reader is referred to more detailed expositions (Iwazumi 1970, Oosawa 1970, O'Konski 1960, Schwarz 1962) and only a summary of the dielectric behaviour of the thin filament is given below.

In an aqueous medium of proper ionic composition the thin filament binds cations on its surface with a density of about 10^{13}/cm^2. These cations (which are mostly divalent) neutralize the negative surface charges of the thin filament. When an electric field is applied, these bound ions (often referred to as 'counter ions') are slightly displaced from their average locations. The net effect of the charge displace-ment is identical to the effect of the induced charge on a body with a high dielectric constant; the thin filament with a cation layer thus appears as if it has a high dielectric constant, which is called the effective dielectric constant. When an electric field is applied and if the effective dielectric constant is greater than that of water, both positive and negative ions tend to accumulate on the surface to form a layer of high conductivity, which appears from outside as if nonconductive macromolecules turned conductive. This is known as surface conductance. It is noted here that high effective dielectric constant alone is not sufficient, but high surface conductance is also necessary to explain the dielectric behaviour of the thin filament.

The effective dialectric constant is found to be proportional to $e^2\sigma$ where e is the charge of each bound ion and σ is the surface density of the bound ions. Therefore, divalent cations are four times more effective than monovalent cations for the same surface density. Moreover, K$^+$ has much smaller affinity for the thin filament than have divalent cations; hence, the effective dielectric constant is dependent mostly upon the concentration of divalent cations in the solution. Sufficient concentration (at the mM level) of divalent cations must therefore exist in the solution in order to attain a high effective dielectric constant. In muscle this requirement is satisfied by Mg^{++}. The measured dielectric properties of the thin filament are more complex than those described here because of permanent dipoles in G-actin monomers (Minakata 1966, Kobayashi, Asai & Oosawa 1964). However, the effect of these permanent dipoles is not significant at very high field strengths since the interaction energy of a dipole with an applied field is proportional to E (field strength) whereas that of the induced moment is proportional to E^2.

When the thin filament has such dielectric properties, the force acting on the thin filament is always in the direction to maximise the thin filament volume which is exposed to the field; the thin filament is therefore drawn into the field as indicated by the arrow in Fig. 3.3. Theoretical calculation indicates that the magnitude of the force is proportional to the product of the cross-sectional area of the thin filament and the energy density in the medium at the tip. The energy density is defined by $W = \frac{1}{2}\varepsilon E^2$, where ε is the dielectric constant of the medium. The use of energy density, instead of field strength, will afford greater convenience in the discussion of the theory. It is important to note that the magnitude of the force is determined only by the energy density on the *tip* of the thin filament; as the energy density on

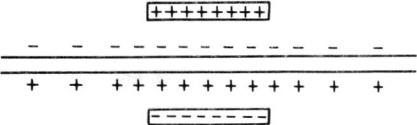

FIG. 3.4. Induced charge distribution on a dielectric cylinder with its tip extending far outside the capacitor. No net axial force acts on the cylinder because of the symmetry of the charge distribution.

the shaft surface does not contribute to the axial force. This fact may seem to violate intuition; however, consider a case in which the tip of the thin filament is far beyond the capacitor field as shown in Fig. 3.4. The induced charges distribute symmetrically about the centre of the capacitor; therefore, no net axial force is developed. The maximum field strength needed to account for the maximum contractile force observed in muscle is of the order of 1 volt/100 Å (or 10^6 volt/cm) which is a value commonly measured at the solid–liquid interface of electrochemical systems.

Since the energy density is maximal at the centre of the capacitor and diminishes in the fringe region, the axial force acting on the tip varies from zero to the maximum depending on the location of the tip. In Fig. 3.5, suppose that the thin filament is axially translated from the far right to the far left passing through the centre of the capacitor. As the tip traverses through the capacitor, the force acting on the filament increases from zero to a maximum (F_{max}) which occurs when the tip is at the centre, and then decreases again to zero. If a constant force is applied to the thin filament in the direction opposed to and less than F_{max}, the force equilibrium is reached always at the location where the tip lies ahead of the centre of the capacitor, i.e. in the left side of the capacitor in Fig. 3.5. The force equilibrium cannot be maintained in the right side since the force balance is unstable in this region. We shall see later

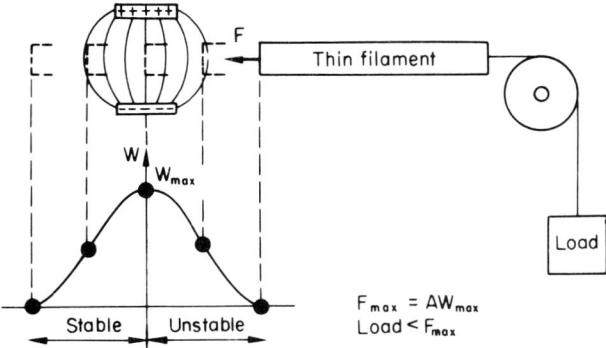

FIG. 3.5. The stability of force balance on the thin filament. The electrostatic force acting on the thin filament is a function of the tip location. The slope of the energy density distribution is equivalent to the modulus of elasticity of the force source. The positive slope gives rise to a stable force equilibrium with the load, and the negative slope to an unstable equilibrium.

that these stable and unstable regions result in profound effects on sarcomere dynamics.

4. The energy source

According to the capacitor model, an energy source is required to separate the charges over a certain distance and thus generate an electrostatic field in the capacitor. It is well known that myosin, a major component of the thick filament, is an ATPase and that ATP hydrolysis accompanies energy liberation. The biochemical and molecular events associated with myosin ATPase activity are still obscure, but it is known that the presence of the thin filament, divalent cations and other molecules greatly affect the activity (Taylor 1972). We shall then introduce the following hypothesis.

Hypothesis 2. The myosin-ATP complex forms an electro-chemical cell so that positive and negative charges are separated over some distance and an electromotive force (EMF) is established.

An immediate implication of this hypothesis is that the electrostatic field is generated by the association of myosin and ATP and not by the dissociation of ADP and phosphate from myosin.* In other words, the adsorption energy of ATP to myosin is equal to the field energy, and a part of this energy is recovered by ADP when it leaves myosin. The other fraction of the field energy is available for either work or heat. Work is done by the field when a dielectric body (the thin filament) is pulled into the field and thereby increases the capacitance. The amount of work extractable from the field depends on the time course of the movement of the dielectric body. Heat is generated when the field causes charged particles to acquire kinetic energy in the form of vibration and translation. Another fraction of the field energy is stored as potential energy of the orientation of polar molecules, such as the formation of structured water. Quantitative energetic arguments will be given later since they require additional information which cannot be derived directly from this hypothesis.

Another consequence of this hypothesis is that the ATP hydrolysis rate is equal to the rate of charge generation. From the capacitor model, it is clear that an initial energy expenditure is required to set up the field, and that a continuous supply of energy is needed for subsequent maintenance of the field to supplement the charge loss to the aqueous medium in the form of ionic current (i.e., heat loss). Hence, we conclude that the time course of ATP hydrolysis must have a large burst initially and then settle down to a low sustained level.

---

* Dissociation of ADP probably occurs when charges are lost to the medium. But this assumption is unnecessary for the development of theory.

5. The role of calcium ions

It has been known that myosin ATPase is affected by many kinds of ions and molecules, and among these the most important one in intact muscle is calcium ion (Ebashi & Endo 1968). Upon activation of the muscle membrane, Ca^{++} concentration in the sarcoplasm increases from 10^{-8} M to 10^{-6} M, and correspondingly myosin ATPase activity increases by about a factor of ten (Weber & Herz 1963). We saw in the previous section that the EMF of the myosin-ATP complex must be in some way related to the ATPase activity. Since Ca^{++} modifies the ATPase activity, we see that there is a relationship between Ca^{++} concentration and the EMF. This relationship is experimentally determined since the EMF is directly related to the force (section 3). The molecular mechanisms whereby calcium ions and other molecules affect the ATPase activity is presently unknown. Fortunately it is not necessary to know the mechanism in order to develop this theory further. At this point we shall describe the function of Ca^{++} in controlling the EMF by the following hypothesis.

Hypothesis 3. The EMF of myosin-ATP complex is controlled by Ca^{++} in such a way that ATP binding to the ATPase site is suppressed by the field strength at the site and that this suppression is removed by Ca^{++} binding to the myosin.

The field intensity is then self-regulated since the higher the Ca^{++} concentration in the medium, the greater the EMF and the greater the suppression of further ATP binding.

An important consequence arises from the principle of force generation and the above hypothesis. Since the force is determined only by the energy density at the tip, it follows that only the capacitor (i.e., myosin-ATP complex) near the tip of the thin filament is relevant. From the above hypothesis, the EMF of this myosin-ATP complex is under the control of the local Ca^{++} concentration; hence, we conclude that only the Ca^{++} concentration at the tip of the thin filament determines the force.

6. Biochemical implications of field theory

At this stage it may be worthwhile to digress from the development of the theory to discuss the process taking place in model muscle systems *in vitro*. The biochemical investigations of muscle proteins, and in particular, the interaction of myosin and actin, are usually done on isolated systems in which the original steric relationships of molecules have been destroyed. Because of this structural destruction it is impossible to measure contractile force in a test tube; therefore, several different methods have been used to indicate interactions between molecules, such as changes in turbidity (optical scattering), viscosity, optical birefringence, and fluorescence. These methods do not specifically indicate what kind of interactions are taking place; therefore, the interpretation of experimental results is ambiguous. What, then, can the field theory say about the interaction between isolated myosin and actin?

Let us first consider a case in which the heavy meromyosin (HMM), the head part of myosin with ATPase, is suspended in an aqueous medium of low ionic strength. The reason for using HMM instead of whole myosin is that light mero-myosin (LMM), the tail part of myosin, has a strong permanent dipole moment which causes myosin to aggregate in a low ionic strength medium (< 0.3 M), thus forming precipitates (Noda & Ebashi 1960). HMM without ATP also has some permanent dipole moments (a weak one in S-1 and a stronger one in S-2 sub-fragment of HMM) but is soluble in a very low ionic strength medium.

It is not known whether HMM actually generates a dipole moment upon binding ATP as hypothesis 2 implies; however, the permanent dipole moment of HMM has been shown to disappear upon ATP binding (Kobayashi & Totsuka 1975). The measurement of the dipole moment of HMM is not trivial, for, when HMM generates a dipole moment in a low ionic strength medium, two HMM's will immediately form a dimer by electrostatic attraction. The individual dipole moment, therefore, cannot be measured properly in the steady state. This also explains the disappearance of the permanent dipole moment. If the ionic strength of the suspend-ing medium is increased to prevent dimer formation, then ionic screening prevents the observation of dipoles. A possible way to circumvent this difficulty is to very quickly mix HMM and ATP and measure the dipole moment before dimer forma-tion. The dipole moment can be deduced by measuring either the dielectric dispersion or birefringence change with impulsive electric fields. The dimer formation may be observed by light scattering fluctuation spectroscopy. This measurement should be carried out at very low ionic strength. To observe the effect of Ca^{++} and Mg^{++}, their concentration should be in the range of mM; the reason for using these seemingly unphysiological concentrations will become clear later.

An essential requirement in maintaining the dipole moment is to retain the charges on HMM. In other words, both positive and negative charges must be bound to HMM with sufficient binding energies. This requirement can be met by introducing the hypothesis below.

Hypothesis 4. The binding energies of charges generated by the myosin-ATP complex increase with the binding of Mg^{++} to HMM.

This hypothesis is not necessary for the theory of sarcomere dynamics, but needed only in this section. The action of Ca^{++} is, as indicated previously, to control the EMF of the myosin-ATP complex; therefore, once the EMF reaches a value determined by the local Ca^{++} concentration after the initial burst of ATPase activity, the steady state activity is reached only to supplement lost charges. This steady state loss decreases when Mg^{++} is present through the mechanism of the above hypothesis. However, the charge loss itself is a function of many variables, for instance, temperature, irradiation, those of mechanical origin (e.g. proximity of a dielectric body and structural deformation), and those related to the medium (e.g.

water molecule orientations, ionic strengths, and divalent cations). In this respect, the behaviour of ATPase activity is very similar to the current flow from a battery connected to various loads; the current can be changed by external factors, but the EMF of the battery is unchanged.

Now consider the effect of the actin monomer on the ATPase activity. The aqueous solution of G-actin cannot contain any significant amount of K^+ or divalent cations since these ions and ATP polymerize G-actin to form F-actin (Martonosi, Molino & Gergely 1964). This means that G-actin has no surface ion layer (except that due to protons), and its effective dielectric constant is probably less than that of water. Therefore, its interaction with the electrostatic field of HMM must be primarily by the G-actin permanent dipole moment, and not by the induced moment. When no ATP is in the solution, HMM cannot generate an electrostatic field except for one from its own permanent dipole. Since G-actin is able to make the so-called rigor bond to HMM,[*] we expect to see G-actin and HMM bound together in this situation (Martonosi & Grouvea 1961). When ATP is in the solution, HMM and G-actin dissociate, and an electrostatic field is generated upon myosin-ATP complex formation. At a basal rate of ATPase activity, it is estimated that the EMF is about 0·1 volt, which results in a dipole moment[†] comparable to that of the HMM permanent dipole. Thus, it is possible that the field from the permanent dipole and that from the myosin-ATP complex counteract such that the resultant field in the aqueous medium is nearly zero. On the other hand, it is also possible that the two moments sum. Even in such a situation, the potential energy of HMM and G-actin interaction is only several kT; hence, the ATPase activity is hardly affected by the presence of G-actin in the solution (Offer, Baker & Baker 1972).

Let us next consider the interaction between HMM and the thin filament (or F-actin). The aqueous solution is assumed to contain a mM level of Mg^{++}, without which the thin filament cannot develop a high effective dielectric constant. If no ATP is present in the solution, HMM and the thin filament form a rigor bond, resulting in arrowhead-like decoration of HMM molecules on the filament (Huxley 1963). When ATP is added to the solution, HMM and the thin filament dissociate (Eisenberg & Kielly 1973). Since no Ca^{++} is assumed to be present in the solution, the EMF of the myosin-ATP complex is lowest (about 0·1 volt), and the ATPase activity is at a basal rate. The interaction energy in this case is only several kT, not enough to form electrostatic aggregations against thermal agitations.

The last case to consider is the effect of Ca^{++}. When Ca^{++} is added to the solution containing HMM, thin filaments, ATP and Mg^{++}, then the EMF and ATPase activity are much greater than those expected from HMM alone with the same concentration of Ca^{++}. This is because the thin filament now has some Ca^{++}

---

[*] Rigor bond might be related to the attraction of dipoles of G-actin and HMM, but the energy involved is only several kT, not enough to explain the tightness of the binding.

[†] This calculation requires more information about the charge distribution and this can be obtained from the theory of lateral stability.

in its ionic layer, particularly abundant around troponin (Yasui, Fuchs & Briggs 1968). If the thin filament is far away from HMM, the EMF is increased from the basal value only by the amount determined by the concentration of Ca^{++} in the medium. When a thin filament with Ca^{++} is drawn into the field, the local Ca^{++} available to the ATPase site is increased. According to hypothesis 3, this increases the EMF further and the thin filament is pulled harder into the field. This process repeats until HMM and the thin filament nearly touch each other, though they do not chemically bind; the proximity depends on the concentration of Ca^{++} in the medium and is typically less than 100 Å (within the fringe field of HMM). At the maximum EMF (about 1·5 volts) the interaction energy reaches about 400 kT (the potential energy in an induced dipole is proportional to E^2), enough to hold HMM and the thin filament tightly together.

In addition to the EMF increase, the effect of thin filament proximity to the ATPase site (to increase the capacitance) brings about increased ATPase activity (to increase the charges to maintain a constant EMF). The proximity of a dielectric body also increases the field strength markedly at the same EMF. This increased field strength on the surface of HMM reduces the potential energy barriers of charges. Consequently, charge loss increases sharply and the ATPase must be greatly accelerated to compensate for the loss.

When Mg^{++} is removed from the solution, then from hypothesis 4 the energy barriers of charges on HMM are reduced, thus resulting in increased charge loss and ATPase activity. The thin filament loses Mg^{++} from its surface layer, but, if enough Ca^{++} is around, it still maintains a high effective dielectric constant. Therefore, the interaction between HMM and the thin filament continues. However, the rate of ATP hydrolysis cannot be increased indefinitely, and this rate-limiting process reduces the EMF, which in turn reduces a force between HMM and the thin filament. This situation is analogous to the terminal voltage drop of a battery under heavy load.

It should be noted that only energy density (or EMF^2) determines the force acting on the thin filament, and that the ATPase activity which compensates for the charge loss has no relation to the force.

The situation that occurs *in vivo* is more complex than described here because of water molecule orientation and steric arrangement of thick and thin filaments. We shall discuss some aspect of these topics in later sections.

7. The ionic distribution in the aqueous medium under high field strengths

An argument against electrostatic theory has been that free ions in the sarcoplasm would act as counter-ions, limiting the field to very short range (only about 10 Å), thus no appreciable force could be generated by such a mechanism (Huxley 1974). There are two reasons for this argument being incorrect in the case of the capacitor model. First, a basic assumption of double layer counter-ion theory is the fixed charge system based upon Poisson's equation, that no current flow (or discharge) is allowed across the layer. The myosin-ATP complex of the capacitor model supplies charges continuously as ATP is hydrolysed to maintain the EMF, i.e. a current flows across the boundary, thus invalidating the basic assumption of double layer theory. Note however, that the double layer theory is applicable on the surface of the thin filament since it is a fixed charge system. Second, the theory of solute exclusion (Ling 1969) is applicable to the capacitor model since the latter satisfies the requirement of a bifacial-dipolar surface for the formation of multi-layer polarised water. In such water solutes tend to be driven out, in the similar way that ice drives solute out, thus creating a local ion depletion. To visualise how such a process could take place, let us look at the medium around a myosin ATPase site. At first the medium is filled with many K^+ and Cl^- ions. When ATP binds myosin and the myosin-ATP complex generates a basal dipole moment, the field energy is not sufficient to instantly orient all surrounding water molecules. Because of the ionic screening, the line of force between the positive and negative charges (which are about 100 Å apart) cannot be established; therefore, the region between them has no field gradient (i.e. zero field strength). This is felt by the ATPase site as zero EMF, thus by the mechanism of hypothesis 3, more ATP is allowed to bind. As more charges appear on the surface, the water molecules around them become oriented along the field lines. Two such oriented regions grow at positive and negative poles, and finally meet at the centre, thus establishing the line of force between these two poles. Once these two separate regions unite to form one connected region, free ions tend to escape from it by the mechanism of solute exclusion. The reduction of ionic concentration in the connected region helps to orient more water molecules in the fringe region, thus extending the ion depleted region to the fringe field of the dipole.

This region of structured water changes its size depending on the field strength and ionic strength. It is noted here that a proper concentration of Mg^{++} is essential for this process to take place, since, according to hypothesis 4, charges readily escape from binding sites without Mg^{++}, and this makes it impossible to build up enough field energy to orient water molecules in the neighbourhood.

The experimental confirmation of the structured water is at present in dispute (Hazlewood 1973). What is now known is that a substantial fraction (about 1/5) of muscle intracellular water is very different from free water in terms of NMR* relaxation times (Cope 1969, Belton, Packer & Sellwood 1973), viscosity (Gamaley & Kaulin 1974) and diffusion (Cleveland *et al.* 1976). The interpretation of NMR data poses some ambiguity since it is not clear whether the changes of relaxation times arise from the bound water or structured water. On the other hand, diffusion coefficients of solutes would be interpreted more straightforwardly. According to the mechanism explained above, if no ATP exists, nor does structured water; hence, solute (e.g. K^+) diffusion ought to be the same as in free water. If ATP is present, structured water develops around each projection which excludes K^+ ions, thus forming a diffusion barrier; hence, there is a significant reduction of diffusion coefficient. Experimental support for this prediction is quite convincing (Ling 1973).

* Nuclear magnetic resonance.

A direct test of ionic exclusion could be performed by electron microprobe analysis of K^+ and Cl^- in the vicinity of projections, but the spatial resolution requirement (much less than 100 Å) is quite formidable.

8. *Theoretical synthesis of ultrastructure*

We now continue the development of the theory. Our objective here is to deduce an ultrastructure of thick and thin filaments which is consistent with the hypotheses concerning the principle of force generation and the energy source, and the two fundamental physical requirements (longitudinal and lateral stabilities). The details are quite involved (Iwazumi 1970) and only the basic ideas will be explained below.

From the longitudinal stability condition, we have seen that the force between the thick and thin filaments is related to the overlap length in such a way that less overlap results in more force. In terms of electrostatic fields, as the thin filament tip proceeds away from the thick filament centre the energy density encountered becomes greater. Combining this statement with the capacitor model one readily finds a solution as shown in Fig. 3.6. In order to satisfy the requirement, it is only necessary to require that the EMF of the myosin-ATP batteries increase towards the right end, i.e. $V_1 < V_2 < V_3 < V_4 < V_5$. Since it was mentioned previously that the EMF increases with Ca^{++} concentration, it follows that the local Ca^{++} concentration at each myosin-ATP battery in Fig. 3.6 must also vary similarly with the EMF. In other words, the longitudinal stability condition requires that the Ca^{++} concentration along the thick filament increase symmetrically towards both ends and be lowest at the centre. Note, however, that this statement implies nothing about the value of concentration; it merely states the slope of the Ca^{++} distribution curve. Therefore, it is possible to have a high average Ca^{++} concentration along the thick filament when the tip of the thin filament is near the centre (i.e. large overlap), thus resulting in a large force. Conversely, a small force is obtained at long sarcomere

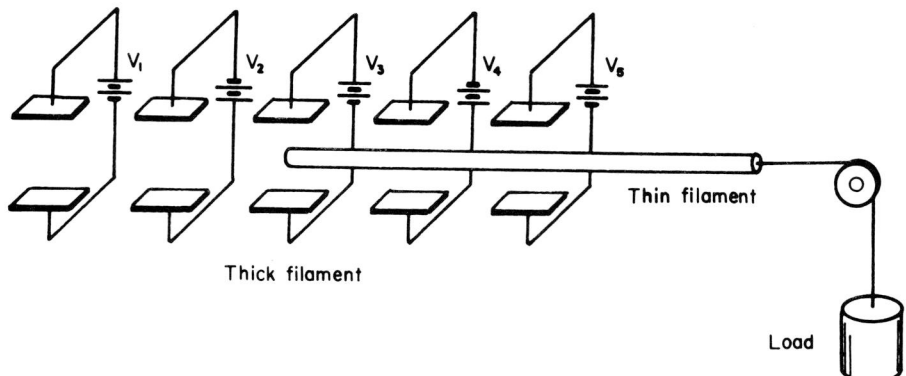

FIG. 3.6. A series of capacitors along the thick filament. The thick and thin filament here represent one half of a sarcomere. The EMF of each myosin-ATP battery is independently controlled by the local Ca^{++} concentration at the battery.

lengths if the average Ca^{++} concentration along the thick filament is low. We shall discuss more about the force-length relationship in another section. It is pointed out here that the slope requirement of Ca^{++} distribution does not prohibit the existence of stepwise changes. In fact, if one considers the proximity effect of the thin filament on the distribution of Ca^{++}, there ought to be a large change at the tip of the thin filament. The symmetry of the Ca^{++} distribution in the A-band is important; if an asymmetry exists, as the case may be when Ca^{++} release from the sarcoplasmic reticulum is nonuniform, e.g. because of damage done by over-extension, then the A-band will not be at the centre of the sarcomere even when it is returned to the rest length.

We have now translated the longitudinal stability condition into two separate requirements: that the longitudinal distribution of Ca^{++} be concave upward, and that the capacitors be arranged in series along the axis of the thick filament.

As the force acting on the thin filament is determined only by the field which is generated by a capacitor near the tip of the thin filament, and since no other capacitors generating fields along the shaft contribute to the axial force, it may appear that this is a very wasteful design. We shall see below that these fields along the shaft are necessary to secure the lateral stability condition. We observed previously that the thin filament is located approximately equidistantly between adjacent thick filaments. This provision is necessary to prevent thick and thin filaments from rubbing each other while sliding past. The question is then whether a thin filament could be suspended in space by an electrostatic field. It turns out this is possible if the field vector is perpendicular to and helically rotating along an axis, and also satisfies some conditions on the gradient and curvature of the energy density. The field that satisfies these requirements surrounds the thin filament with a spiral wall, somewhat like a screw in a threaded hole.

Having obtained all requirements for an electrostatic field, we require a spatial charge distribution which results in this field. This is a field synthesis problem, and no further discussions about it will be made here since it is too involved. Only the result of the synthesis is described below.

In most synthesis problems there are many solutions, and one chooses a particular solution according to a set of criteria which are often selected subjectively. Our synthesis problem, however, turns out to be very tightly constrained, and without any subjective choice only one solution emerges. The three dimensional distribution of charges is illustrated in Fig. 3.7 in a transverse cross-section of the ultrastructure of thick and thin filaments. Each cross-projection of the thick filament has clusters of positive and negative charges. The pointed end of the cross-projection is to indicate that it does not connect two thick filaments. The cross-projections point to the adjacent thick filaments and are distributed along the shaft helically with 60° turn per advance. The direction of the helix is left-turn (anti-clockwise), and the resulting field vector rotates around the thin filament in right-turn (clockwise). It has been argued that the cross-projections of the thick filament could take one of many different configurations depending upon the type of muscle

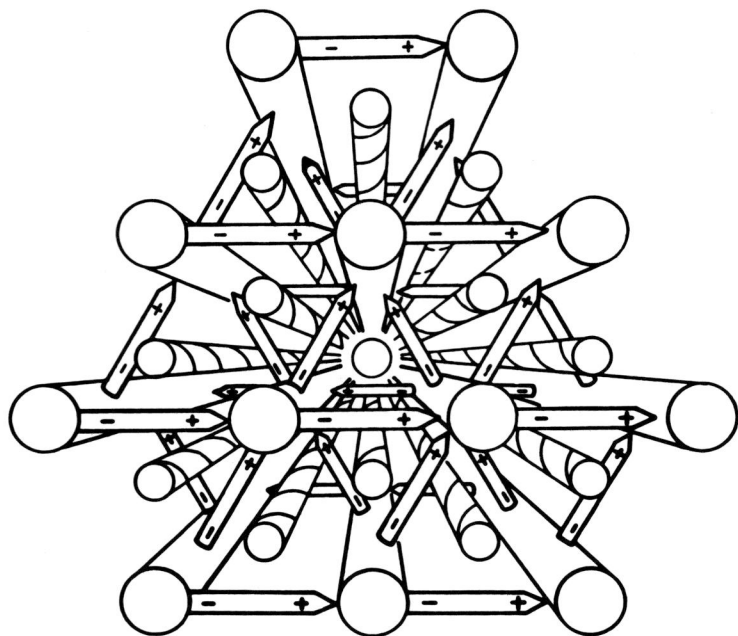

FIG. 3.7. Transversal view of the theoretically synthesised ultrastructure. The pointed end of each projection is to indicate the orientation, not its actual shape. The left hand helical array of projections generates right hand helical electrostatic fields.

(Squire 1975), but this field theory predicts that there exists only one configuration, shown in Fig. 3.7, that can generate a field which satisfies the lateral stability condition. This means that the ultrastructural features of the thick filament are common to all striated muscles, including insect flight muscle (but not necessarily for non-striated muscle). The ultrastructural difference between different types of striated muscle is the number of thin filaments. The theory predicts the stable locations of the thin filament depending upon the number in a unit cell, and we shall come back to this topic later.

One of the many interesting properties of this ultrastructure is the potential energy associated with the assembly. The slope of this potential energy as a function of the inter-filament distance between two thick filaments varies from positive at short distance to negative at long distance. In other words, the thick filament ultrastructure experiences a transverse compressive force when the sarcomere length is long, and an expansive force when it is very short. Of course, at rest length the ultrastructure experiences no transverse force.

Another interesting property is the dependency of the lateral stability upon the distance between positive and negative charges on a cross-projection. It turns out that the ratio of the charge separation distance to the projection separation distance (about 143 Å in muscles) must be less than 0·8 in order to secure the lateral stability, i.e. the distance between positive and negative charges must be about 100 Å. This

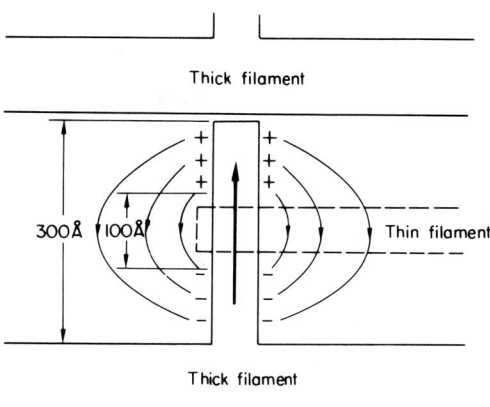

Thick filament

300 Å 100 Å   Thin filament

Thick filament

FIG. 3.8. Theoretically inferred charge distribution on a projection. The ATPase site is likely located in the middle of the projection and able to generate a dipole moment upon binding ATP. Dimensions are approximate.

is the value used in the calculations of biochemical and field energy. Fig. 3.8 summarises the conclusions on the geometry and charge distribution of a cross-projection from the field synthesis.

Once the geometry of the capacitor is known, it is possible to calculate its capacitance, field energy at maximum EMF, and charge density. They are: 5×10^{-18} F, 3.5×10^{-18} J and $4 \times 10^{13}/cm^2$ respectively. The ATP hydrolysis energy converted to field energy amounts to about 14 kcal/mol.

There are many features of this synthesised ultrastructure which are very different from those constructed from the interpretation of the cross-bridge theory. An outstanding difference is the length and direction of a cross-projection: this theory predicts it is about 300 Å long and oriented towards the adjacent thick filament, whereas cross-bridge theory predicts that it is less than about 120 Å and oriented towards the thin filament. Considering the great difference of these features, one might expect to see clear evidence in electron micrographs supporting one and rejecting the other. If one closely examines an electron micrograph in Fig. 3.9, it will become apparent that both features can be observed; particularly in the H-zone where there is no thin filament, bridges are seen between thick filaments rather than oriented towards the trigonal points. The field theoretical explanation for the co-existence of bridges between thick and thick filaments and thick and thin filaments is as follows. During the fixation process of live muscle in either rest or activated states, most of the ATPase sites exhaust the available ATP. The thin filaments which were suspended in space by electrostatic fields when ATP was present are now free to move by thermal agitation. As a result, some cross-projections and thin filaments come into contact and are able to form rigor bonds. On the other hand, in the H-zone, the cross-projections suffer no large disturbance, and remain approximately in the original orientation.

An interesting consequence of the ionic exclusion may be observed in electron

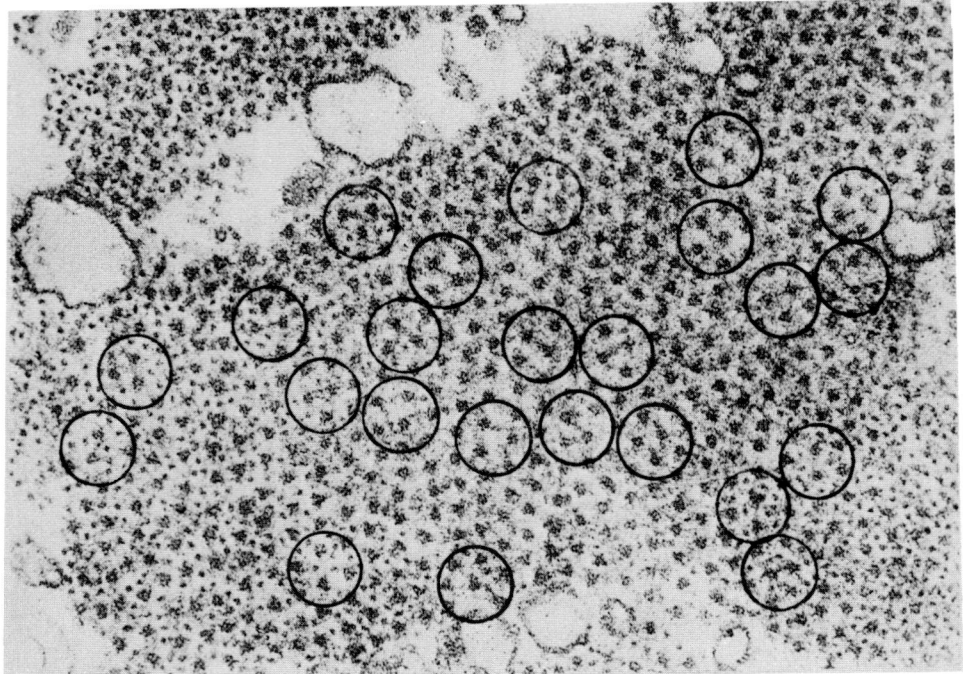

FIG. 3.9.   Electron micrograph of transverse section of skeletal muscle. The section was made near the tips of thin filament; therefore, we see no thin filament in some areas. Note that many lines can be seen between the thick filaments in the area without thin filaments. On the other hand, such lines are harder to find in the area with thin filaments.

micrographs. Since excluded K^+ and Cl^- must migrate towards the thick and thin filaments during the activated state, they form a layer of high ionic strength region over the shafts of the filaments. It is well known that the shaft of the thick filament is formed by an electrostatic aggregation of LMM and can be dissolved at high ionic strength (Noda & Ebashi 1960). Consequently, one would expect to see a swelling of thick filaments during contraction.

   Having obtained a detailed charge distribution in the three dimensional space of the synthesised ultrastructure, we are now in a position to develop a theory of sarcomere dynamics. In four sections that immediately follow we examine the properties of the field generated in the synthesised ultastructure. The sarcomere dynamics will be discussed in the subsequent sections.

9. *Three-phase distribution of energy density*

According to the synthesised ultrastructure, each projection has positive and negative charges, and the helical arrangement of these charge pairs (dipoles) results in a helical electrostatic field whose helix axis is located at the midline between and in parallel with two thick filaments. We shall call this helix axis the primary stability

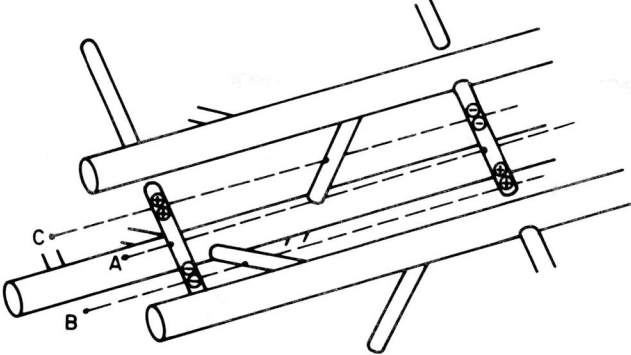

FIG. 3.10. Three dimensional illustration of the orientation of projections and associated primary stability lines. The projection spacing is disproportionately made longer so as to avoid cluttering. Each primary stability line, *A*, *B* and *C*, passes through the centre of dipole on the projection.

line. Thus, there are six primary stability lines around each thick filament, and these lines bisect cross-projections (henceforth called simply 'projections'). Fig. 3.10 shows three thick filaments and three primary stability lines in three dimensional perspective. The distance between succeeding projections is depicted disproportionately longer so as to avoid cluttering the figure. The three primary stability lines are designated *A*, *B* and *C*. In Fig. 3.11 the distribution of the energy density along the three primary stability lines is shown. Let us suppose that we are on the line *A* of Fig. 3.10 walking to the right starting from the projection which points upward. Evidently, at this location we experience the greatest field strength; hence, the energy density is greatest as shown in Fig. 3.11. As we walk to the right, the field strength rapidly diminishes and at the same time the field vector rotates clockwise.

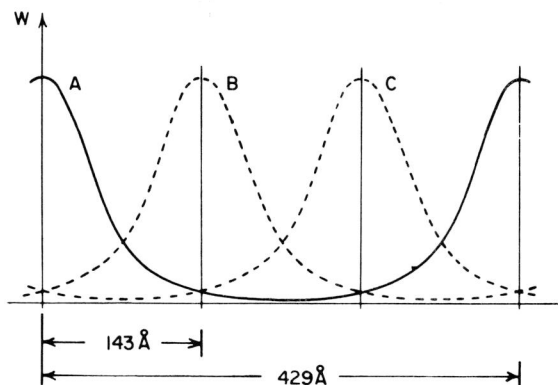

FIG. 3.11. Three-phase distribution of the energy density along the primary stability lines. *A*, *B*, and *C* correspond to the respective lines in Fig. 9. Note the fairly straight portion of the down slope and the distance of fringe field extending about 150 Å. Recall that this slope is equivalent to the modulus of elasticity of the force source.

Note that the direction of projections rotates counterclockwise. At the midpoint to the next projection, the field strength is nearly zero. As we walk further to the right, the field strength begins to increase, and at the next projection it is again greatest. The direction of the field is now 180° from that of the starting point. If one repeats the same process for lines B and C, the energy density distribution along each line will be found to be the same as that of line A except that the distribution curve is shifted axially by 143 Å as indicated by dotted lines in Fig. 3.11. We have now found that the energy density distribution in the synthesised ultrastructure is a three-phase system. This interesting spatial distribution of energy density will be shown to cause extremely complex dynamic behaviour of the sarcomere.

10. *Paired thin filaments*

When thin filaments are introduced into the synthesised ultrastructure they tend to settle down at most stable locations which vary depending on the number of thin filaments in the hexagonal array of thick filaments. If the number of thin filaments is exactly equal to the number of primary stability lines, each thin filament occupies the location of primary stability line as shown in the left side of Fig. 3.12. This thin filament pattern has been seen in insect flight muscle and is most stable out of all other possible patterns. In this case the ratio of the number of thick filaments to thin filaments is 1 : 3.

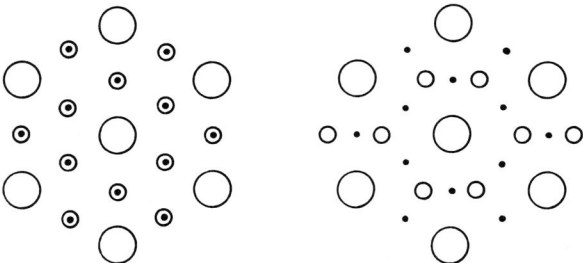

FIG. 3.12.   The location of the primary stability lines and thin filaments in the transversal section of ultrastructure. The left pattern is most stable and found in insect flight muscle. The right pattern is found in cardiac and skeletal muscle.

When the ratio of filaments is other than 1 : 3, the stable locations of thin filaments vary. In the case of cardiac and skeletal muscle the ratio is 1 : 2, and the stable locations are indicated in the right side of Fig. 3.12. Note that each primary stability line is juxtaposed by two thin filaments. This situation arises because of mutual repulsion of thin filaments (due to the ionic surface layer and also to the permanent dipole moment) in balance with the attractive force towards the primary stability line. The reason that two thin filaments are juxtaposed perpendicularly to the line connecting two thick filaments is that the curvature of the potential energy well in this direction is less than the one in any other direction.

A consequence of two thin filaments competing for a position becomes apparent when one of these filaments is missing due to structural defect. The remaining one obviously occupies the position of the primary stability line, and this phenomenon can readily be seen in electron micrographs. The converse to this is an excess of thin filaments; occasionally one can observe paired thin filaments in insect flight muscle.

Another consequence is that paired thin filaments do not occupy the trigonal positions, but are closer together. Pairing need not occur between the same two thin filaments. It may occur with different neighbours at different locations along the shaft of a thin filament.

11. Electrostatic induction

When the value of a capacitance is suddenly changed by moving a dielectric body in an electrostatic field of a capacitor, a reactive force acts on the body. This is analogous to the magnetic induction in which a conductor moving in a magnetic field experiences a reactive force due to eddy currents induced in the conductor.

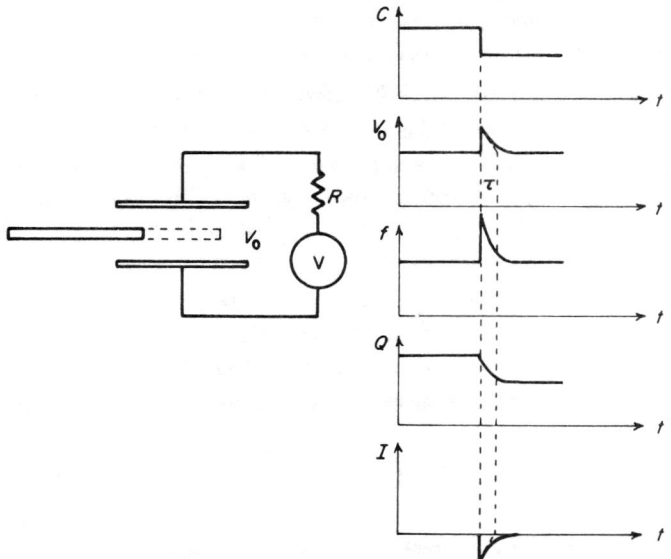

FIG. 3.13.   Electrostatic induction associated with a sudden pull-out of a dielectric cylinder. R represents a rate limiting process, not a resistive element. C = Capacitance; V_0 = Voltage across capacitor; f = Force; Q = Charge; I = Current; and V = Voltage (EMF) of an ideal source.

Referring to Fig. 3.13, when the thin filament is quickly pulled out of the capacitor, the capacitance drops in stepwise fashion. Due to the rate-limiting chemical process in the myosin-ATP complex, during the very short time of the step change of capacitance, the charge Q remains constant. From the relationship, $Q = CV_0$, where V_0 is the potential difference between the capacitor plates (equal to the EMF if no current flows), a step decrease of C must be counteracted by a step increase of V_0. Afterwards, a finite current flows which removes the excess charges from the plates, thus causing V_0 to go down as indicated in the figure. The relaxation time constant is given by $\tau = RC$, but this does not imply the existence of a resistive element since R represents a rate limiting process. The force f acting on the thin filament changes in proportion to $(V_0)^2$.

When the thin filament moves into the capacitor, the capacitance increases, and the reactive force appears to decrease the force acting on the thin filament. A more quantitative treatment may be found elsewhere (Iwasumi 1970).

Some important aspects of electrostatic induction need to be emphasised here. First, as in a viscous situation, the induced force is also a function of relative velocity between thick and thin filaments, but it is approximately linear only in the range below 0·1 μm/s. The induced force becomes virtually independent of velocity above 10 μm/s. Second, for the same velocity, the magnitude of induced force is proportional to the force that existed before the motion, i.e. the normalised induced force appears to have the same time course. Third, the induced force has a relaxation time constant which is determined by the chemical processes and geometrical factors such as the number of thin filaments in the field of one projection. Although the relaxation time is definable, the time course cannot be approximated by a single time constant. Since the forward and backward rate constants of chemical reactions are usually different, the shortening time constant and lengthening time constant should differ significantly. It is also necessary to take the rate of charge loss to the medium into consideration. Fourth, since the rate limiting process of ATPase, which is not a resistive element, is the major contributor to the relaxation time constant, the induced force is not accompanied by an energy loss. Fifth, the range of travel in which the electrostatic induction is clearly observable is limited. As we have already seen the fringe field of the projection extends only about 150 Å (Fig. 3.11). When thin filaments travel across many successive projections, the induction effects from individual projection become fused, and only force ripples will be seen.

12. Tip alignment effects

In the course of the molecular assembly of thick and thin filaments, some variations of filament lengths and misalignment of ultrastructure inevitably occur. Also, none of the elements of the ultrastructure are perfectly rigid. This is clearly demonstrated in electron micrographs of sarcomeres as skewed and curved Z-lines and A-bands. What effects do we expect to see from the structural variance and elasticity on the dynamic behaviour of sarcomeres?

Let us observe a sarcomere at rest. Initially the tips of thin filaments are not well aligned with respect to the projections. This is true even if both A-band and Z-lines are perfectly straight and no length variations of filaments exist since the projections are helically arranged. Let us next infuse Ca^{++} while holding the sarcomere length constant. As the field develops around each projection a force acts on each thin filament with a magnitude dependent upon the position of its tip. Those filaments with tips close to the projections feel a great force and are pulled forward, while those with tips between projections feel no force. These forces are transmitted to the projection, Z-line and M-line and strain their structures. The greatest strain will appear in the Z-line because of its network-like structure. The result is the relative movement of tip positions: those in high fields move forward to lesser fields and those in low fields are pulled back to higher fields. Fig. 3.14 illustrates the relative movement of filaments and resulting strains in the Z-line. The strains in the Z-line and M-line are mostly of shear, whereas that of the projection is of bending.

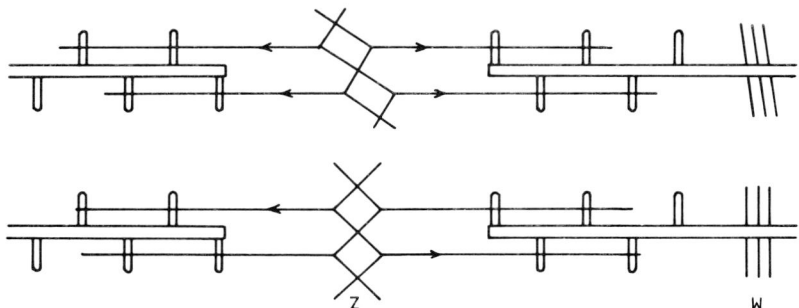

FIG. 3.14.   Thin filament tip alignment with projection. Shear strains at the Z-line and M-line allow the tip of thin filament to align with the projection. The projection itself also suffers a bending strain which is not shown here.

Besides these strains, there will be small strains in the thick and thin filament. We shall now summarize the above in a hypothesis.

Hypothesis 5. The shear strains in the Z-line and M-line at the maximal force level are sufficient to allow the majority of the tips of the thin filament to be aligned with the projections.

As the isometric force becomes stronger, the greater proportion of the thin filament tips are closely aligned with the positions of the projections. From this argument we would expect to see two phenomena. One is a vigorous relative motion between the thick and thin filaments during the position adjustment period; this is discussed further at a later point. The other is a discrete sarcomere length distribution. Since the positions of the projections are spatially discrete, the distance from the tip of the thin filament in the left half of the sarcomere to the tip of the thin filament in the right half is also discrete. Hence, the sarcomere lengths tend to assume values whose differences are integral multiples of 429 Å (the distance between two peaks of energy density distribution).

It is essential to the observation of this discrete sarcomere length distribution in muscle that the contraction be extremely steady; if sarcomeres either shorten or lengthen during contraction, there is little possibility of seeing this phenomenon. In the muscle fibres which were able to contract exceptionally steadily the discreteness has indeed been observed (Iwazumi, ter Keurs & Pollack 1977).

13. Quick release from a steady isometric contraction

Suppose that a sarcomere is in a steady and maximally activated state. Most of the thin filament tips are then aligned with projections. If we suddenly let the sarcomere shorten freely, what will be the time course of force as a function of shortening distance? (Huxley & Simmons 1973). Since the shortening velocity in this case is limited only by viscosity and electrostatic induction (mass effect is negligible), it readily reaches 10 μm/s relative velocity between thick and thin filament. Therefore, the induced force is essentially independent of velocity and depends only upon the change of capacitance. For example, if a 10% increase of capacitance occurs for a given shortening distance, the force is reduced to $1/(1\cdot1)^2$ or 82·6% of the force that would have existed at the shortened position if there were no electrostatic induction. Since the capacitance change and the shortening distance are not linearly related because of the complex projection geometry, an exact expression for the induced force is difficult to obtain. However, for very small shortening, the induced force is approximately proportional to the shortening distance. To explain the above description more graphically the time course of force is shown on the left side of Fig. 3.15 and the geometrical relationship on the right. F_i is the magnitude of an induced force (negative in this case), and F_r is the force reached after shortening.

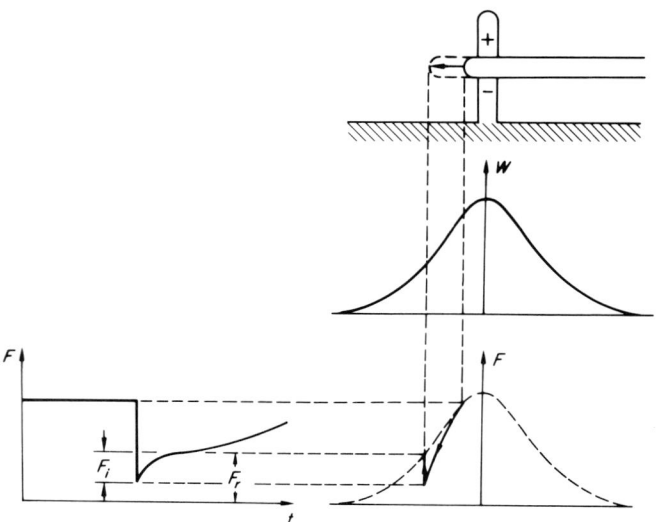

FIG. 3.15.   Quick release from a steady isometric contraction. On average the tip of thin filament is slightly ahead of the projection at a maximum steady state force. Upon quick release over a small distance, the tip moves forward at the velocity limited primarily by viscosity. The capacitance increase due to the forward movement of thin filament brings about a momentary reduction of the field strength by the electrostatic induction effect. The induced force F_i decays and the force approaches F_r which is the value determined by the fringe energy density at the new tip location. Afterwards, force tends to recover towards the previous level through redistribution of tip locations if the shortening did not disturb Ca^{++} distribution to a great extent.

The force will not remain at F_r since the tips of thin filaments begin to redistribute so as to settle at the most favourable positions to bear the maximum force again. Therefore, during this force recovery phase one would expect to see a vigorous movement of filaments. The time course of recovery becomes complicated by the fact that the tip redistribution accompanies Ca^{++} distribution changes and resulting changes in the EMF of projections near the tips (more about this later). A corollary to this statement is that if the shortening distance is very small, the amount of spatial tip redistribution is also very small; therefore, one would observe only the induction effect.

Since the synchronous movement of thin filament tips is possible only at high force levels so as to produce enough strains in the projection, Z-line, and M-line for the tip alignment, the quick release from low force levels, such as those in the early phase and relaxing phase of contraction, will not result in the responses proportional to steady state responses. At low force levels, F_r approaches the initial force since the tip locations are not well aligned with projections.

It is clear from Fig. 3.15 that the quick release response strongly depends upon the distribution curve of energy density. If, for example, the ionic strength of the medium is elevated, the peak height and the width of the energy density distribution curve diminishes. The consequence is a diminished maximum force and zero force shortening distance.

As mentioned previously, the relaxation time of the induction is a function of many variables: ATPase activity (related to charge generation and absorption), ionic strength (related to charge loss to the medium), temperature, and capacitance. The last item is an important factor when thin filament double-overlap at short sarcomere lengths is considered. This topic is discussed separately in a later section. The sarcomere dynamics of slow and long range shortening is much more complex even in the single-overlap region and is discussed in another section.

14. Quick stretch responses

Let us suppose that sarcomeres are fully activated and most thin filament tips are aligned with cross-projections. If sarcomeres are suddenly stretched what will be the time course of force? We already know that the electrostatic induction will result in a time course of force which sharply rises and then decays with a time constant. If we consider the steric arrangement of projections, the situation is quite a bit more complicated. Referring to Fig. 3.16, when the thin filament is pulled to the right, it is able to move some distance to the right without losing the force since the force increase by electrostatic induction will compensate for the force reduction due to decreasing energy density. But beyond a certain distance the induction effect becomes insufficient to compensate for the reduction of energy density, and the force acting on the thin filament suddenly falls. This causes the thin filament to lose a force balance with the load applied at the Z-line; hence, the tip position suddenly jumps to the right until the tip enters a sufficiently strong field to counteract the load.

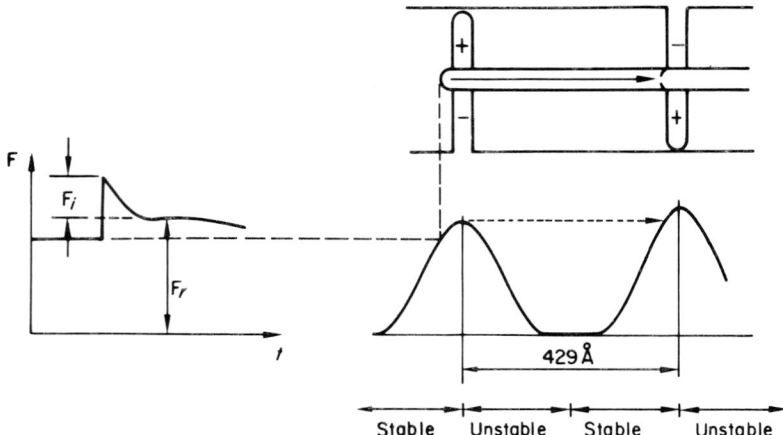

FIG. 3.16.   Quick stretch from a steady isometric contraction. On average, tip of thin filament is slightly ahead of the projection at a maximum steady force. When thin filament is pulled quickly with a force that overcomes the electrostatic induction at the left projection, then the tip jumps backward to the right projection. This is because the tip is unstable in the negative slope of the energy density distribution.

The jump distance depends upon the elasticity of the thin filament and the Z-line. (If the compliance is infinitely large, the jump proceeds as shown in Fig. 3.16.) If the stretch distance is small enough not to cause this 'give' phenomenon to happen, the time course of force consists of a sharp spike with a decay and a plateau which is slightly higher than the force before stretch. When the stretch distance is large and the thin filament has made a jump, the time course of force appears much the same except for greater spike and plateau height since these are determined by the field which the tip has entered after the jump. The distance of jump is not in general limited to one inter-projection distance such as depicted in Fig. 3.16 but is dictated by the stretch.

Let us next consider the case of multiple thin filaments in a sarcomere. The average tip position of the thin filament is always ahead of the projection. This is because tip positions have some distribution, even at the maximum sarcomere force, and this distribution cannot include the region behind the projection since thin filaments are unstable there. Now if we stretch the sarcomere slightly, some of the thin filaments which were supporting a maximum possible force exactly at the centre of the projection must give and jump back to the next projection. As we increase the stretch distance more and more thin filaments make jumps until a distance is reached at which all thin filaments in the sarcomere have made backward jumps.

After a quick stretch a redistribution of tip positions takes place regardless of the number of jumped thin filaments because those thin filaments that have just made backward jumps must necessarily bear less forces than before. Even during the redistribution period some thin filaments will be forced to jump either forward or backward until no thin filament tip is in the unstable region.

It is important to note that filament jumping does not imply sarcomere length jumping. In order to observe the latter, simultaneous tip alignment with the projections is necessary.

The exact time course of force during the redistribution period after a transient is difficult to predict quantitatively since it involved elastic properties of the projection, Z-line, and M-line, sarcomere geometry, and nonuniformity of activation. The same argument also applies to the redistribution after quick shortening.

We are now led to conclude that there will be a vigorous axial movement of filaments during and immediately after a transient, that this movement will subside slowly as thin filament tips settle down, and that the magnitude of activity is related to force being generated. This filament 'jumping' can be characterized by the distribution of filament relative velocities. When a large fraction of thin filaments are jumping, the velocity distribution has a peak at high velocities (about 20 μm/s). As the jumping subsides the peak moves to lower velocities. Such a statistical property of the thin filament jumping can be measured by light intensity fluctuation spectroscopy. The results of actual measurement (Bonner & Carlson 1975) agree very well with the expected behaviour of thin filament jumping.

15. The role of troponin

Biochemical investigations of isolated troponin have established that each troponin molecule can selectively bind several calcium ions. It is also known that it distributes along the entire length of the thin filament at an interval of about 400 Å (Ohtsuki, Masaki, Nonomura & Ebashi 1967). Because of the fact that some muscle lacks troponin, it has been thought that troponin plays a regulatory role in the Ca activation process of muscle. What, then, can the field theory say about the role of troponin in contraction?

As already discussed in section 6, the thin filament is essentially a Ca^{++} carrier, and Ca^{++} is transferred to myosin through the proximity effect. The distribution of Ca^{++} in the medium along the thick filament is concave, and this distribution also dictates the distribution of Ca bound to the thin filament. Now, let us assume that there are discrete Ca binding sites along the thin filament at 400 Å intervals beginning near the tip,* as shown in Fig. 3.17. Because of the slight difference of the intervals of projections and Ca sites, the distance between the projection and Ca site varies from location to location. It is clear that, if the tip is aligned with a projection, then the next projection is further away from the Ca site by about 29 Å and so on, until the 15th projection where the Ca site becomes closest again; this 'vernier' effect continues all along the overlap region. The furthest Ca site occurs at the 8th projection. This situation is shown in Fig. 3.18. The top figure shows the

* It is advantageous to have a Ca site slightly away from the tip for alignment purposes. The antitroponin staining however, appears to show the first troponin site about 250 Å from the tip (Ebashi, Ohtsuki & Mihashi, 1973). But this value seems to include an artifact arising from tropomyosin.

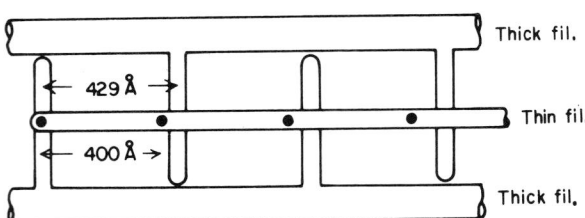

FIG. 3.17.   Interference arrangement of projection and troponin (Ca source). The distance between the projection and troponin (filled circle) increases by an integral multiple of 29 Å.

distribution of Ca^{++} concentration in the medium along the thick filament. The average number of Ca^{++} ions that bind the projection in a unit time (assumed to be proportional to the field strength at the Ca site) is indicated by the height of each bar in the bottom figure. The local energy density at each cross-projection is approximately proportional to the height of the bar. What then are the consequences of this undulated distribution of energy density peaks?

Let us first consider only one sarcomere. If this sarcomere is quick stretched over a long distance, the thin filament tip will jump all the way to the 13th or 14th projection. The time course of force would look much the same as the one we discussed previously, namely, having a sharp spike with a decay leading to an elevated plateau. Now let us quick stretch the sarcomere by such a length that the

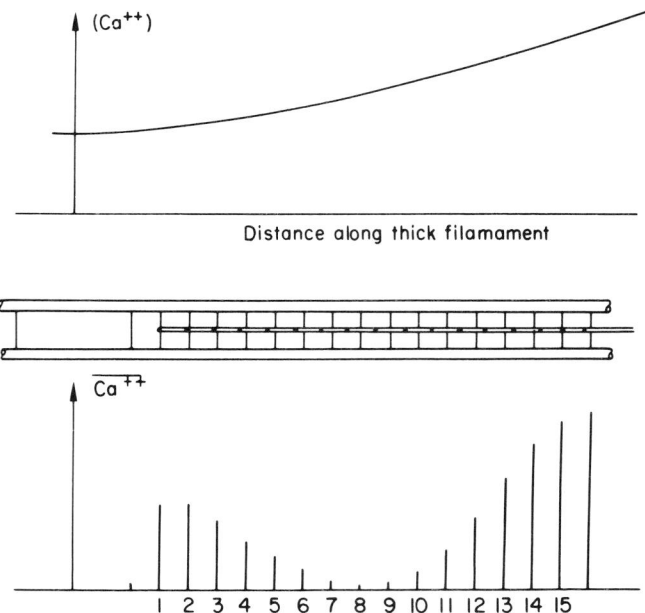

FIG. 3.18.   Vernier effect of projections and troponin sites. At 8th projection, troponin sites (Ca sources) are about 215 Å away. Hence, the 8th projection is least activated by Ca^{++}. $[Ca^{++}]$ = Ca^{++} concentration in the medium; $\overline{Ca^{++}}$ = average number of Ca^{++} that binds projection in a unit time.

tip of thin filament stops at the 8th projection. Since the charges on the 8th projection cannot be increased instantaneously, at the moment the thin filament tip enters the field of the projection the energy density is still very small, and accordingly the magnitude of the induced voltage is also small. Hence (immediately after a very sharp spike which arises from the induction at the 1st projection and the viscous force during jump), the time course of force suddenly falls, then creeps up to a higher level than before the stretch. This is because the Ca^{++} concentration of the medium at this location is greater than that of the initial location. The time course of force for this case is shown in Fig. 3.19.

We have just arrived at one of the most striking predictions of the field theory. Is it really possible to observe this transient reversal phenomenon in actual muscle? Let us first consider a case in which many sarcomeres are connected in series and parallel just as in actual muscle fibres. If these sarcomeres were identical in length

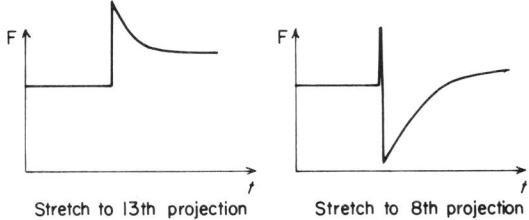

FIG. 3.19. Time course of forces acting on a thin filament in Fig. 3.18. Depending upon the distance of very high velocity stretch, force responses vary. The transient reversal is greatest at the 8th projection. A sharp spike in the right figure is due to the induction at the first projection and the viscosity during stretch.

and also in activation (i.e. in Ca^{++} distribution), and assuming the muscle length to be short enough for the force propagation time to be much less than the relaxation time, then this muscle should behave in exactly the same way as a single sarcomere. However, if there were some nonuniformity in sarcomere length and activation, weaker sarcomeres would be stretched all the way and stronger ones only half way. The resulting time course of force will be a composite of the two types shown in Fig. 3.19. In other words, the force response to large quick stretch is strongly dependent upon the uniformity of sarcomeres, and if one sees a transient reversal, it is an evidence of very high degree of sarcomere uniformity. On the other hand, if a muscle with poor sarcomere uniformity is stretched quickly beyond several thousand Å per average sarcomere, then the force response is unpredictable and the sarcomere nonuniformity becomes extremely enhanced, since some sarcomeres will be stretched beyond overlap length. It is reemphasized here that the stretch time and force propagation time must be shorter than the relaxation time in order to observe the transient reversal phenomenon. A corollary is that as the stretch time increases the time course of force shows less reversal and reverts to an ordinary shape. The transient reversal phenomenon has actually been observed experimentally

(Sugi 1972) and demonstrated to be associated only with very high velocities (i.e. short stretch time).

For the quick shortening in the single overlapped region, the effect of troponin distribution is nil. However, in the double overlapped region, there will be an interesting phenomenon which will be explained in the section dealing with the double overlap.

It might appear from Fig. 3.18 that the undulated distribution of energy density peaks violates the longitudinal stability condition. That this is not the case will become clear when one realises that the Ca^{++} concentration distribution in the medium has a coordinate fixed with respect to the thick filament; therefore, when the thick filament is moved from the centre of the sarcomere, the Ca^{++} distribution also moves with it, thus resulting in the increased Ca^{++} concentration at the tip of the thin filament on one side and the decreased Ca^{++} concentration on the other side, which results in a restoring force.

When one looks at the undulated distribution of energy density peaks, it becomes apparent that due to the interference between the projection and troponin site the energy consumption becomes much less than without such sites. The interference arrangement of troponin is perhaps nature's way of saving energy without jeopardising the essential requirement for structural integrity.

16. *Slow shortening and stretch*

Thus far we have been concerned with the dynamics of sarcomeres in synchronised transients. Synchronisation was made possible by aligning the tips of thin filaments with projections taking advantage of strains in the various parts of the ultrastructure (primarily in the Z-line) as explained in section 12. The average behaviour of the thin filaments in a sarcomere can then be approximated very well by that of a single thin filament.

In the non-steady state, even if the sarcomere length is held constant, filament tips are continually jumping as they attempt to settle down at most favourable positions. Is it then possible to describe the sarcomere dynamics on the basis of *average* tip positions in order to evaluate the force from the corresponding *average* energy density? If so, the calculation of sarcomere dynamics will be greatly simplified.

It turns out that this averaging (approximation) method is valid only for isometric and lengthening sarcomeres but not for shortening ones. Implicit to the averaging method is the assumption that all projections in the sarcomere are fully activated in accordance with the local Ca^{++} concentration. This assumption is certainly valid along the shaft of the thin filament which exerts the proximity effect upon the projections to enhance the Ca^{++} activation.

In the case of shortening, since the projections ahead of the thin filament are not activated by the proximity effect, their fields are not fully developed yet. The averaging method therefore fails to predict the dynamics of shortening. It is, however, possible to modify the averaging method by introducing terms to the Ca^{++}

distribution function to account for the delayed activation by the proximity effect. The theoretical derivation of such terms appears to be very difficult at present, but empirical expressions will be sufficient for practical calculations.

To see what physical processes take place during slow shortening, let us first consider a case in which an isometric sarcomere is fully activated, and the applied force is slightly reduced so that the sarcomere begins to shorten. In the initial isometric state all tips are assumed to have settled in the stable regions of the nearest projections. The distribution of tip locations depends upon the elastic properties of the projection, Z-line and M-line relative to the force. If the total elasticity is low (i.e. compliant), most of the tips will settle close to the peak of the energy density distribution curve with very few in the valley regions. If the force is low or the elasticity is relatively high, then the tip distribution will be more spread.

When the load is slightly reduced, all tips move slightly ahead, and those tips which were located at regions of zero energy density now move into the front (and therefore unstable) regions of the next projections. Although these tips are in the unstable region, they do not immediately jump forward since the next projections are not yet fully activated.* So, they keep moving ahead and bear more and more force; this changes the strain distribution in the elastic structure, particularly of the Z-line (see Fig. 3.14), and some tips at the peak of energy density distribution suddenly give. This initiates jumping. Now, a small number of thin filament tips can reach the projections ahead and activate them. This process continues and more and more tips jump ahead. Those tips that have jumped must necessarily bear a much greater load than before, thus relieving those tips which bear a heavy load and letting them advance to a region of zero energy density.

Compared with the complexity of the processes involved in the slow shortening at a heavy load, unloaded shortening (V_{max}) is much simpler. In this case the tip positions are randomly distributed, and when some tips move ahead in the stable region, those tips in a zero energy density region are pushed along with them and eventually come close to the next projection and activate them. The time it takes for a tip to jump forward is very short since the velocity is limited only by viscosity; therefore, the time it takes to move from one projection to one further ahead is limited essentially by the time that is required to develop a field, which is directly related to the shortening relaxation time of electrostatic induction, and in turn is a function of several variables as discussed in sections 11 and 13.

17. Double overlap

As the sarcomere length shortens below twice the length of the thin filament, thin filaments from the opposite side meet at the centre of sarcomere, and then overlap with one another. This is commonly referred to as double overlap.

---

* The condition for jump is determined by the slope of the energy density distribution and the total elastic modulus.

There is one important question that must be answered before discussing the effect of double overlap. Electron micrographs of any striated muscle show a bare zone of the thick filament at the centre containing no projections, except for the *M*-lines, over the length of about 1500 Å. According to the field theory, if the thick filaments and thin filaments are well registered, there is no possibility that the thin filaments can cross the bare zone. This is certainly true, and insect flight muscle apparently takes advantage of this situation to synchronise the oscillatory movement of thin filaments (note that the simultaneous tip alignment with a projection is an essential condition for any synchronous movement of sarcomeres). In cardiac and skeletal muscle the centre bare zone is something that must be coped with by means of structural alterations. There are basically two ways to cross the bare zone. One is to make the thin filament length non-uniform. If the difference between the longest and shortest ones is greater than 1500 Å, which is about 15% of the average thin filament length, then the bare zone can be crossed even if thick filaments are perfectly in register. Another is to make thick filaments out of register or skewed with respect to the *Z*-line by about 10% of their length. In muscle both situations seem to occur simultaneously. It may appear, however, that the longitudinal stability condition is violated by the longitudinal skewing or misregistration of thick filaments. That this is not the case is readily understood by referring to Fig. 3.2. The ball is stable in the potential well, but at the centre the slope of the well wall is zero, and the ball can readily be agitated by a small disturbance. By the same token, the thick filament can easily be offset a small distance by a slight force imbalance which always exists during contraction as explained in section 14 (filament jumping).

Once the thin filament tips cross the bare zone, they meet with the thin filaments from the other side. Since they have divalent cation surface layer, they repel each other as they overlap. This repulsive force is proportional to the length of double overlap and counteracts the contractile force. A quantitative treatment of the forces acting on the thin filament in double overlap has yet to be worked out, but some qualitative statement can be made by extending the results obtained from the case of single overlap.

The electrostatic induction effect of the doubly overlapped thin filament will be much less than that of the single overlap. Since the projection near the tip of the thin filament is already occupied by the shaft of another thin filament, the relative change of capacitance by introducing the second tip is therefore much less than in single overlap. This will result in an induced force of lower magnitude than in single overlap. Both shortening and stretch relaxation times will also be affected by double overlap because of a greater effect of proximity which increases capacitance and ATPase activity. Since increased capacitance causes longer relaxation times, whereas increased ATPase activity results in shorter relaxation times, the combined effect will vary from case to case.

More significant differences will be found in the transient behaviour immediately after the electrostatic induction. The presence of the thin filament shaft near the projection changes the field distribution substantially and results in a narrower energy density distribution curve along the thick filament. The distance which a thin filament jumps becomes much greater because of the bare zone, the flat Ca^{++} distribution near the centre, and diminished electrostatic induction. A consequence of all these is a more frequent jumping of filaments with double overlap.

As the extent of double overlap is increased, another interesting phenomenon shows up. We have seen before that the longitudinal stability condition requires the Ca^{++} distribution curve in the *A*-band to be concave. This distribution assures the stability when the thin filament maintains a single overlap with the thick filament. However, as the tip of thin filament enters the other half of the *A*-band, it sees a greater and greater field as it advances and this will result in longitudinal instability. Fortunately, because of mutual repulsion of thin filaments, which counteracts contractile forces, the net force acting on the thin filament still diminishes for a certain distance, thus the stability is maintained. Beyond this point, however, the sarcomere becomes longitudinally unstable and contracts maximally. As it does so, the inter-filament distance of thick filament greatly increases, and this in turn causes the potential energy of the thick filament assembly to fall into the negative slope region (section 8), which results in a transversal expansive force. Now the ultrastructure has completely lost its integrity and can never return to the original form.

As mentioned before, the effect of troponin distribution is nil in the single overlap region but not so in the double overlap region. This is because all projections in the doubly overlapped sarcomere are in close proximity with the thin filament. The extent of activation of individual projections depends upon the proximity of the Ca site (troponin) to the projection. In section 15 it was seen that the 8th projection from the one at the tip was least activated. In other words, those projections situated within 3000 ± 1000 Å from the tip are so far away from the Ca sites that they are not well activated by Ca^{++} even though thin filament shafts are very closely located to them. Now, let us assume that the central bare zone length is exactly integral multiples of 429 Å (say, 1287 Å), then thin filament tips, just after crossing the bare zone, see the projections already partially activated. Therefore, these tips can jump forward more readily than they could in the single overlap region; they then activate projections ahead more strongly upon reaching them. However, since these projections are already occupied by other thin filaments, the tips which have just arrived cannot fully exert their proximity effect; therefore, these projections cannot be fully activated unless they have been fully activated by those Ca sites of the already existing thin filaments. As tips move more deeply into the other side of the *A*-band, the projections ahead are less and less activated. When the length of double overlap is about 0·3 μm (about 1·7 μm sarcomere length), the projections ahead are least activated. Let us consider another possibility. If the bare zone length is integral multiples and a half of 429 Å (say, 1501 Å), the tips again see projections which are partially activated after crossing the bare zone. As the tips advance, they now see the projections ahead more and more strongly activated until the maximally activated projections are found at the sarcomere length of about 1·7 μm. We have now reached an interesting conclusion: as sarcomere shortens below double overlap length (about 2 μm), the force will decrease or increase depending upon the length of the bare zone assuming that the Ca^{++} concentration in the *A*-band is unchanged.

Although both intact cardiac and skeletal muscle show diminished force as sarcomere length shortens below 2 μm, one cannot conclude that the bare zone length takes integral multiples of 429 Å because it has been known that the Ca^{++} release from the sarcoplasmic reticulum diminishes with sarcomere length below 2 μm (Taylor, Rudel & Blinks 1975). Also, some skinned fibres did not show much force reduction at short sarcomere lengths (Schoenberg & Podolsky 1972). Therefore, it still remains to be tested whether the bare zone length has a critical effect on the force.

18. Force-length relationship

In section 8 it was mentioned that the distribution of Ca^{++} concentration along the thick filament is concave upward. It was pointed out that the value of concentration is arbitrary as far as the longitudinal stability condition is concerned. In other words, there is no restriction nor requirement on the level of Ca^{++} concentration in the *A*-band; therefore, the Ca^{++} concentration at the tip of the thin filament can be varied from zero to the saturation level at any sarcomere length below the limit of overlap. Hence, the field theory does not predict any fixed relationship between sarcomere length and force unless Ca^{++} concentration is specified. In actual muscle, however, there exist additional mechanisms which control the release and uptake of Ca^{++} by the sarcoplasmic reticulum. Of course, these Ca control mechanisms are entirely outside the field theory. But, given an isometric force–sarcomere length relationship, it is possible to say something about the characteristic of Ca^{++} control mechanisms.

In Fig. 3.20 the top figure is an example of a force–length relationship commonly observed in skeletal muscle: the force is high at short sarcomere lengths but diminishes at long lengths. In order to attain a high force the Ca^{++} concentration at the tip must be high; therefore, the Ca^{++} concentration in the *A*-band is high at short sarcomere length (l_5). On the other hand, a low force is obtained at long sarcomere length (l_1) because of low Ca^{++} concentration in the *A*-band.

Although the field theory can predict the Ca^{++} concentration in the *A*-band as a function of sarcomere length from a given force–length relationship, it can say nothing about the concentration of Ca^{++} in the *I*-band. Complete sarcomere dynamics can be solved only if all the boundary conditions (e.g. Ca^{++} source and sink), diffusion coefficients, and geometry of the sarcomere are given in the Ca^{++} diffusion equations (Iwazumi 1970). At present, none of these quantities is known with a reasonable certainty.

The time course of sarcomere isometric force is obtainable from the solution of the Ca^{++} diffusion equations evaluated at the projection nearest to the tip of thin filament. Although it is not possible to obtain a quantitative solution, the qualitative behaviour of the solution is readily understood. In fast muscle, such as fast skeletal muscle, the time course of force of a twitch contraction is strongly dependent upon the diffusion process. However, in slow muscle, such as cardiac muscle, diffusion

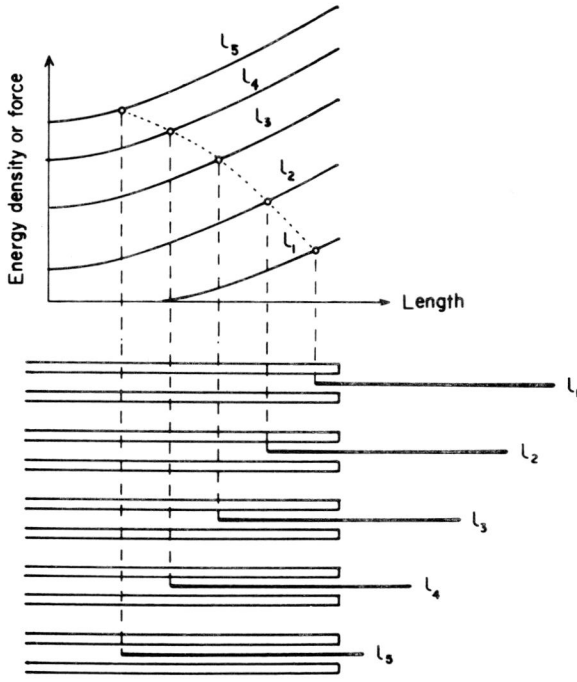

F I G. 3.20. Force-length relationship and the Ca^{++} distribution in the A-band. The Ca^{++} concentration in the A-band is not only non-uniform but also dependent upon the sarcomere length. High force at short sarcomere lengths is due to high Ca^{++} concentration, not due to large overlap length.

time is not a limiting factor, and the time course of a twitch contraction is primarily determined by the time course of Ca^{++} release and uptake. This means that in cardiac muscle the time course of sarcomere isometric force should follow closely with that of Ca^{++} concentration in the sarcoplasm.

19. Concluding remarks

In this chapter we have discussed some selected topics in the fundamental aspects of muscle contraction in terms of field theory. Emphasis was placed on theoretical predictions which solicit experimental tests. It is hoped that this chapter will stimulate the interest of investigators in this field and result in new experiments to test the field theory.

REFERENCES

BELTON P.S., PACKER K.J. & SELLWOOD T.C. (1973) Pulsed NMR studies of water in striated muscle. II. Spin-lattice relaxation times and the dynamics of the non-freezing fraction of water. *Biochim. Biophys. Acta*, **304**, 56–64.

BONNER R.F. & CARLSON F.D. (1975) Structural dynamics of frog muscle during isometric contraction. *J. Gen. Physiol.*, **65**, 55–581.

CLEVELAND G.G., CHANG D.C., HAZLEWOOD C.F. & RORSCHACH H.E. (1976) Nuclear magnetic resonance measurement of skeletal muscle. *Biophys. J.*, **16**, 1043–1053.

COPE F.W. (1969) Nuclear magnetic resonance evidence using D_2O for structured water in muscle and brain. *Biophys. J.*, **9**, 303–319.

DELEZE J.B. (1961) The mechanical properties of the semitendinosus muscle at lengths greater than its length in the body. *J. Physiol.*, **158**, 154–164.

EBASHI S. & ENDO M. (1968) Calcium ion and muscle contraction. *Prog. Biophys. Mol. Biol.*, **18**, 123–183.

EBASHI S., OHTSUKI I. & MIHASHI K. (1973) Regulatory proteins of muscle with special reference to troponin. *Cold Spring Harb. Symp.*, **37**, 215–223.

EDMAN K.A.P., ELZINGA G. & NOBLE M.I.M. (1978) Enhancement of mechanical performance by stretch during tetanic contractions of vertebrate skeletal muscle fibres. *J. Physiol.* **281**, 139–155.

EINSENBERG E. & KIELLY W.W. (1973) Evidence for a refractory state of heavy meromyosin and subfragment-1. *Cold Spring Harb. Symp.*, **37**, 145–152.

GAMALEY T.A. & KAULIN A.B. (1974) Some properties of muscle water. *Physiol Chem. & Physics*, **6**, 445–456.

HAZLEWOOD C.F. (ed.) (1973) Physicochemical state of ions and water in living tissues and muscle systems. *Ann. N.Y. Acad. Sci.*, **204**.

HUXLEY A.F. (1974) Muscular contraction. *J. Physiol.*, **243**, 1–43.

HUXLEY A.F. & NIEDERGERKE R. (1954) Interference microscopy of living muscle fibres. *Nature*, **173**, 971–973.

HUXLEY A.F. & SIMMONS R.M. (1971) Proposed mechanism of force generation in striated muscle. *Nature*, **233**, 533–538.

HUXLEY A.F. & SIMMONS R.M. (1973) Mechanical transients and the origin of muscular force. *Cold Spring Harb. Symp.*, **37**, 669–680.

HUXLEY H.E. (1963) Electron microscope studies on the structure of natural and synthetic protein filaments from striated muscle. *J. Mol. Biol.*, **7**, 281–308.

HUXLEY H.E. (1969) The mechanism of muscular contraction. *Science*, **164**, 1356–1366.

HUXLEY H.E. & HANSON J. (1954) Changes in the cross-striations of muscle during contraction and stretch and their structural interpretation. *Nature*, **173**, 973–976.

IWAZUMI T. (1970) A new field theory of muscle contraction. *Ph.D. Thesis, Univ. Pennsylvania.* University Microfilms Inc, Ann Arbor, Michigan.

IWAZUMI T., ter KEURS H.E.D.J. & POLLACK G.H. (1977) Do sarcomeres assume discrete lengths? *Biophys J.*, **7**, 199a

KOBAYASHI S., ASAI H. & OOSAWA F. (1964) Electric birefringence of actin. *Biochim. Biophys. Acta*, **88**, 528–540.

KOBAYASHI S. & TOTSUKA T. (1975) Electric birefringence of myosin subfragments. *Biochim. Biophys. Acta*, **376**, 375–385.

LING G.N. (1969) A new model for the living cell: a summary of the theory and recent experimental evidence in its support. *Int. Rev. Cytol.*, **26**, 1–61.

LING G.N. (1973) Mobility of potassium ion in frog muscle cells, both living and dead. *Science*, **181**, 78–81.

MARTONOSI A. & GOUVEA M.A. (1961) Studies on actin. VI. The interaction of nucleoside triphosphates with actin. *J. Biol. Chem.*, **236**, 1345–1352.

MARTONOSI A., MOLINO C.M. & GERGELY J. (1964) The binding of divalent cations to actin. *J. Biol. Chem.*, **239**, 1057–1064.

MINAKATA A. (1966) Dielectric dispersion of G-actin. *Biochim. Biophys. Acta*, **126**, 570–577.

NOBLE M.I.M. & POLLACK G.H. (1977) Molecular mechanisms of contraction. *Circulation Res.*, **40**, 333–342.

NODA H. & EBASHI S. (1960) Aggregation of myosin A. *Biochim. Biophys. Acta*, **41**, 386–392.

OFFER G., BAKER H. & BAKER L. (1972) Interaction of monomeric and polymeric actin with myosin subfragment 1. *J. Mol. Biol.*, **66**, 435–444.

OHTSUKI I, MASAKI T., NONOMURA Y. & EBASHI S. (1967) Periodic distribution of troponin along the thin filament. *J. Biochem.*, **61**, 817.

O'KONSKI C.T. (1960) Electric properties of macromolecules. V. Theory of ionic polarization in polyelectrolytes *J. Phys. Chem.*, **66**, 605–619.

OOSAWA F. (1970) Counterion fluctuation and dielectric dispersion in linear polyelectrolytes. *Biopolymers*, **9**, 677–688.

OPLATKA A., GADASI H. & BOREJDO J. (1974) The contraction of "ghost" myofibrils and glycerinated muscle fibres irrigated with heavy meromyosin subfragment-1. *Biochem. Biophys. Res. Commun.*, **58**, 905–912.

SCHOENBERG M. & PODOLSKY R.J. (1972) Length–force relation of calcium activated muscle fibres. *Science*, **176**, 52–54.

SCHWARZ G. (1962) A theory of the low-frequency dielectric dispersion of colloidal particles in electrolyte solution *J. Phys. Chem.*, **66**, 2636–2642.

SQUIRE J.M. (1975) Muscle filament structure and muscle contraction. *Ann. Rev. Biophys. & Bioeng.*, **4**, 137–163.

SUGI H. (1972) Tension changes during and after stretch in frog muscle fibres. *J. Physiol.*, **225**, 237–253.

TAYLOR E.W. (1972) Chemistry of muscle contraction. *Ann. Rev. Biochem.*, **41**, 577–616.

TAYLOR S.R., RUDEL R. & BLINKS J.R. (1975) Calcium transients in amphibian muscle. *Fed. Proc.*, **34**, 1379–1381.

WEBER A. & HERZ R. (1963) The binding of calcium to actomyosin systems in relation to their biological activity. *J. Biol. Chem.*, **238**, 599–605.

YASUI B., FUCHS F. & BRIGGS F.N. (1968) The role of sulfhydril groups of tropomyosin and troponin in the calcium control of actomyosin contractility. *J. Biol. Chem.*, **243**, 735–743.

CHAPTER 4
THE MECHANICS OF CARDIAC CONTRACTION

CARDIAC CONTRACTION AS AN OSCILLATORY PHENOMENON—
A PULSATION

The heart beat has been a favourite object of study by physiologists and physicians over the years. Papers continue to appear in the medical journals presenting new ways of describing this physical phenomenon and advocating different variables for its quantification. This surprising state of affairs reflects the fact that the approaches used in the past have limitations. There are three main aspects of the heart beat which should be taken into account when characterising cardiac contraction:
(1) The heart is a muscle which has similar contractile properties to other striated muscle.
(2) The heart is a pump which needs to be characterised in terms of pump function.
(3) Cardiac contraction is pulsatile requiring analysis in terms of an oscillatory phenomenon.

The history of this subject is a story of apparent conflict between the first and second approaches. Frank analysed cardiac contraction in muscle terms, Starling analysed it in pump terms. Both realised the importance of the initial length of the muscle fibres as a determinant of the strength of the subsequent beat (now usually referred to as the Frank-Starling mechanism) but the descriptive methods used were different and the relationship between their descriptive variables is frequently misunderstood. There is even greater difficulty in finding common ground between the more modern approaches of applied muscle mechanics (as used by Sonnenblick's group) and of ventricular function curves (as used by Sarnoff's group). It is not my intention to present a detailed critique and comparison of these approaches, but rather to explain how the method I have adopted solves problems of describing both muscle and pump properties.

The correct description and handling of oscillating pressures and flows in the cardiovascular system has only recently been achieved and has been confined largely to the arterial system (see Chapters 7–9). Application of the same methods to ventricular contraction has been slow, probably because the mathematical and physical concepts come easier to the engineer than to the physiologist. I will therefore explain first how oscillating physical phenomena are measured and analysed and apply this to pressures and flows in the heart. This method will then be applied to a pump and pump function of the heart characterised. The method will then be applied to a muscle and the relationship between the pump function and muscle function characteristics explored.

Analysis of oscillating pressure and flow

Pressure is a measure of potential energy and must always have a reference zero pressure. Flow of fluid occurs when there is a difference in potential (pressure) between two points, i.e. pressure gradient. In the heart and arterial system we are concerned with the driving pressure gradient across the peripheral resistance and back to the great veins. The pressure in the great veins is assumed to be sufficiently near zero to be ignored. Thus whenever we use left ventricular or aortic pressures we really mean the pressure difference between left ventricle or aorta and great veins. Sometimes, as when considering force in the wall of the ventricle, we mean the pressure difference between left ventricle and thoracic cavity (transmural pressure gradient). It is often useful to consider the equivalents of the hydraulic variables and elements of the cardiovascular system in electrical terms. Thus pressure (gradient) is equivalent to electrical potential difference (i.e. voltage) and this produces fluid flow which is equivalent to electrical current.

The simplest oscillation of pressure and flow is the sine wave (Fig. 4.1). In panel (a) of Fig. 4.1 there is an oscillation of both pressure and flow between a maximum value and zero. Horizontal dashed lines have been drawn through the middle of the sine waves; these are the average (mean) values of pressure and flow. In this case the pressure and flow go up and down exactly together—this is called 'in phase' (no phase shift, zero phase shift) and occurs when the hydraulic element across which the pressure (gradient) is measured is a simple resistance. This is equivalent to an electrical resistor. Under these circumstances at any given instant of time, pressure divided by flow is given by the same ratio which is the value of the resistance. The same value is given by the ratio of mean pressure to mean flow.

In panel (b), a more realistic situation is presented. Now there is a time lag between the peaks and troughs of pressure and flow, i.e. there is now a phase shift due to the fact that the element across which the pressure is measured is not now a pure resistance. Now at any given instant of time, pressure divided by flow is not given by the same ratio. All the instantaneous values are different. The value of the resistance is *only* given by the ratio of mean pressure to mean flow. The use of instantaneous values is invalid. In the cardiovascular system, one never has a pure resistance. Therefore *characterisation of cardiovascular phenomena by relating instantaneous values of pressure and flow is invalid.*

In the cardiovascular system, the pressure and flow waveforms are not sinusoidal and the shapes of the waveforms are different (Fig. 4.2). The reason why aortic pressure has a different shape of waveform from aortic flow is that the arterial system is not a pure resistance. There are so-called reactive components to the system resulting from elasticity of vessel walls (equivalent to electrical capacitative reactance) and the inertia of blood (equivalent to electrical inductance). The details of this complicated relationship (the aortic input impedance) can be elucidated by breaking the flow and pressure waves into component sine waves of different frequency and phase shift (Chapter 7). However, the resistive part of this impedance is still given

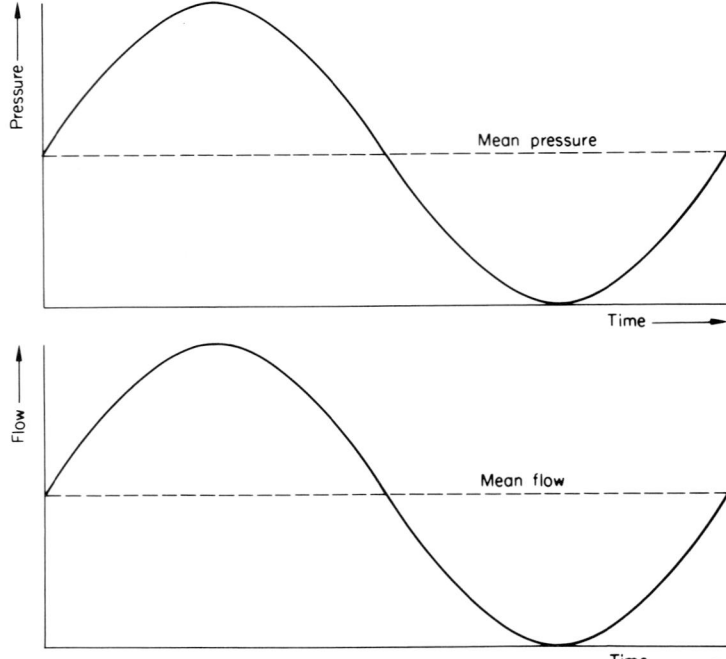

FIG. 4.1(a)

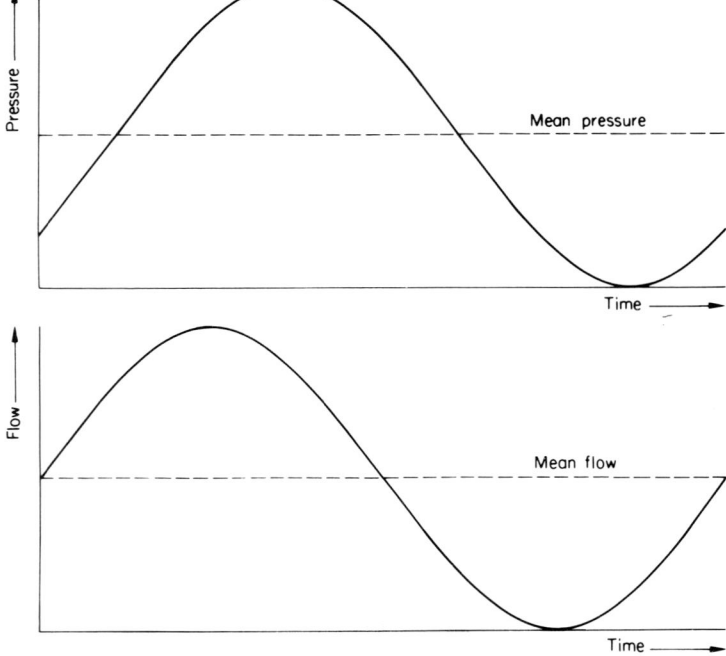

FIG. 4.1(b)

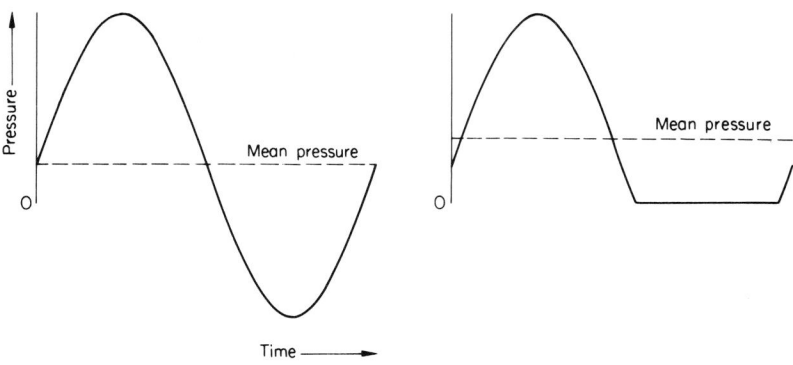

FIG. 4.1(c)

FIG. 4.1. (a) Sine waves of pressure and flow in phase. (b) Sine waves of pressure and flow out of phase with flow leading pressure. Instantaneous pressure/flow is not the same as mean pressure/mean flow. (c) Effect of introducing a valve to stop backflow. Note increase in mean pressure.

by the ratio of mean pressure to mean flow, i.e. the peripheral resistance. The analysis of oscillating physical phenomena by means of a mean term plus a number of component sine waves is called analysis in the 'frequency domain'. The simplest feature which must be understood at this stage and applied to the heart is the use of mean pressure and mean flow.

A further difficulty which must be resolved before applying this method to the heart is the effect of a non-linear element like the aortic valve; this is equivalent to a diode in the electrical case. In panel (c) of Fig. 4.1 is illustrated the effect of such a valve. Note that there is now a profound effect on the mean values in contrast with the effect shown in panel (b). Therefore mean values for a whole system cannot be used if

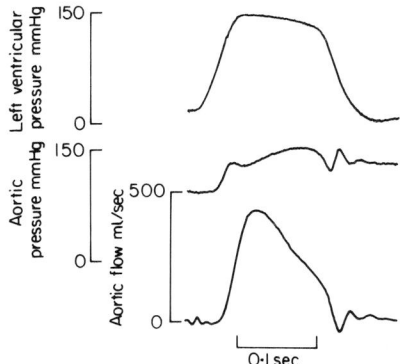

FIG. 4.2. Aortic flow measured distal to the aortic valve by electro-magnetic flowmeter is the same as left ventricular outflow. Pressure on the ventricular side of the valve (left ventricular pressure) is quite different from pressure distal to the valve (aortic pressure). Mean aortic pressure is much higher than mean left ventricular pressure because of the much higher diastolic pressure in the aorta.

there is a valve in the system. One has to divide the system into two parts on either side of the valve and study each separately using measurements made on the corresponding sides of the valve only. The arterial system is studied by analysing aortic pressure and aortic inflow, the left ventricle by analysing left ventricular pressure and left ventricular outflow. Aortic inflow and left ventricular outflow are the same (the same fluid goes through the two parts of the system) but the pressures are different (Fig. 4.2).

It should now be apparent that in order to characterise the left ventricle, mean left ventricular pressure must be related to mean left ventricular outflow.

Pump function of the ventricles

The flow delivered by hydraulic pumps depends on the pressure they have to overcome. It is not possible to deliver the same flow against a high pressure as can be pumped against a low pressure. In order to specify the capabilities of a hydraulic pump, a 'head capacity' curve is derived. An example is given in Fig. 4.3 of a roller pump which does not occlude the tubing and has a constant speed of rotation. It can raise fluid in a vertical column to a certain height; at this point flow is zero. If the outflow tube is lowered below this height some fluid is pumped out and the flow rate can be measured by measuring the volume delivered in a set time. A series of values of

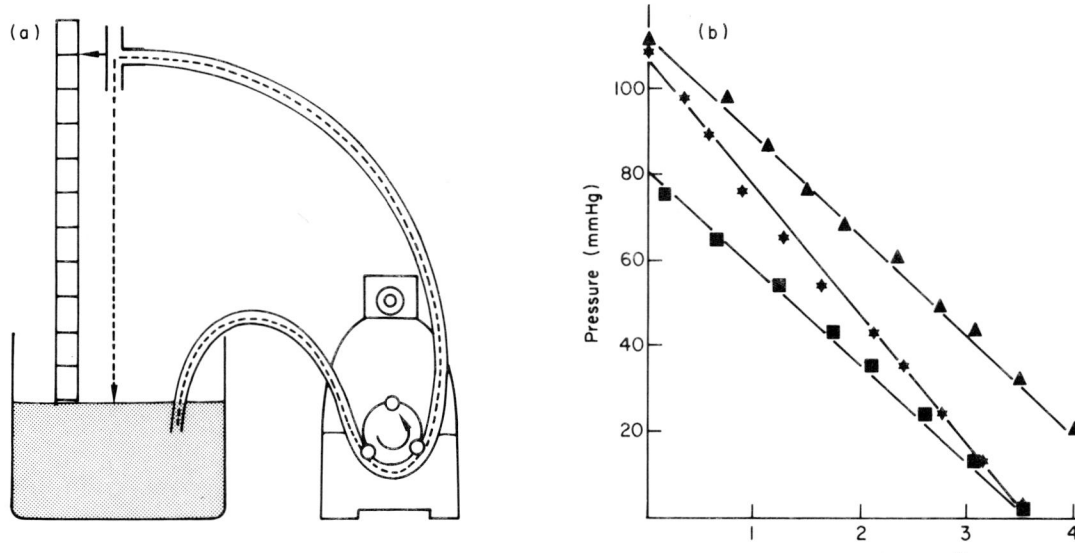

FIG. 4.3.   (a) Non-occlusive roller pump set to maintain a height of fluid. At different heights of the outflow tube the fluid overflow can be measured. Pump performance can be changed by increasing rotation speed or making rollers more occlusive. (b) Plots of pressure in the outflow tube against outflow. ■ control, ★ increased occlusiveness of the rollers ▲ increased roller speed. Data from Elzinga G. & Westerhof N. (1979) *Circulation Res.*, **44**, 303.

flow are then obtained at a series of corresponding heights (pressures). An inverse relationship between pressure and flow is obtained (panel (b)) which is the 'head capacity' curve. This specifies to the engineer what flow will be delivered at any desired pressure and what pressure can be developed at any given flow—a complete description of the pumping ability.

The roller pump in this example is by its nature pulsatile and the values plotted in panel (b) are means. At certain positions of the rollers, fluid can leak backwards past them since they are not occlusive. This backflow can be prevented by placing a one way valve in the outflow tube. The pressure maintained beyond the valve will now be higher for any given flow than without the valve. However the same curve as that in panel (b) will be obtained if pressure is measured proximal to the valve. This situation is analogous to a ventricle, the pumping ability of which is measured in the same way, i.e. by measuring a series of mean ventricular pressure and mean flow values and plotting them as in Fig. 4.3. A ventricle, e.g. left ventricle in the body, is more complicated because as one raises aortic and left ventricular pressure, the ventricle dilates and this produces an increase in the strength of the pump due to the Frank-Starling mechanism (Chapter 5). This is like having a transducer and feedback circuit which senses increases in pressure in the outflow tube which are made to produce an increased speed of rotation of the motor. The effect of this on the 'head capacity' curve is to steepen it so that there is a greater ability to maintain nearly the same flow and greater maximum pressure can be obtained. The opposite effect might be expected with the left ventricle in the body as a result of stimulating the baroreflex. In Fig. 4.3 is shown the effect of increasing pump speed (equivalent to an increase in end-diastolic volume in the heart) and of making the rollers more occlusive (equivalent to increasing contractility of the heart—see Chapter 5).

In order to characterise these separate effects, it is necessary to isolate the heart first and determine its pumping ability with the left ventricular end-diastolic size and pressure constant; this has been achieved most elegantly by Elzinga and Westerhof. Subsequently the effects of increased heart size and other influences can be determined; these will be described in Chapter 5.

Before describing the isolated heart preparation, a few more points concerning the pump function curve (Fig. 4.3b) require to be made. The slope of the line has dimensions of resistance (pressure/flow) and is referred to by engineers as the apparent source resistance of the pump or, in the electrical analogy, the apparent source resistance of the generator. It is not actually a resistance but exactly the same rules apply to its analysis as in the case of a resistance as outlined in the first part of this chapter. Its value is given by the slope of the inverse mean pressure/mean flow relationship. There are phase lags and differences in waveform between pressure and flow when it is not a pure resistance, i.e. when there are reactive components to the impedance. In this case the full characterisation of the apparent source impedance requires, in addition, determination of the relationship between a series of component sine waves of different frequencies exactly as in the case of the aortic input impedance (Chapter 7), i.e. full analysis in the frequency domain. In addition to the slope of the line in Fig 4.3b one requires knowledge of the intercept on the pressure axis called the mean hydromotive pressure. This is equivalent to the electromotive force of an electrical generator. This also has higher frequency terms or harmonics.

Determination of the pump function curve of the left ventricle

The analysis of the mean pressure/mean flow curve of the left ventricular pump has been achieved by Elzinga and Westerhof using an isolated ejecting cat heart perfused with a red cell suspension. The root of the aorta is connected to an artificial hydraulic

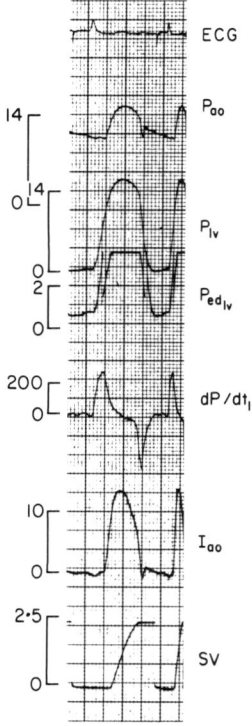

FIG. 4.4a.   Waveforms obtained from an isolated ejecting cat heart. Pao = aortic pressure. Plv = left ventricular pressure. Ped$_{lv}$ = left ventricular pressure at high gain to show diastolic part. dP/dt = rate of change of left ventricular pressure. Iao = aortic flow. SV = stroke volume. Pressures in kPa flow in ml/sec, SV in ml. Tracings kindly provided by Gijs Elzinga.

model of the arterial system which has the same input impedance as the cat's own arterial system. This ensures that the left ventricle ejects into a normal load with normal aortic flow, aortic pressure and left ventricular pressure waveforms (Fig. 4.4a). The aortic pressure is varied by adjusting the artificial peripheral resistance (Fig. 4.4b). Larger changes are introduced for single beats by opening the artificial aorta to an external pressure source (Fig. 4.4c). Isovolumic beats are obtained by occluding the artificial aorta with a shutter (Fig. 4.4d). Left ventricular end-diastolic volume is kept constant by maintaining a constant level of fluid in the reservoir connected to the left atrium. Heart rate is kept constant by electrical pacing. Thus everything is kept constant except the pressure against which the left ventricle ejects.

The mean pressure*/mean flow curve obtained is shown in Fig. 4.5. This is a complete pump function curve similar to that derived for a mechanical roller pump (Fig. 4.3) except that the inverse relationship is curved. For any given load, as defined by mean left ventricular pressure, the flow delivered by the pump is specified. The pressure which can be generated against a total obstruction is given by the intercept at zero flow or mean hydromotive pressure. This is a similar pressure to that exerted by a column of fluid in a vertical tube attached to the pump outflow (Fig. 4.3).

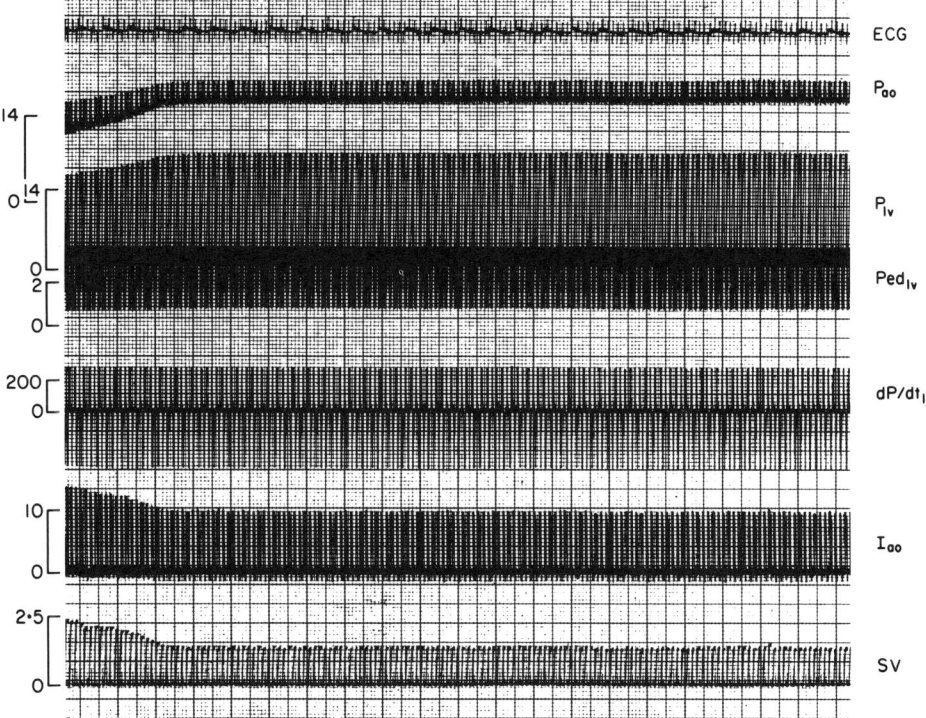

FIG. 4.4b. Slower time base to show effect of increasing peripheral resistance.

It is apparent from this result that the left ventricle has similar characteristics to man made pumps, i.e. an inverse relationship between pressure and outflow or 'head capacity' curve. Since the outflow is very dependent on load pressure the pump function cannot be adequately described by outflow (i.e. cardiac output) alone. The power output is obtained by multiplying *aortic* pressure by flow. This is shown in Fig. 4.6 which demonstrates that power output is also very dependent on load pressure. Also different curves are obtained for each setting of arterial compliance as in Fig. 4.7b below. Similar considerations apply to work output. Therefore the pump function cannot be adequately described by power or work output. Power and

* Mean left ventricular pressure is the same as Sarnoff's tension time index per minute.

work are much less satisfactory variables to use for this purpose than flow because all work outputs except the maximum are produced at two completely different load pressures.

The comprehensive nature of the mean pressure/mean flow curve as a description of pump function can be further illustrated by seeing what happens if one produces a

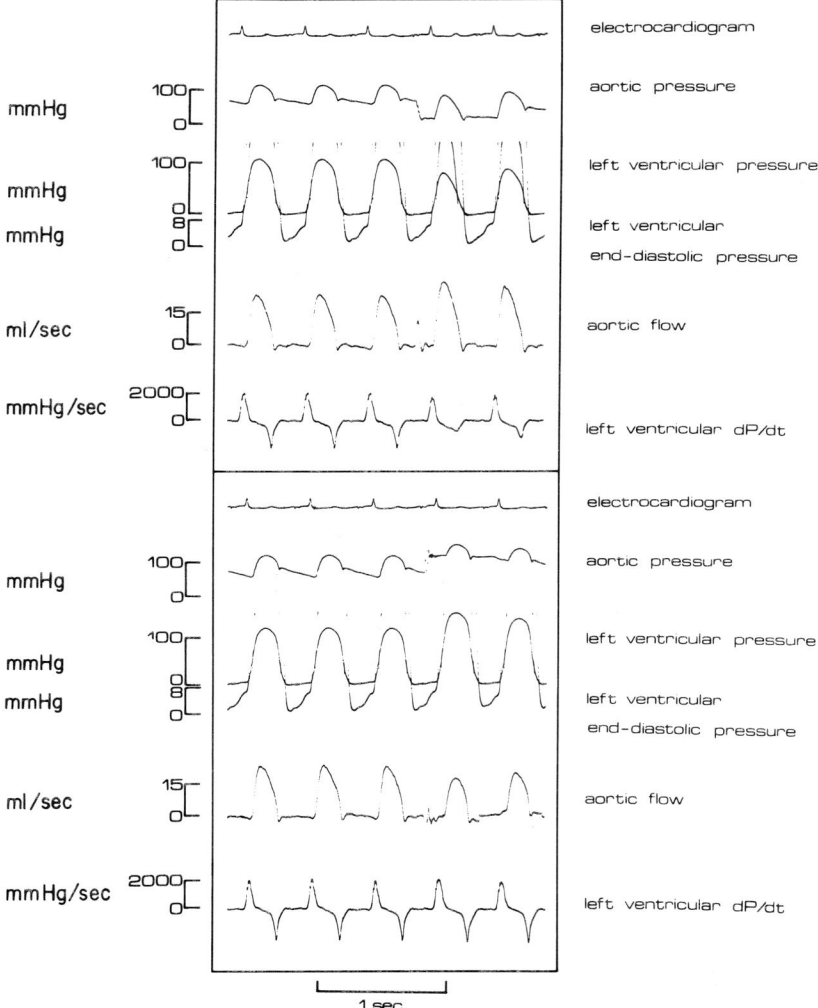

FIG. 4.4C.   On the fourth beat of each panel, aorta is connected to pressurised bottle. Above at low pressure, below at high pressure.

large change in the nature of the aortic load. In Fig. 4.7a the artificial arterial system into which the isolated left ventricle ejects has been adjusted so that it is much stiffer, as if the arterial walls had been made inelastic. This intervention produces a large change in the pressure and flow waveforms (Fig. 4.7a) and in the relationship between any instantaneous pressure value (e.g. peak left ventricular pressure) and flow. There is also a shift of the relationship between pressure distal to the valve (aortic pressure) and flow (Fig. 4.7b). Only the relationship between mean left ventricular pressure and mean left ventricular outflow (Fig. 4.7c) is constant. This must follow from the underlying theory (above), but is a practical demonstration of the fact that this relationship characterises the pump and does not change if the pump is the same.

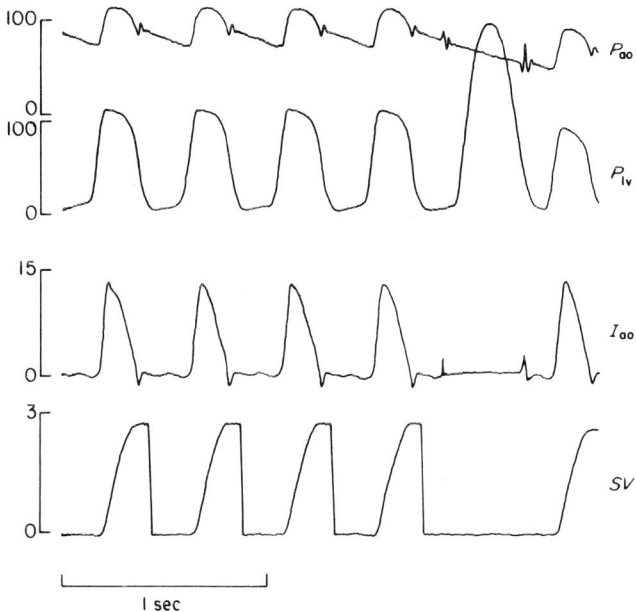

F I G. 4.4d.   On the fifth beat the aorta is occluded and an isovolumic beat recorded.

Contractile performance of cardiac muscle

The mechanical performance of skeletal muscle is characterised by the inverse relationship between force and velocity. In order to determine this relationship, an isolated single muscle fibre is tetanised into prolonged contractions of relatively constant contractile activity during which shortening against a series of loads is studied (Fig. 4.8a). The slope of the length change during shortening is plotted against the corresponding load (Fig. 4.8b).

   There are a number of reasons why it is impossible to apply the same analysis to the heart beat:

(1) The method of obtaining the force-velocity curve of skeletal muscle cannot be applied to the heart, i.e. to tetanise it into a prolonged steady state of contractile activity during which controlled shortenings can be applied. During a cardiac contractile pulse the contractile activity (and therefore the entire force-velocity curve) rises from zero to a peak and back in a manner determined by the rise and fall of calcium activator and its interaction with the contractile proteins (Chapters 2 and 3).

(2) The instantaneous force-velocity curve at any particular time in the contraction

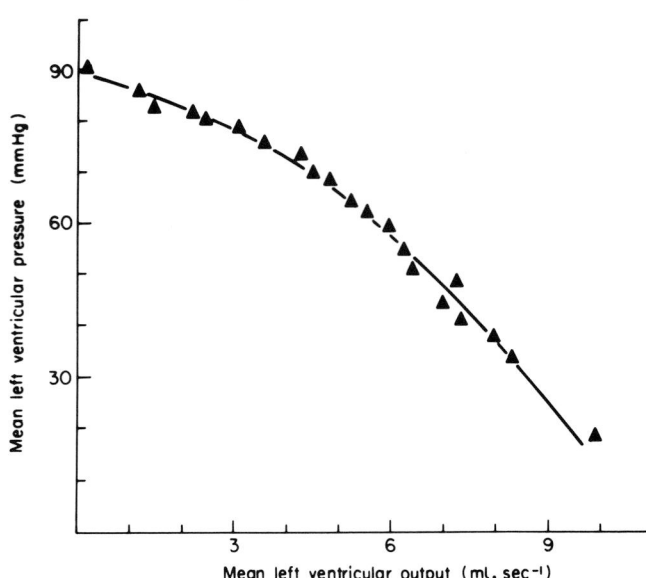

FIG. 4.5. Mean left ventricular pressure plotted against mean output in an isolated ejecting cat heart. Data from Elzinga G. & Westerhof N. (1977) *J. Physiol*, 266, 46P.

must be determined by the quick-release technique (as used by Edman & Nilsson) which cannot be used in the intact ventricle. In any case this curve does not take into account the time course of the contraction. However the time course is an important determinant of the overall mechanical performance of a cardiac contraction, i.e. a sustained cardiac contraction produces greater flow than a very brief one.

(3) Cardiac muscle (like skeletal muscle) has some properties analogous to those of a spring. If a strip of muscle is stimulated to contract and develop force isometrically (no shortening) there will be a sudden recoil of length and force if one end of the

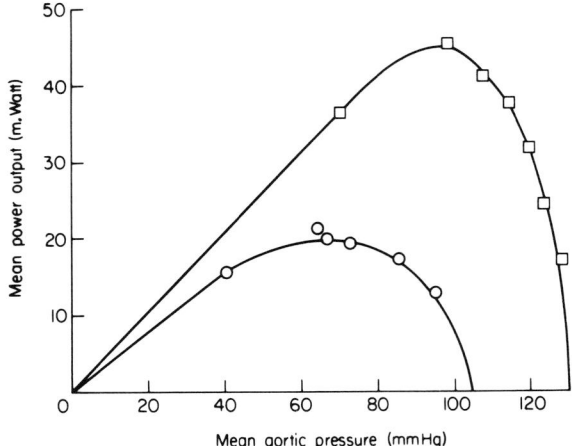

FIG. 4.6. Mean power output as a function of pressure calculated from data in Fig. 4.7b. Different curves are obtained for different settings of arterial compliance.

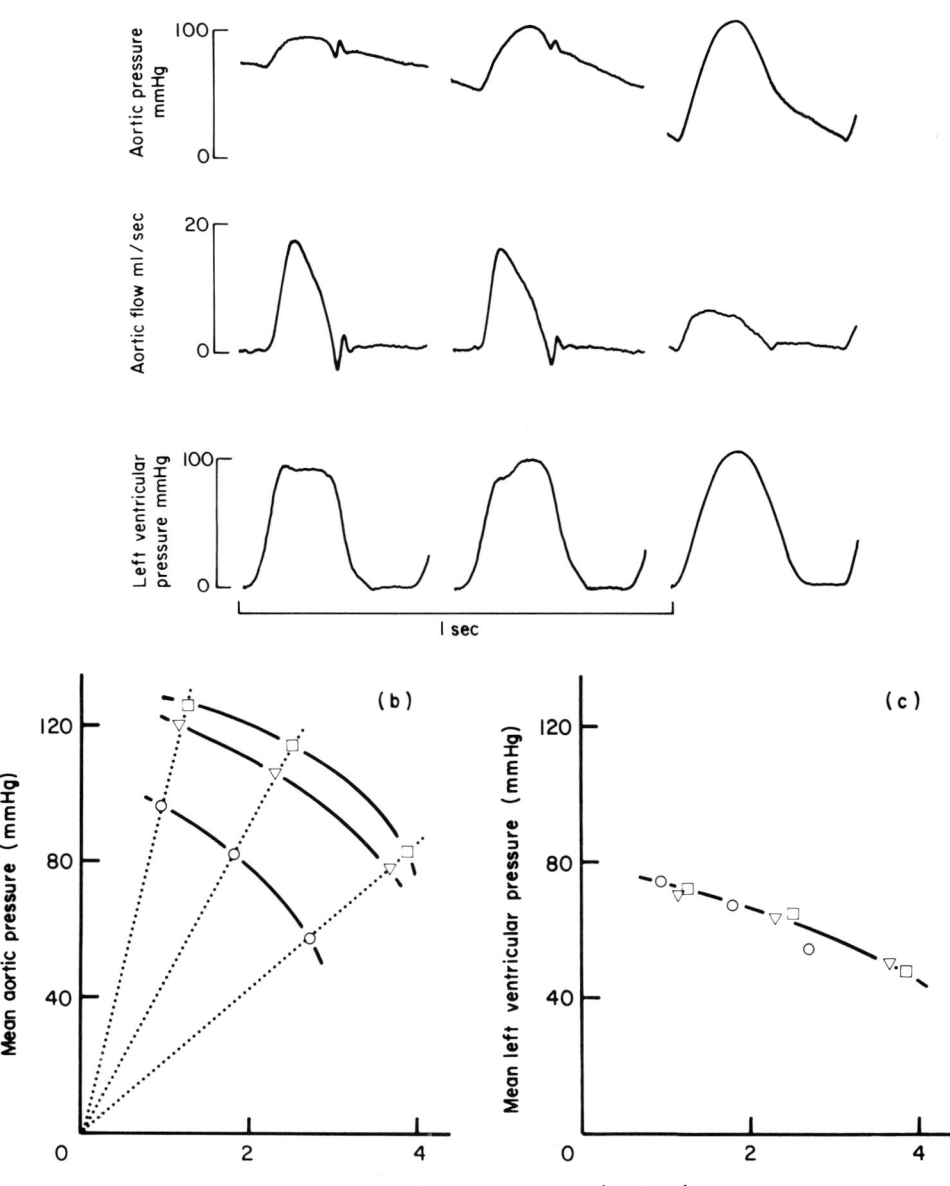

FIG. 4.7. (a) Pressures and flows generated by the left ventricle against 3 different arterial compliances (increasing stiffness towards the right). Top = aortic pressure in mm Hg, Middle = aortic flow in ml/sec, bottom = left ventricular pressure in mm Hg. Peripheral resistance constant at $28\cdot5 \times 10^3$g/cm^4 sec^{-1}. Data abstracted from Fig. 3 of Elzinga G. & Westerhof N. (1973) *Circulation Res.*, **32**, 182. (b) Data from panel (a), together with similar data obtained at two higher settings of peripheral resistance (slope of dotted lines = peripheral resistance). Mean aortic pressure/mean outflow plots yield three different curves for the three settings of arterial compliance. (c) Data superimposes when plotted as mean left ventricular pressure against mean outflow. Data from Elzinga G. & Westerhof N. (1979) *Circulation Res.*, **44**, 303.

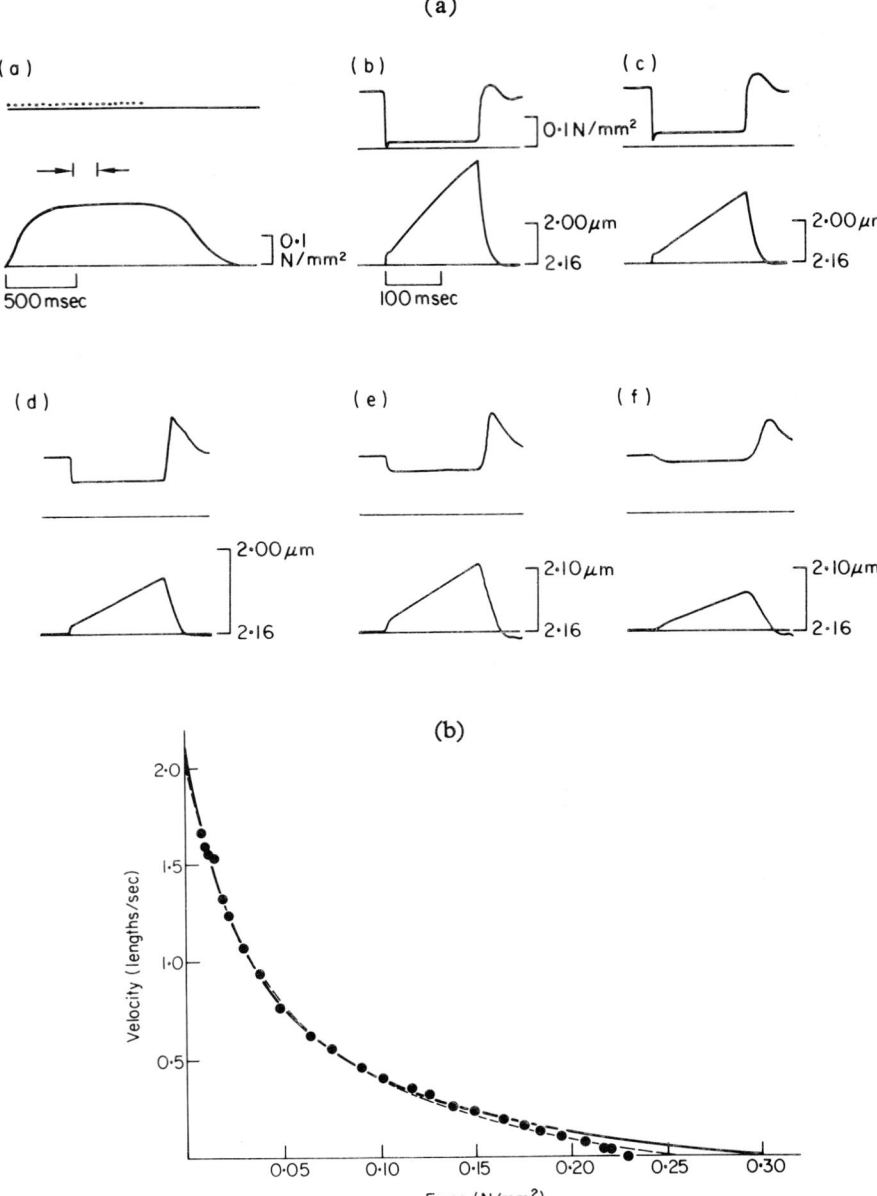

FIG. 4.8.   (a) Oscilloscope records illustrating: *a*, fused isometric tetanus and *b–f*, active shortening against various loads in a single fibre from frog skeletal muscle. The loads were applied during the interval of tetanus indicated by horizontal arrows in (a). The shortening records indicate actual sarcomere length (gain is increasing from *b* to *f*). The force calibration is the same in *a–f*. Progressive fall of the slope of length change with time (velocity) as force increases from *b* to *f*. (b) Plot of velocity against force from a similar experiment. From Edman K.A.P. & Hwang J.C. (1977) *J. Physiol.*, **269**, 259.

muscle is released (the so-called quick-release phenomenon). These spring-like properties constitute a reactive element, an elastance. The behaviour is as if there is a shortening element connected to a spring. These are usually thought of as the contractile element (CE) and series elastic element (SE). The velocity of shortening will be different when the length of the SE is changing from when it is constant. The only load which ensures constant SE length is one which maintains force constant during shortening, i.e. the classical isotonic afterload as used in skeletal muscle experiments (Fig. 4.8a). The force in the wall of the ventricle is not constant during shortening. When such time varying loads are applied to isolated strips of cardiac muscle, the relationship between instantaneous force and velocity changes. This shows that the construction of a *force-velocity curve from instantaneous values is invalid*; this conclusion must follow from the presence in the system of reactive elements. This problem was discussed in connection with fluid resistance. The same considerations apply to mechanical reactance (masses and springs).

These problems are overcome by relating mean velocity and mean force. The

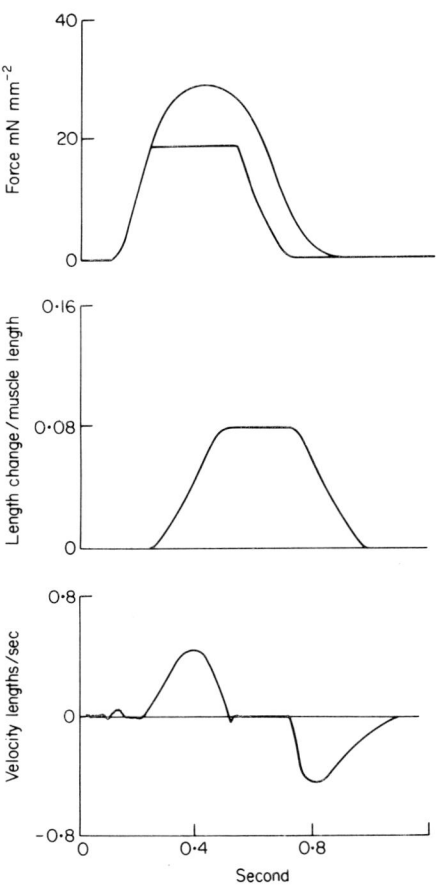

FIG. 4.9a. Record of tension (force) and length in a physiologically sequenced cat papillary muscle contraction. Data kindly provided by Gijs Elzinga.

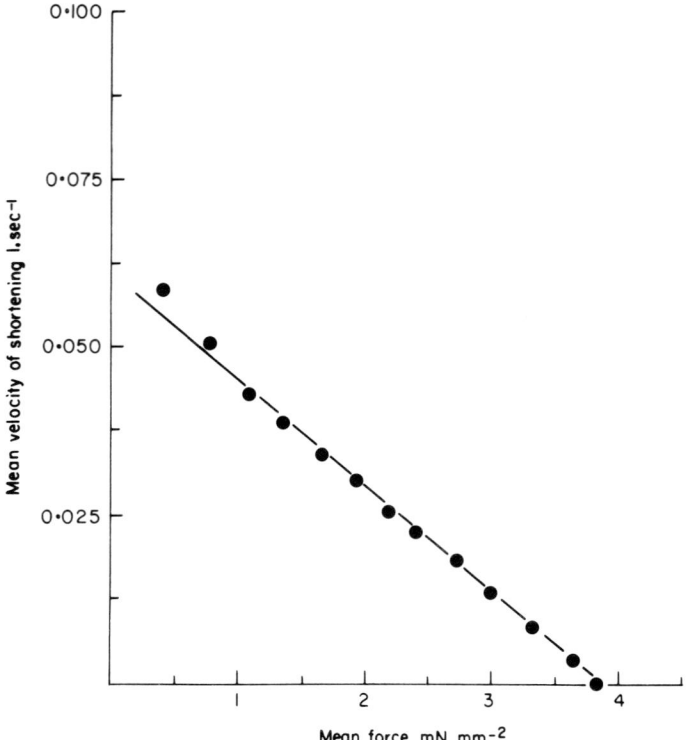

FIG. 4.9b.   Mean velocity plotted against mean force from contractions similar to (a) at various loads.

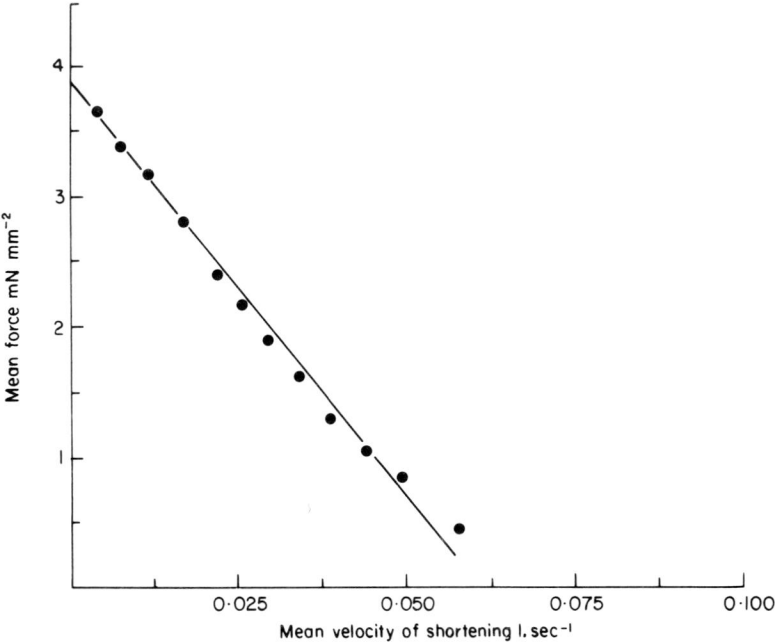

FIG. 4.9c.   As (b) plotted as mean force against mean velocity.

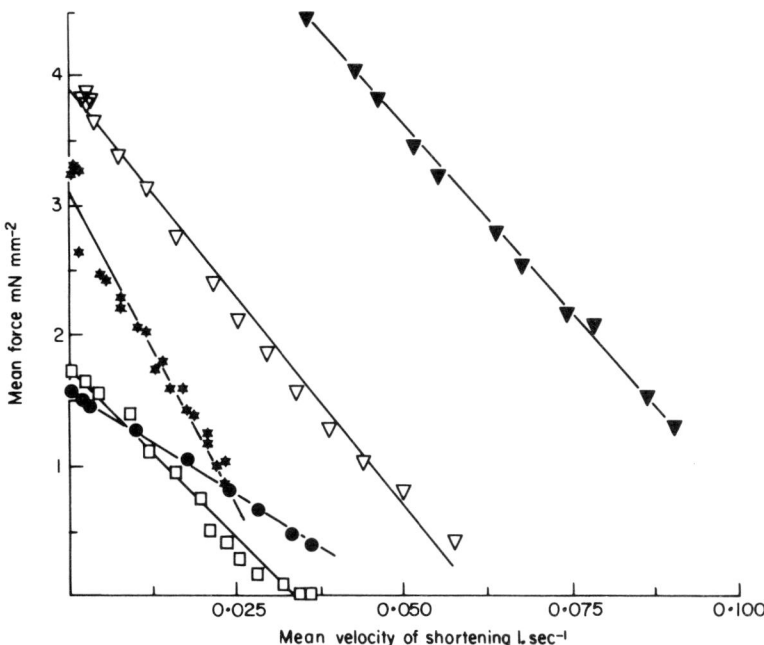

F I G. 4.9d.   Mean force/mean velocity curves from five different muscles.

instantaneous variations caused by time varying contractile activity, time varying load and reactive elements are then eliminated. The resultant force-velocity curve defines the contractile performance of the muscle by specifying the mean velocity achieved against any given load (mean force) and the mean load lifted at any given mean velocity of contraction. This force-velocity curve is determined by the mean contractile activity. Longer duration contractions move the curve outwards (higher mean velocity at any mean load) and shorter contractions move the curve downwards (lower mean velocity at any mean load). The curve is unaffected by the nature of the load, i.e. whether the load is inertial, viscous, elastic or an isotonic force.

Force-velocity curves of this type have been determined for isolated papillary muscles by Elzinga and colleagues. In order to simulate the sequence of events in the heart, the apparatus was arranged so that the muscle first developed force isometrically in a manner equivalent to the isovolumetric contraction period of the ventricles. Shortening then occurred against a variable load as during the ejection period. At peak shortening the muscle length was held constant while force relaxed to zero as during the isovolumetric relaxation period. Then length was allowed to relax back to the initial value as during ventricular filling (Fig. 4.9a). When the load is varied over a range from zero to peak isometric force, mean velocity of shortening can be plotted against mean force to obtain an inverse force-velocity relation (Fig. 4.9b). Since force and velocity are interdependent variables, they can also be plotted on the alternative axes (Fig. 4.9c). The mechanism of this inverse interrelationship in both cardiac and skeletal muscle lies in the mechanism of contraction which is itself uncertain (Chapter 3).

Some examples of mean force-mean velocity curves in cat papillary muscles are shown in Fig. 4.9d. The position of the curves varies widely indicating widely varying contractile performance. These muscles were studied at unphysiologically low temperatures and stimulation rates. The position of the curves was primarily a function of the duration of the contractile activity. Would the muscles with the highest force-velocity curve make the best pumps if incorporated into a ventricle?

Relationship of pump and muscle function in the ejecting heart

It is clear that the development of contractile force in the ventricular wall causes the build-up of pressure within the cavity during the isovolumic contraction period. The

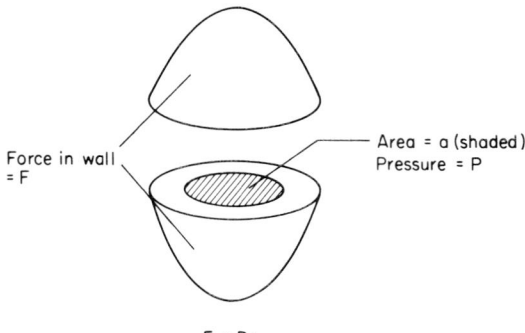

FIG. 4.10a.   When the left ventricle (in the imagination) is cut into two halves, the force tending to pull the two halves apart is the left ventricular pressure multiplied by the cross-sectional area of the cavity. After Lloyd Hefner.

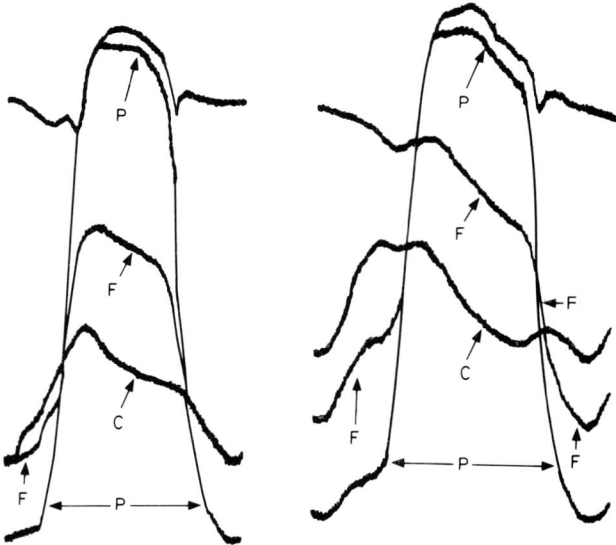

FIG. 4.10b.   Left ventricular pressure (P), circumference (C) and wall force (F) recorded from a dog heart. From Hefner L.L. *et al.* (1962) *Circulation Res.*, **11**, 65.

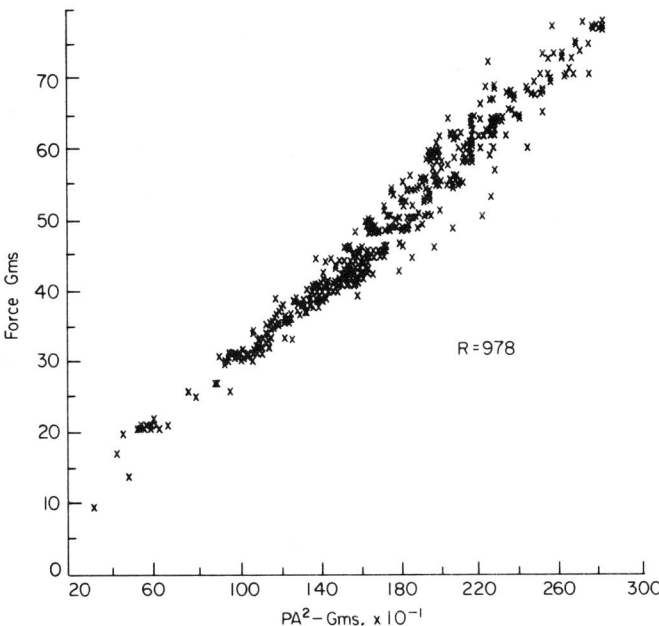

FIG. 4.10c. When force obtained from records similar to (a) is plotted against pressure times cavity cross-sectional area (calculated from circumference), a close correlation is obtained. From Hefner L.L. *et al.* (1962) *Circulation Res.*, **11**, 660.

relationship between wall force and ventricular pressure has been the subject of many studies. The study of Hefner and colleagues remains the most useful conceptually because their basic approach makes no assumptions about the shape of the left ventricle. If, in the imagination, the ventricle is cut through its equator into two halves (Fig. 4.10a), the force tending to pull the two halves apart (exerted over the cut surface area of muscle) is equal to the intraventricular pressure multiplied by the cross-sectional area of the cavity. In order to verify this relationship it was necessary

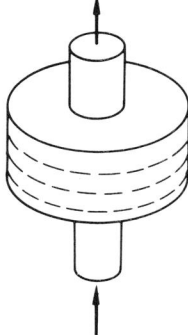

FIG. 4.10d. Cylindrical model of left ventricle in which all shortening is assumed to take place in the circumferential direction. From Elzinga G. & Westerhof N. (1979) *Circulation Res.*, **44**, 303.

to make assumptions about the shape of the cross-section of the cavity. The simplest assumption is that it is a circle and that the cross-sectional area is πr^2 where r is the radius. Hefner calculated this from measurements of external circumference. Wall force and intraventricular pressure were measured directly. During ejection, when left ventricular pressure is relatively constant, wall force falls due to the decreasing heart size (decreasing circumference and cavity cross-sectional area, Fig. 4.10b). A good correlation was found between measured force (F) and pressure (P) times cavity cross-sectional area, a (Fig. 4.10c), i.e. $F = P \cdot a$ (Hefner's equation).

This study shows the value of using the fewest and simplest possible assumptions. This is more difficult when trying to take this approach further to find the relationship between the force exerted by a fibre in the wall of the ventricle and ventricular pressure. The geometry of the ventricle is extremely complex and realistic models of it yield rather impractically complicated equations for this purpose. However if one assumes the simplest possible situation—i.e. that the ventricle is a cylinder (Fig. 4.10d), a useful relationship emerges which helps understanding. If the cylinder is thought to be of fixed length during ejection and contracts by shortening of fibres of equal length and force arranged in rings around its circular circumference (Fig. 4.10d), the force developed by each fibre is found to be proportional to the ventricular pressure times the fibre length:

$$F = K \cdot P \cdot l$$

$$\text{i.e.} \quad P = F/K \cdot l$$

The proportionality constant K depends on the assumptions as to the length of the cylinder, the number of fibres in each circumferential ring and the total number of fibres. Throughout the cardiac cycle, a continuous derivation of fibre force from pressure and fibre length or of pressure from fibre force and length can be carried out using this equation.

It is clear that shortening of muscle fibres in the ventricular wall causes the decrease in volume of the chamber, i.e. outflow during ejection. The relationship between outflow and shortening velocity is more difficult to establish for the real heart. The most successful approach to this problem was that of Fry but the mathematical procedure required was complex and the method has not therefore been applied to any great extent.

A much simpler method can be applied if one again makes the gross assumptions implied in the cylindrical model (Fig. 4.10d). For this model, the outflow at any instant turns out to be proportional to both the length of each fibre (l) and its velocity, dl/dt:

$$q = M \cdot l \cdot dl/dt$$

The proportionality constant M depends on the assumptions made about the length of the cylinder and the number of fibres in each circumferential ring.

With the equations for P and q in the cylindrical model, data can be taken from an isolated muscle strip experiment (e.g. Fig. 4.9) and the corresponding pressure and outflow curves obtained for the cylindrical model. These curves are then averaged over the cardiac cycle to yield mean pressure and mean outflow for any particular load. These values are plotted for a series of loads in the familiar pump function curve (Fig. 4.11).

A number of important points emerge from this simple exercise:

(1) The inverse nature of the relationship between ventricular pressure and outflow is due to the inverse nature of the force-velocity curve of the myocardium.

(2) The pump function curve is directly related to the mean force–mean velocity curve through factors describing the geometry of the ventricle so that with constant

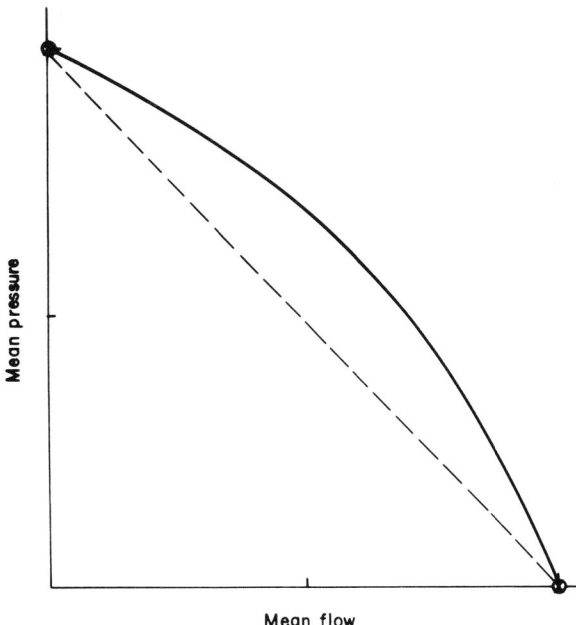

FIG. 4.11. Continuous line—mean pressure/mean force curve obtained from the model in Fig. 4.10b assuming that the muscle in the wall behaves as in Fig. 4.9. Dashed line is obtained if the shortening in the cylinder takes place only in the lengthwise direction with constant circumference. Curvature is due to circumferential shortening. From Elzinga G. & Westerhof N. (1979) *Circulation Res.*, **44**, 303.

heart size, changes in the force-velocity curve can be shown by measuring changes in the pump function curve.

(3) It is possible, by making the assumption that the ventricle is a cylinder (Fig. 4.10d) of specific dimensions and fibre composition, to calculate back from the pump function curve to the force-velocity curve. Similar calculations can be done for spherical and spheroidal models. The results of such calculations depend heavily upon the geometric assumptions used.

(4) These exercises (2 and 3 above) are not valid for instantaneous values of pressure and outflow, force and velocity because of the changing nature of the load (Fig. 4.10b), the different waveforms of the variables concerned and the changing with time of contractile activity. This re-emphasises the need to use mean values.

(5) A curvilinear pump function relationship is obtained for a cylindrical model made from fibres with a straight mean force-mean velocity curve (Fig. 4.11). A straight pump function curve is obtained from the same cylinder if it is assumed that it shortens lengthwise with a constant cavity cross-sectional area (dashed line in Fig. 4.11). It is known that the ventricle contracts circumferentially during ejection (Fig. 4.10b). It is therefore reasonable to conclude that the curvature of the pump function curve of the heart (Fig. 4.5) is due to the circumferential shortening.

Indices of speed of onset of contraction

In the approach to characterisation of ventricular contraction given above, the overall performance is expressed in what appears to me to be the only meaningful quantification, i.e. mean force or pressure—mean velocity or flow. In terms of time course of contraction, these relationships are influenced by the duration of contraction; when reduced to force developed by an isometric muscle strip, they reflect the area under the curve (Fig. 4.12A). The same area can occur under different types of contraction, e.g. Fig. 4.12B and C. These two contractions may give identical pump function

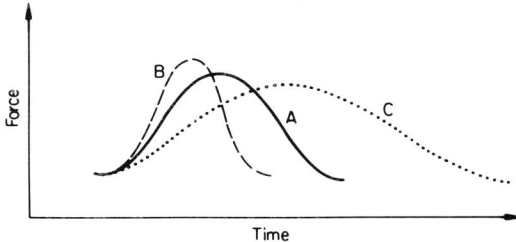

FIG. 4.12.   (A) Control contraction. (B) Rapid contraction, e.g. under catecholamine influence. (C) Slowed relaxation, e.g. under caffeine influence.

curves when the corresponding fibres are incorporated into a ventricle. Nevertheless they are different; contraction B clearly has a faster onset than contraction C. While this difference in character of the contraction makes no difference at all to mean pump function, it does nevertheless give information about the physiological state of the muscle. In particular, inotropic interventions markedly affect speed of onset of contraction (Chapter 5).

In the isometric isolated heart muscle strip (Fig. 4.12), this aspect of the contraction can be expressed by measuring the maximum rate of rise of isometric force— dF/dt max. How can this same quality be expressed in an intact ejecting heart? If the isolated muscle shortens against zero load, no force is developed and dF/dt max is zero. As the load is increased there is a longer and longer period of isometric force development before shortening occurs (Fig. 4.13a) and dF/dt max consequently increases. Above a certain load the isometric contraction period extends beyond the time of peak dF/dt of the totally isometric contraction. Subsequently dF/dt max is independent of load (Fig. 4.13b). Exactly the same considerations apply to the

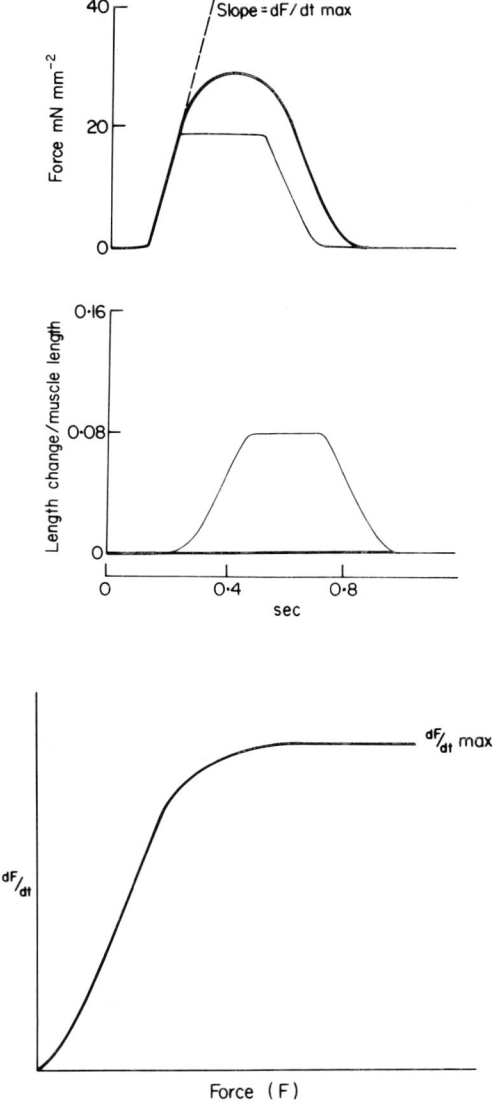

F IG. 4.13. (a) Length and tension in a papillary muscle contraction to illustrate the maximum rate of rise of force which occurs before shortening begins. (b) Above a given load, dF/dt max is independent of load.

isovolumetric contraction period of the left ventricle. The aortic pressure must be high enough for the load independent region of Fig. 4.13b to be applicable. This is checked by raising aortic pressure between beats and ensuring that the maximum rate of rise of left ventricular pressure (dP/dt max) is unchanged.

In the ventricle, it is impractical to measure dF/dt in the wall. dP/dt max is measured instead. If one takes Hefner's equation and assumes that in the isovolumetric contraction period the fibres contract isometrically (not true but a reasonable approximation in this circumstance) the relationship obtained is:

$$dP/dt = \frac{dF/dt}{a}$$

where a is the cavity cross-sectional area. Thus for a given heart size (a), dP/dt max is a very reasonable index of dF/dt max. It is by far the most useful index of the early velocity of contraction. It should be pointed out that dF/dt and dP/dt indicate the speed of contraction of the organ as a whole. The introduction of extra series elasticity (e.g. an infarcted area) will reduce them as well as reductions in the speed of contraction of the contractile tissue.

The use of indices in which dP/dt is divided by left ventricular pressure is to be condemned. The only meaningful pressure which could be used for this purpose is the transmural pressure, i.e. the pressure difference between inside and outside the ventricle. This is impractical. To use conventional left ventricular pressure for this purpose is nonsense. The ratio $dP/dt/P$ merely becomes a function of the reference zero—different for mid-chest and angle of Louis, fluctuating with breathing etc.

The question remains as to whether it is possible to gain information about early contraction speed when aortic pressure is low and dP/dt max unreliable. The best index under these circumstances is the maximum acceleration of blood from the ventricle. This arises from an intuitive idea of Guz that the faster cardiac contraction takes off, the greater will be the accelerating force applied to the blood. The idea was elaborated as the 'initial ventricular impulse' by Rushmer. The considerable limitations in theory and practice of this index were enumerated by Van den Bos and colleagues. The index has some usefulness but it should be used with caution in full knowledge of its limitations.

Before it is possible to decide how the various measurements of ventricular contraction should be used in physiological and clinical practice, it is necessary to know how the heart responds to various controlling influences. This problem will therefore be discussed in the next Chapter after these influences have been described.

REFERENCES

ABBOTT B.C. & MOMMAERTS W.F.H.M. (1959) A study of inotropic mechanisms in the papillary muscle preparation. *J. Gen. Physiol.*, **42**, 533–551.

BRADY A.J. (1965) Time and displacement dependence of myocardial contractility problems in defining the active state and force-velocity relations. *Fed. Proc.*, **24**, 1410–1420.

BLINKS J.R. & JEWELL B.R. (1977) The meaning and measurement of myocardial contractility. In *Cardiovascular Fluid Dynamics*. Vol. 1. D.H. Bergel, Ed. 225–260. Academic Press, London.

BRUTSAERT D.L. & PAULUS W.J. (1977) Loading and performance of the heart as muscle and pump. *Cardiovasc. Res.*, **11**, 1–16.

BURTON A.C. (1957) Importance of shape and size of heart. *Am. Heart J.*, **54**, 801.

EDMAN K.A.P., MULIERI L.A. & SCUBON-MULIERI B. (1976) Non-hyperbolic force-velocity relationship in single fibres of the frog muscle. *Acta Physiol., Scand.*, **98**, 143–156.

EDMAN K.A.P. & NILSSON E. (1972) Relationships between force and velocity of shortening in rabbit papillary muscle. *Acta Physiol., Scand.*, **85**, 488–500.

ELZINGA G. & WESTERHOF N. (1979) How to quantify pump function of the heart. The value of variables derived from measurements on isolated muscle. *Circulation Res.*, **44**, 303–308.

ELZINGA G. & WESTERHOF N. (1973) Pressure and flow generated by the left ventricle against different impedances. *Circulation Res.*, **32**, 178–186.

ELZINGA G. & WESTERHOF N. (1976) The pumping ability of the left heart and the effect of coronary occlusion. *Circulation Res.*, **38**, 297–302.

FRANK O. (1895) Zur Dynamik des Herzmuskels. *Z. Biol.*, **32**, 370. Translated by Chapman C.B. & Wasserman E. (1959) *Am. Heart J.*, **58**, 282 and 467.

FRY D.L. (1962) Discussion of a paper by Sonnenblick E.H. *Fed. Proc.*, **21**, 991–993.

FRY D.L., GRIGGS D.M. JR. & GREENFIELD J.C. JR. (1964) Myocardial mechanics: tension-velocity-length relationships of heart muscle. *Circulation Res.*, **14**, 73–85.

HEFNER L.L. & BOWEN T.E. (1967) Elastic components of cat papillary muscle. *Am. J. Physiol.*, **212**, 1221–1227.

HEFNER L.L., SHEFFIELD L.T., COBBS G.C. & KLIP W. (1962) Relation between mural force and pressure in the left ventricle of the dog. *Circulation Res.*, **11**, 654–663.

HUISMAN R.M. (1977) Forces in the wall of the left ventricle. Ph.D. Thesis. Free University of Amsterdam.

LEWARTOWSKI B., SEDEK G. & OKALSKI A. (1972) Direct measurement of tension within left ventricular wall of the dog heart. *Cardiovasc. Res.*, **11**, 654–663.

MCDONALD D.A. (1974) *Blood Flow in Arteries*. Edward Arnold, London.

MITCHELL J.H., HEFNER L.L. & MONROE R.G. (1972) Left ventricular performance. *Am. J. Med.*, **53**, 481–494.

NOBLE M.I.M., TRENCHARD D. & GUZ A. (1966) Left ventricular ejection in conscious dogs. I. Measurement and significance of the maximum acceleration of blood from the left ventricle. *Circulation Res.*, **19**, 139–147.

NOBLE M.I.M., GABE I.T., TRENCHARD D. & GUZ A. (1967) Blood pressure and flow in the ascending aorta of conscious dogs. *Cardiovasc. Res.*, **1**, 9–20.

PATTERSON S.W., PIPER H. & STARLING E.H. (1914) The regulation of the heart beat. *J. Physiol.*, **48**, 465.

REEVES T.J., HEFNER L.L., JONES W.B., COGHLAN C, PRIETO G. & CARROLL J. (1960) The hemodynamic determinants of the rate of change in pressure in the left ventricle. *Am. Heart J.*, 745–761.

RUSHMER R.F. (1964) Initial ventricular impulse. A potential key to cardiac evaluation. *Circulation*, **29**, 268.

SARNOFF S.J. & MITCHELL J.H. (1962) The control of the function of the heart. *Handbook of Physiology*, Sec. 2. Circulation 1, 489.

SONNENBLICK E.H. (1962) Implications of muscle mechanics in the heart. *Fed. Proc.*, **21**, 975–990.

VAN DEN BOS G.C., ELZINGA G., WESTERHOF N. & NOBLE M.I.M. (1973) Problems in the use of indices of myocardial contractility. *Cardiovasc. Res.*, **7**, 834–848.

CHAPTER 5

THE CONTROL OF
CARDIAC CONTRACTILE PERFORMANCE

Unlike skeletal muscle, all myocardial fibres contract all the time. A stronger contraction cannot be obtained by recruiting more fibres as in skeletal muscle. A stronger contraction is obtained by increasing the contractile strength of each fibre.

There are two principal ways in which the strength of the heart beat can be increased. One is by an increase in the length of the fibres at the end of diastole, i.e. an increase in the end-diastolic volume. This is the Frank-Starling mechanism. The other mechanism is a so called 'increase in contractility' or 'positive inotropic response'.

The Frank-Starling mechanism

The simplest way to demonstrate this phenomenon is to take an isolated strip of heart muscle and allow it to contract isometrically (without shortening). Having recorded the force during a control twitch, the length of the muscle is varied and the resulting twitches recorded (Fig. 5.1a). Stretching the muscle results in an increase in force during diastole called resting force. This resting force, the total force during systole, and the increase in force from the resting to total level (the developed force) can be plotted against muscle length (Fig. 5.1b). This plot illustrates the increasing force obtained by stretching the muscle.

A similar study can be done on the isovolumetrically contracting heart as was done by Frank. In this case isovolumetric pressure is plotted against end-diastolic volume (Fig. 5.1c and d). However, this is not quite the same as the isolated muscle experiment (Fig. 5.1a and b). Volume along the abscissa is proportional to the square or cube of the fibre length. Pressure on the ordinate is the muscle force divided by the cavity cross-sectional area (Hefner's equation) which is increasing with volume. Therefore isovolumetric pressure rises less steeply with increasing volume than force with increasing fibre length.

Similar conclusions about the control of contraction by end-diastolic volume are frequently drawn in the ejecting heart from the changes in outflow with increasing end-diastolic volume. However this is much more complicated. Starling arranged for the heart to eject into a 'Starling resistor' which allows blood through only when it exceeds a certain predetermined pressure. Thus the aortic pressure was controlled and constant. However the true load on the muscle fibres was not held constant and the aortic input impedance was made alinear and very unphysiological.

The setting of aortic pressure is indicated by the horizontal dashed line in the pressure-volume diagram (Fig. 5.2a). In a heart beat beginning from point *A* on the

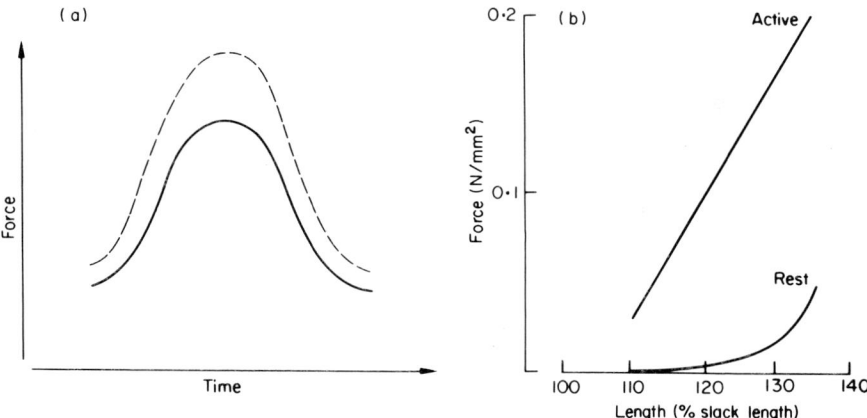

FIG. 5.1 (a). Schematic diagram of isometric cardiac muscle twitch: continuous line = control, dashed line = effect of increase in muscle length. (b). Relationship between twitch height (see a), i.e. active force, resting force (between twitches) and length of isometric cardiac muscle.

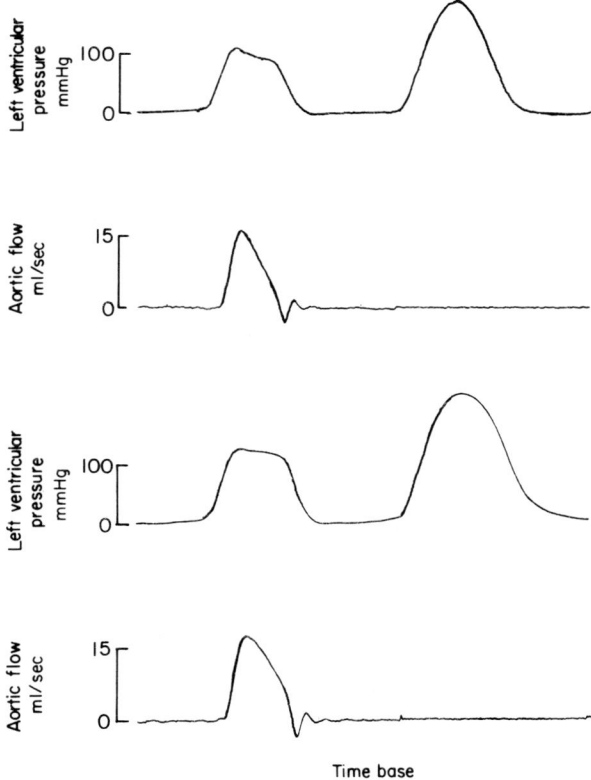

FIG. 5.1C. Left ventricular pressure and outflow from an isolated ejecting cat heart. The second beat is isovolumetric. Control above, increased end-diastolic volume and pressure below. Note increase in peak isovolumetric pressure. Tracings kindly provided by Gijs Elzinga.

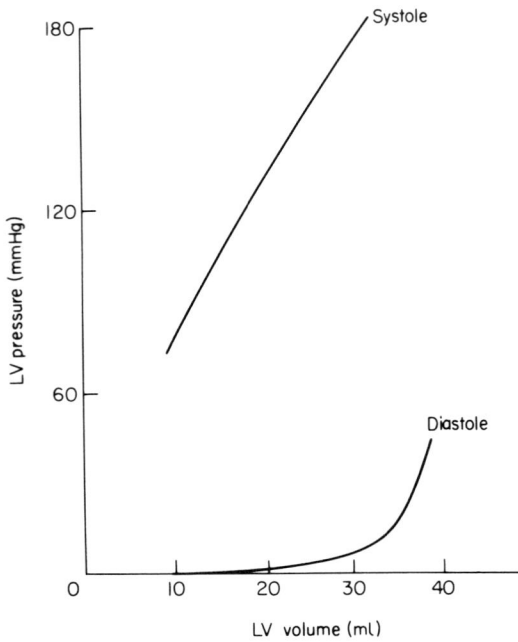

FIG. 5.1d. Relationship between isovolumic systolic pressure (see c), diastolic pressure and volume of isolated dog heart. Data adapted from Weber, Janicki and Hefner (1976).

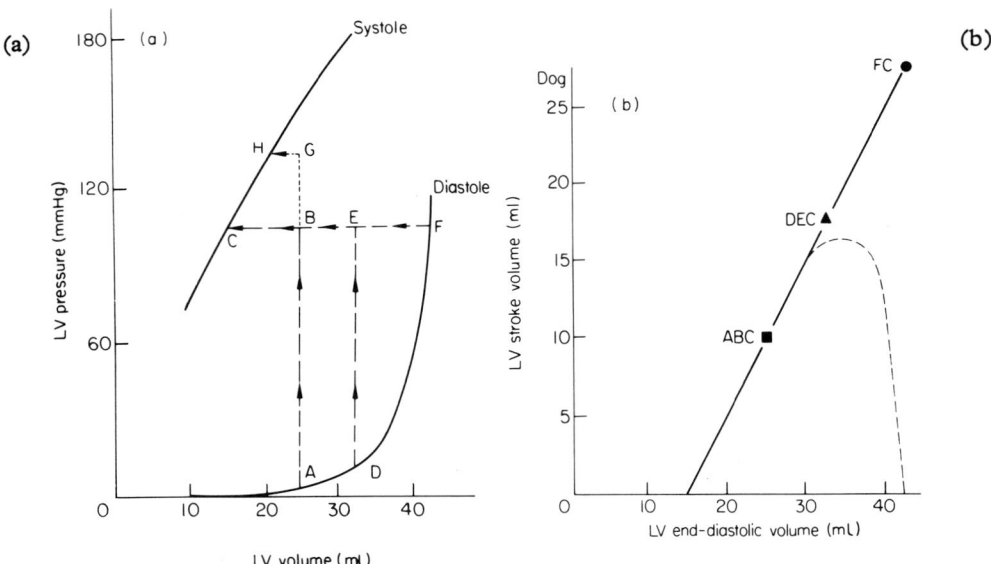

FIG. 5.2.   (a) Left ventricular (LV) pressure-volume curve of the dog. Upper continuous line: isovolumetric systolic pressure developed from corresponding volumes. Lower continuous line: diastolic pressure arising from increasing volume. Data from Fig. 5.1d with extrapolation of diastolic curve at upper end. Dashed lines indicate course of ejecting beats at a systolic pressure of 100 mm Hg (hypothetical in the case of contraction *FC*.) Dotted line indicates course of an ejecting beat at a systolic pressure of 135 mm Hg. The stroke volume of this beat (*GH*) is reduced as pressure increases. From Noble (1978). (b) Stroke volumes achieved at increasing left ventricular (LV) end-diastolic volumes ■ contraction *ABC* in (a), ▲ contraction *DEC* in (a), ● contraction *FC* in (a). Dashed line indicates actual performance in an overdistended ventricle.

116

resting pressure-volume relation, the ventricle contracts isovolumically to point *B* where the preset aortic pressure is reached and ejection begins. The ventricle then empties down to the systolic pressure-volume line at point *C*. The aortic valve then closes and isovolumic relaxation takes place. The stroke volume is *BC*. In Starling curves or 'ventricular function curves' as used by Sarnoff, this or some other variable determined by stroke volume is plotted against end-diastolic volume or pressure (Fig. 5.2b). In the case of cardiac output, stroke volume multiplied by heart rate is used, heart rate being constant; in the case of stroke work, stroke volume multiplied by aortic pressure is used, aortic pressure being constant. When the end diastolic volume is increased, the heart begins to contract from another point *D* on the resting pressure-volume diagram, contracts isovolumetrically to the same aortic pressure at point *E* and then again empties down to point *C*. The stroke volume is now *EC* and gives a point on the rising Starling curve in Fig. 5.2b.

An important point is now apparent. *The Starling curve gives no information whatever about the length-tension curve of the muscle.* It is readily apparent that the same Starling curve will be obtained whether the pressure-volume curve rises steeply or hardly at all, as long as it goes through the point *C*. The muscle length-tension curve can only be obtained from the pressure-volume diagram by making assumptions about geometry (see above). The points on the Starling curve are solely determined by the volume above that at point *C* to which the ventricle is distended in diastole. This is because of the property of the heart of contracting down to the same end-systolic volume for any given systolic pressure.

The Starling curve can be extended to the right as far as the heart can stand being distended without failing. One could imagine an extreme case when the end-diastolic volume was increased to point *F* where the end-diastolic pressure is the same as the aortic pressure. The heart would again eject down to *C* giving a maximum stroke volume of *FC* which is the value at the absolute limit. It is impossible to go any higher than this because when left atrial and left ventricular end-diastolic pressures exceed aortic pressure, both mitral and aortic valves are permanently open and blood pours through the heart in diastole. In fact, it is not possible to go as far as point *F* because there is no pressure gradient for the coronary circulation under these circumstances, the ventricle is ischaemic and fails. Therefore the value for stroke volume of *FC* on the Starling curve is not reached but there is a fall off in cardiac performance to a much lower value as indicated by the dashed line. At high volumes less than *F*, there is subendocardial ischaemia due to the high end-diastolic pressure which becomes progressively more severe. In addition, with increasing dilatation of the ventricle, the mitral valve ring becomes stretched and there is mitral insufficiency. These and other factors induce failure of myocardial contractile performance which is responsible for the experimental result indicated by the dashed line. This is often described as the descending limb of the ventricular function curve which is due to the descending limb of the length-tension curve; this is clearly a misconception.

It must be quite clear from consideration of Fig. 5.2 that *the descending limb of the Starling curve is an artefact* in physiological terms. There is no way that the shortening along the horizontal line in Fig. 5.2a can decrease as one starts from further to the right unless the muscle performance is impaired by some additional factors, i.e. the descending limb is pathological. It is clear that measurement of different shortenings along the horizontal line in Fig. 5.2a to the point C (Starling curve) cannot give information about whether or not there is a descending limb on the pressure-volume diagram (continuous line in Fig. 5.2a) or the muscle length-tension curve on which it depends.

Fig. 5.2a shows that a completely different value for stroke volume (and therefore stroke work, etc) is obtained if the Starling resistor in the aorta is adjusted so that the left ventricle has to achieve a higher pressure before ejection can occur (dotted line BGH, Fig. 5.2a). The stroke volume is now reduced to GH for the same end-diastolic volume that previously produced a stroke volume of BC. Thus we can say that *the Starling curve is critically dependent on aortic pressure.*

The Starling curve therefore has a number of limitations compared with the Frank curve. However, the Frank curve does not give information about pump output. How then should the Frank-Starling mechanism be characterised?

The Frank-Starling mechanism and the pump function curve

In Chapter 4, I advocated the use of a plot of mean ventricular pressure against mean outflow as the best method of describing pumping function. This specifies the mean output at any mean level of pressure and vice versa. It is independent of the nature of the aortic input impedance and this makes it unnecessary to use a Starling resistor in the aorta. Thus more physiological preparations can be used.

The isolated ejecting cat heart preparation of Elzinga (see Chapter 4) is the method of choice for clearly defining the pump function curve under different circumstances. This is because the end-diastolic volume can be held constant while the load is changed in order to delineate the curve.

In Fig. 5.3 are shown two pump function curves at two different end-diastolic volumes. At the higher end-diastolic volume there is a higher output at any given pressure and a higher pressure at any given outflow. The entire pump function curve is shifted outwards indicating (1) an increase in total pump function and (2) an increase in the force-velocity curve of the myocardium (an increase in its mechanical performance). This method demonstrates both the Frank and the Starling aspects of increased heart size. The increase in the pressure intercept is due to the increase in isovolumic pressure (no output) observed by Frank. The increase in the outflow at any given pressure, such as that indicated by the dashed line, is due to the fact that under these circumstances the ventricle contracts down to the same end-systolic volume from a larger end-diastolic volume; this is the mechanism of the ascending part of Starling's curve.

It is clear that the increase in isovolumetric pressure with increasing volume (Fig. 5.2a) is unrelated to the increase in stroke volume (Fig. 5.2b). This is also shown in Fig. 5.3. The mean pressure is related to the peak pressure used in Fig. 5.2a while mean outflow is the stroke volume (Fig. 5.2b) divided by the interval between beats (constant). In order to superimpose the two pump function curves shown in Fig. 5.3a one requires different factors to multiply values along the pressure axis and to multiply values along the flow axis. (Fig. 5.3b). The pressure factor is determined by the slope of the Frank curve (Fig. 5.2a). The flow factor is determined by the slope of the Starling curve (Fig. 5.2b) which is in turn determined by how much the end-diastolic volume was increased as a fraction of the original stroke volume.

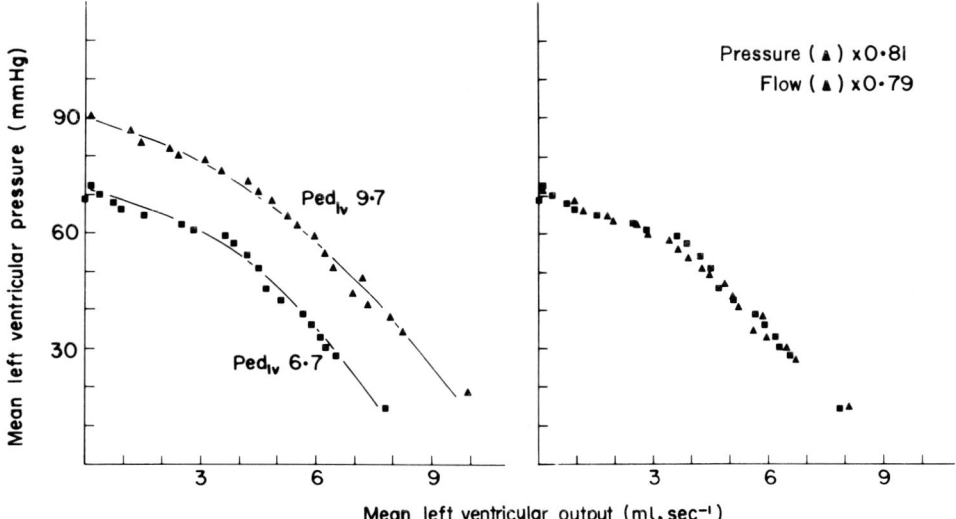

FIG. 5.3.   Relationship between mean left ventricular pressure (P_{lv}) and mean left ventricular output in isolated ejecting cat heart at left ventricular end-diastolic pressures (Ped_{lv}) of 6·7 and 9·7 mm Hg. In the right hand panel the LV pressure values for end-diastolic pressure of 9·7 have been multiplied by 0·81 and the LV output values by 0·79 producing superimposition with the data for an end-diastolic pressure of 6·7 mm Hg. From Elzinga and Westerhof (1977).

The Frank-Starling mechanism and the Weber-Janicki-Hefner curve

The most valuable alternative to the mean pressure-mean outflow curve for characterising the performance of the left ventricular pump is the relationship between stroke volume and pressure resisting ejection advocated by Hefner's group. Changes in stroke volume and mean outflow are the same for a fixed heart rate while mean left ventricular pressure and left ventricular pressure during ejection change together as long as the latter remains reasonably constant as in the experiments of Weber *et al.* Thus both the pump function curve and the Weber-Janicki-Hefner curve (Fig. 5.4) give essentially the same sort of information. In Fig. 5.4a the relationship is plotted in the same way as Weber *et al.* In Fig. 5.4b, I have plotted the same data on reversed axes to show the familiar inverse relation between pressure and outflow that was found in the pump function curve (Fig. 5.3). In Fig. 5.4c I have plotted the same data

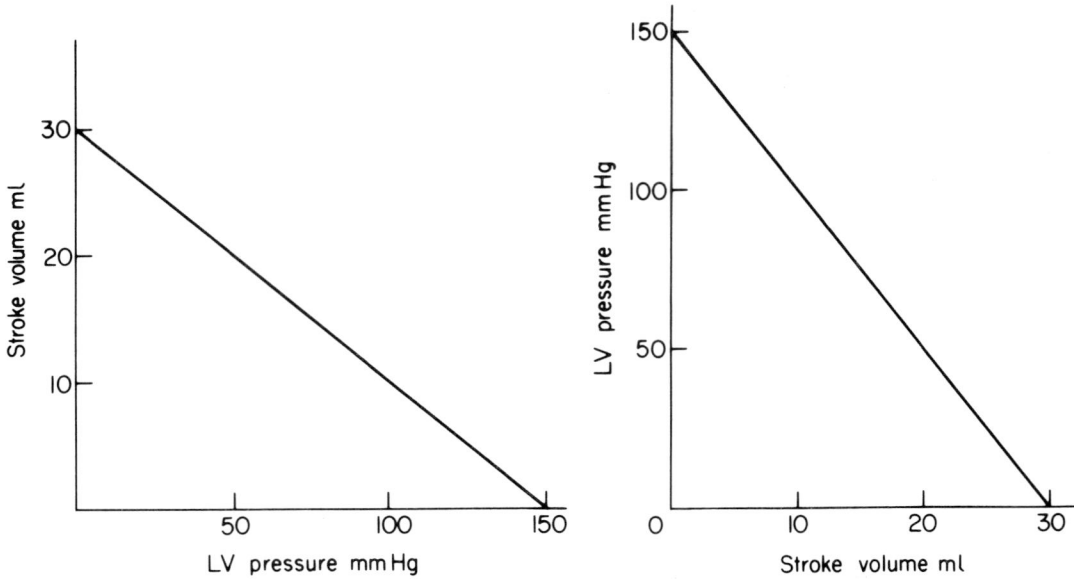

FIG. 5.4. (a) Relationship between stroke volume and left ventricular (LV) systolic pressure at constant LV end-diastolic volume. After Weber, Janicki and Hefner (1976). (b) Data from (a) plotted as pressure-output curve. Compare with Fig. 5.3.

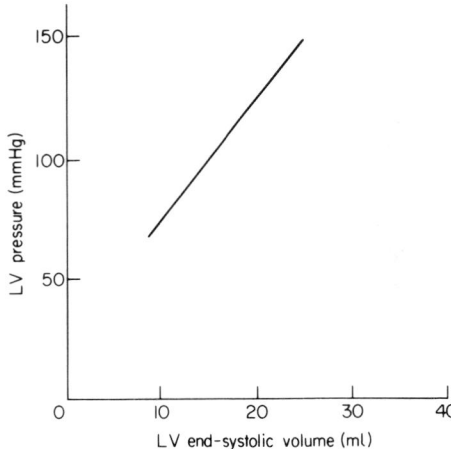

FIG. 5.4c. Relationship between LV pressure and end-systolic volume obtained by subtracting stroke volume values in (b) from constant end-diastolic volume.

but now with end-systolic volume on the abscissa obtained by subtracting the stroke volumes (Fig. 5.4b) from the end-diastolic volume given by the authors. It has been shown by these authors and by Suga and Sagawa that the end-systolic volume for a given left ventricular pressure is the same volume from which that pressure is generated in an isovolumetric beat. Therefore the plot in Fig. 5.4c is identical to the Frank curve (Fig. 5.2a). Thus with knowledge of the end-diastolic volume, *the Weber-Janicki-Hefner curve is easily transformed into the Frank curve.*

The effect of an increase in end-diastolic volume on the Weber-Janicki-Hefner curve is shown in Fig. 5.5a; this is very similar, as expected, to the effect on the pump function curve (Fig. 5.3). The same data in the transformed plot is shown in Fig. 5.5b. Here we see that the different lines for different end-diastolic volumes in Fig. 5.5a become the same line in Fig. 5.5b, the effect of increasing volume being merely to extend the explored range of the Frank curve further to the right. The heart ejects more blood in contracting down to the same end-systolic volume from a larger end-diastolic volume. In the experiments of Weber *et al.* the end-diastolic volume was controlled in an isolated dog heart preparation. However, as long as a continuous

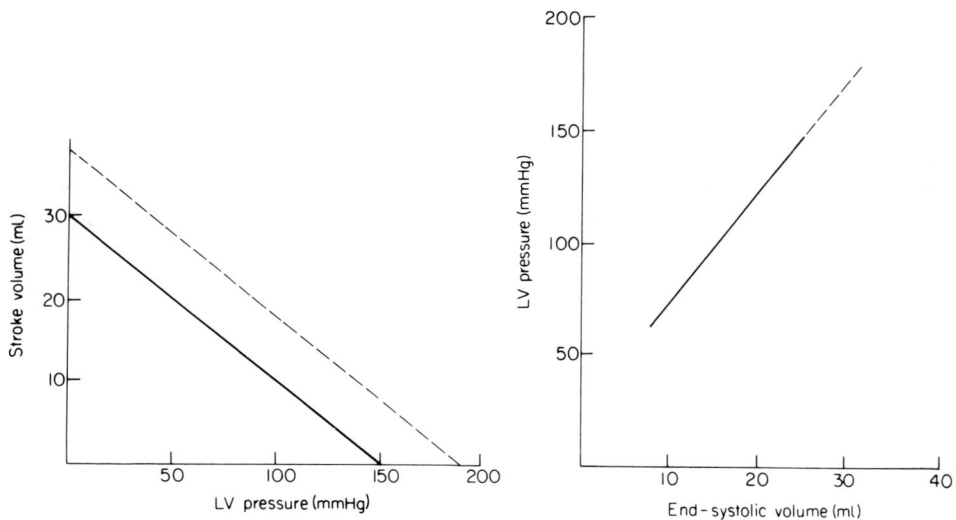

FIG. 5.5. (a) Data from Fig. 5.4a plus the effect of increased end-diastolic volume (dashed line). (b). Data from (a) plotted against end-systolic volume. Compare with Fig. 5.4c.

registration of heart size is made, e.g. left ventricular diameter from a sonomicrometer, the transformed Weber-Janicki-Hefner curve (Frank curve) can be delineated without controlling end-diastolic volume in an intact animal.

Having obtained this data, one can convert it into the length-tension curve of the left ventricular myocardium. Hefner's equation can be used to convert pressure to wall force if one knows the internal radius of the cavity. Volume can be converted to length if one assumes some shape. Weber, Janicki and Hefner did this by assuming a spherical shape so that length was proportional to the cube root of volume. Their results, with length normalised for length at zero filling pressure (L_0) and wall force normalised for the cross-sectional area of muscle in the wall, are shown in Fig. 5.6. Clearly, *there is an ascending force-length relationship over the entire range of heart size that can be explored in the intact heart.*

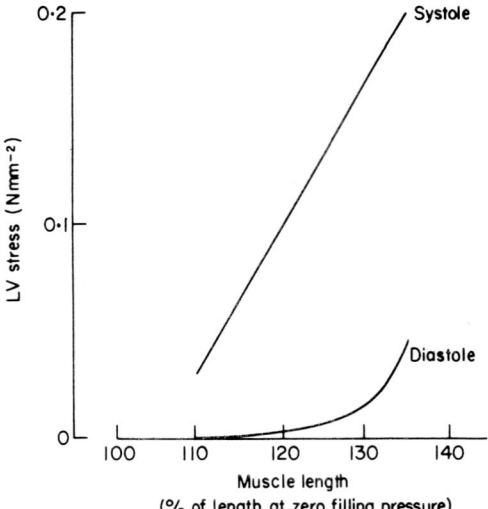

F<small>IG</small>. 5.6.   Relationship between force and length of fibres in the wall of the dog left
ventricle (LV). Data from Weber, Janicki and Hefner (1976). Muscle length is given as
percentage of the unstretched length with no resting diastolic force. Force is normalised by
dividing by the cross-sectional area of muscle; the ratio is stress. From Noble (1978).

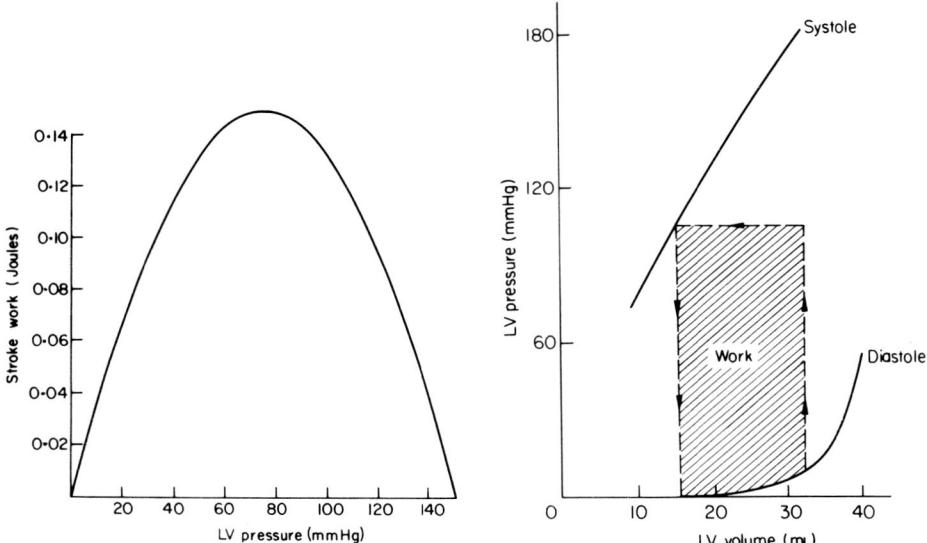

F<small>IG</small>. 5.7.   (a) Relationship between stroke work and left ventricular pressure. Calculated from
Fig. 5.4a. (b) Pressure-volume diagram from Fig. 5.1d. Stroke work is the cross-hatched area
within the course of an ejecting beat indicated by the dashed line.

Work and the Frank-Starling mechanism

The stroke work during these experiments has sometimes been used as an index to plot against end-diastolic volume or end-diastolic pressure following the example of Sarnoff. Stroke work is obtained from the Weber-Janicki-Hefner curve by multiplying each value of pressure by the corresponding value of stroke volume. This is shown in Fig. 5.7a for the data shown in Fig. 5.4a. Stroke work is also mean power (Fig. 4.6) divided by heart rate. Thus, different stroke work/pressure curves are obtained for different settings of arterial compliance as in Fig. 4.7b (mean left ventricular pressure, Fig. 4.7c, cannot be used to calculate work and power output). The use of such a derived variable as stroke work obscures the fundamental underlying relationship between pressure and flow.

In the type of experiment performed by Weber, Janicki and Hefner and Suga and Sagawa, stroke work is given by the area within the pressure-volume loop (Fig. 5.7b). These loops can extend anywhere within the end-diastolic and end-systolic boundary lines of the Frank diagram. There is no consistent relationship between stroke work and end-diastolic volume. I recommend that the use of work be abandoned in favour of its underlying determinants.

Indices of peak velocity of shortening and the Frank-Starling mechanism

The maximum rate of rise of left ventricular pressure (dP/dt max) was shown in Chapter 4 to be approximately governed by the equation:

$$dP/dt = \frac{dF/dt}{a}$$

where dF/dt is the rate of rise of force in the ventricular wall and a is the cross-sectional area of the cavity. If end-diastolic volume is increased, dF/dt rises as a result of the length-tension relationship (Fig. 5.1b). However, the cross-sectional area of the cavity is increased—that is the intervention. Clearly then the resulting ratio, $(dF/dt)/a$ (i.e. dP/dt) may rise, may fall or may not change. The only general statement one can make is that dP/dt max is far less sensitive to change in heart size than dF/dt.

A record of left ventricular pressure and its rate of change is shown in Fig. 5.8. In this case (an intact dog), there is no effect of change in heart size on dP/dt max. However, this is not always the case as one might expect from the equation. If by good luck one has a situation as in Fig. 5.8, dP/dt max can be used for detecting changes in dF/dt due to other causes without the need for careful control of end-diastolic volume. Such causes are the positive and negative inotropic effects (see below).

Similar considerations apply to the maximum accleration of blood from the left ventricle. Acceleration (A) is related to an accelerating force (f) by the equation:

$$f = mA$$

where m = the mass of blood. The fraction of ventricular force dissipated in acceleration is negligibly small compared to that required to generate pressure but it presumably changes in proportion to the total when end-diastolic volume is increased.
However such an increase in heart size involves a greater mass of blood to be accelerated, i.e. the volume increment is added. Thus the ratio f/m which determines the
acceleration may increase, may decrease or may stay the same. The last result is also
illustrated in Fig. 5.8.

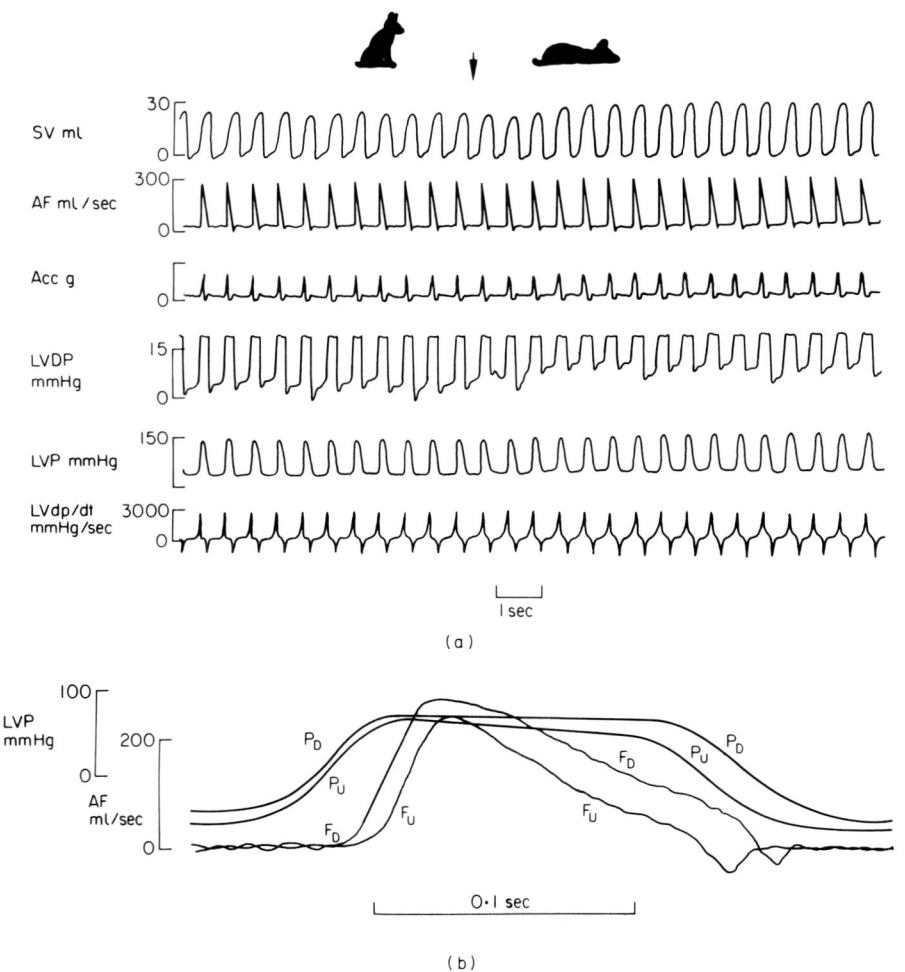

FIG. 5.8. Effect of a change in posture from vertical to horizontal in a dog with denervated
heart (eliminating reflex effects). This intervention is used to produce an increase in
end-diastolic volume and study its effects. (a) Multichannel pen recorder trace showing stroke
volume per beat (SV), aortic flow (AF), acceleration of blood from the left ventricle (Acc),
left ventricular (LV) diastolic pressure (LVDP), LV pressure (LVP) and rate of change of
LV pressure (LV dp/dt). (b) Fast records taken from oscilloscope screen of LVP and AF.
Pu = LVP in vertical posture, P_D = LVP in horizontal posture. Fu = AF in vertical posture,
F_D = AF in horizontal posture. Note increase in LVED and SV at constant heart rate
without change in LV dp/dt max. From Noble *et al.* (1972).

When dP/dt max and maximum acceleration are used as inotropic indices one has to remember that they can also be affected by aortic pressure. When aortic pressure falls to the level where the aortic valve opens before the time when left ventricular pressure would otherwise have reached its maximum, the recorded dP/dt max falls. If aortic pressure is raised, maximum acceleration will fall until one achieves an isovolumic beat (when acceleration and outflow are zero).

The cellular mechanism of the Frank-Starling phenomenon

The relationship between isovolumetric pressure development (Frank) is closely related through geometric factors to the length-tension relation of the myocardium. Much attention has therefore been paid to the mechanism by which increases in muscle length produce increased contractile performance.

A basic piece of information required for the understanding of this is the relationship between contractile force and sarcomere length. Good data on this point is only just beginning to be available because the papillary muscles which were previously used for these studies were too thick to enable sarcomere length measurements to be made. Now, ever thinner preparations are being used giving clearer optical measurements of sarcomere length in the contracting muscle.

Jewell has reviewed this subject and compared studies of Pollack in rat and Julian in rabbit muscle. The former obtained a linear increase in tension with sarcomere length from zero tension at $1\cdot6$ μm to maximum tension at $2\cdot2$ μm, with the maximum value maintained from $2\cdot2$ μm to $2\cdot3$ μm. Julian obtained a linear increase in tension from about 30% maximum tension at $2\cdot0$ μm to maximum tension at nearly $2\cdot4$ μm; there was no plateau in the curve. The difference between the two studies could lie in difference in method, species, inotropic state or temperature. Both used hypothermic muscles superfused with physiological solution in the usual manner so that the length-tension curves are unlikely to apply precisely to the intact heart. This is also true of the more recent study of ter Keurs (Fig. 5.9) using a thinner preparation.

An important conclusion to be drawn from these studies is that over the range of sarcomere length $1\cdot95$ μm to $2\cdot1$ μm where the number of cross-bridges in apposition is constant, there is still an 'ascending limb' or positive length-tension curve. There is no 'descending limb' above $2\cdot1$ μm sarcomere length. There is no correlation between force and cross-bridge number.

Jewell marshalls evidence gleaned from various studies of both skeletal and cardiac muscle to strongly suggest that at shorter sarcomere lengths, muscle is not completely activated by calcium. Since the activation system is dependent on depolarisation of the sarcolemma, the problem of incomplete activation can be overcome by removing it. A crucial piece of evidence in cardiac muscle therefore comes from studies of such 'skinned' preparations by Fabiato. These show that the relationship between tension and sarcomere length is very flat. The tension at $1\cdot6$ μm is still about 85% of the maximum at $2\cdot1$ μm. At sarcomere lengths below $1\cdot6$ μm (the length of the thick filaments) the thick filaments must be compressed but the tension still only falls to about 65% of maximum when one goes down to $1\cdot2$ μm sarcomere length.

This rather flat relationship between tension and sarcomere length therefore represents the effect in the fully activated tissue of the impediment to tension development of double overlap of thin filaments below 1·95 μm and of the compression of the A band below 1·6 μm (Fig. 5.9). Thus *the major part of the decrease in tension with shorter sarcomeres seems to be due to incomplete activation.* This is consistent with direct evidence obtained in skeletal muscle fibres by Taylor showing that calcium release is a function of initial sarcomere length.

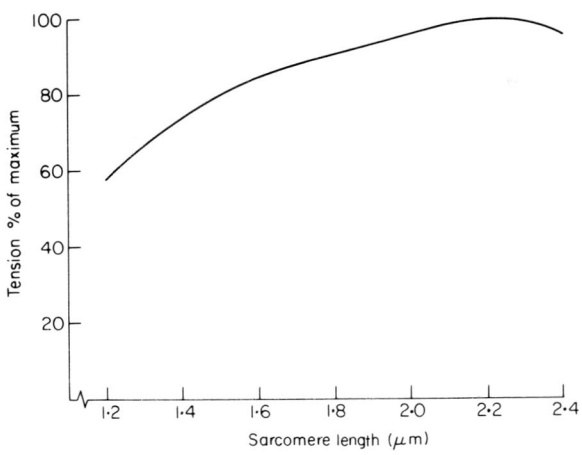

FIG. 5.9. Tension as a function of sarcomere length in 'skinned' cardiac cells. Data replotted from Fabiato A. & Fabiato F. (1975) *Nature,* **256,** 54.

If the decrease in tension with shorter sarcomeres is due to incomplete activation by calcium, it follows that:
(1) There is no fundamental difference between the final mechanism of control at contractile protein level for the Frank-Starling mechanism and for inotropic phenomena.
(2) No index of contraction can be unique for inotropic phenomena (changes in contractility) excluding any possible length dependent effect.
(3) The decreased tension at short lengths will be counteracted by adding an inotropic influence of which the simplest is an increase in calcium ion concentration.

Confirmation of the latter was obtained by Jewell's group who showed that increase in tension with increasing fibre length was different proportionately when the Ca^{++} concentration in the bathing medium was increased. This is confirmed at sarcomere level by ter Keurs (Fig. 5.10) who finds that the effect of Ca^{++} is greater at short than at long sarcomere length.

It is possible that other mechanisms play a role in producing the length-tension curve. These factors and the evidence concerning them are discussed by Jewell. I think that the evidence at the moment is overwhelmingly in favour of his conclusions:
(1) That the ascending limb of the length-tension curve in isolated papillary muscle is almost entirely due to length dependence of activation.

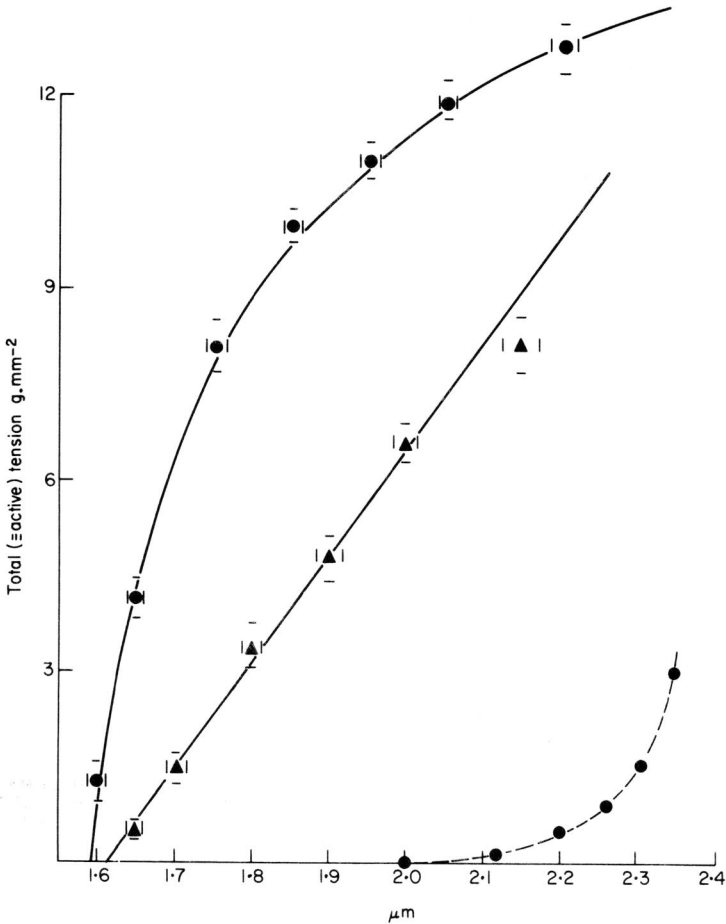

FIG. 5.10. Sarcomere length-tension curve measured in trabeculae from the right ventricle of the rat. Sarcomere length was measured at peak twitch tension by laser diffraction in both muscle isometric and sarcomere isometric conditions. Resting tension (dashed line) is negligible up to sarcomere lengths of 2·1 μm, i.e. total tension is equivalent to active tension. Ca^{++} concentration in the bathing fluid, ▲ = 0·5 mM, ● = 2·5 mM. |•| = s.e.m. Mean results from 14 trabeculae at 25°C. Data kindly provided by Henk ter Keurs.

(2) Since inotropic influences also affect the degree of activation, length and ino-tropism cannot be regarded as independent regulators of cardiac contractile per-formance.

The concept of contractility

Until recently it was always thought that there was some fundamental difference between the influence of length on contraction (Frank-Starling) and changes in contraction at constant length. In view of the considerations above, this idea is no longer tenable. The constancy of length must always be specified when discussing changes in contractility. The property of myocardium which enables it to change contractility at a constant length is important because the whole of the muscle is active all the time. There are no quiescent units which can be recruited as reinforcements as is the case with skeletal muscle.

Before leaving the subject of the Frank-Starling mechanism and going on to examine the factors influencing contractility, it is worth pondering the consequences to the circulation were the Frank-Starling mechanism not to exist.

The physiological importance of the Frank-Starling mechanism

An 'ascending limb' type of length-tension curve renders the muscle stable. If some sarcomeres are stronger than others, they shorten down and stretch the weaker sarcomeres. At the shorter sarcomere length they become weaker according to the length-tension curve. The stretched sarcomeres become stronger. Therefore there is a tendency for sarcomeres always to return towards the average length. If it were not for the length-tension relation, great dispersion of sarcomere length would occur and the myocardium would become more non-homogeneous and unstable.

Similar considerations apply in the intact heart where the important feature is the Starling curve. As we have seen, the ability of the heart to always contract down to the same end-systolic pressure ensures an 'ascending limb' for the stroke volume/end-diastolic volume relationship. If the heart could not do this it would progressively dilate and fail. This is precisely what happens on the 'descending limb' which as I have described above, is always pathological. An increase in end-diastolic volume here leads to a decrease in stroke volume, increase in end-systolic volume and with continued filling at the same rate, further increase in end-diastolic volume and decrease in stroke volume.

Heterometric autoregulation and homeometric autoregulation

Sarnoff introduced this nomenclature. Heterometric autoregulation refers to control of contractile performance by changes in fibre length—in other words the Frank-Starling mechanism. Homeometric autoregulation therefore refers to mechanisms of control at a constant initial length of the myocardial fibres but still intrinsic to them, i.e. not externally imposed inotropic influences like sympathetic stimulation or adrenaline.

One of the mechanisms which Sarnoff included under this heading is the effect of changing heart rate, i.e. the Bowditch effect, the force-frequency relationship (Chapter 2). However the unique nature of this control and the complexities of separating steady state and optimal contractile responses were not realised. These considerations make it essential to treat this mechanism separately as I have done in Chapter 2. In line with most workers, I do not include it under homeometric autoregulation. The other mechanism discussed by Sarnoff was the Anrep effect. However this is also much less straightforward than was thought and is discussed under the heading 'load dependent changes in myocardial performance' below.

Load dependent changes in myocardial contractile performance

The pump function curves and force-velocity curves (Chapter 4) require for their delineation that shortening against a number of different loads be studied. If the change in load affects the contractile state of the muscle, these relationships will be distorted and will not describe one contractile state. However there are well described effects on the contractile state produced by changes in load. In some circumstances an

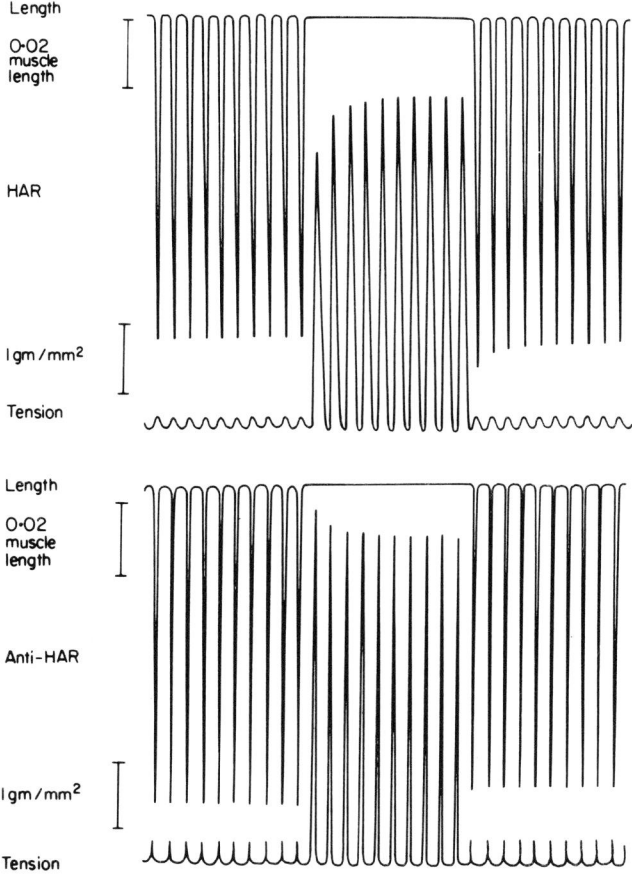

FIG. 5.11a. Dog papillary muscle contracting isotonically with downward deflections of the length record indicating shortening. After 10 isotonic contractions during which muscle reaches a steady state, muscle is held isometric for 10 contractions and then isotonic again for 10 contractions. Top panel shows a positive inotropic response to the increased load (homeometric autoregulation, HAR). Bottom panel shows negative inotropic response (anti HAR). From Donald *et al.* (1976).

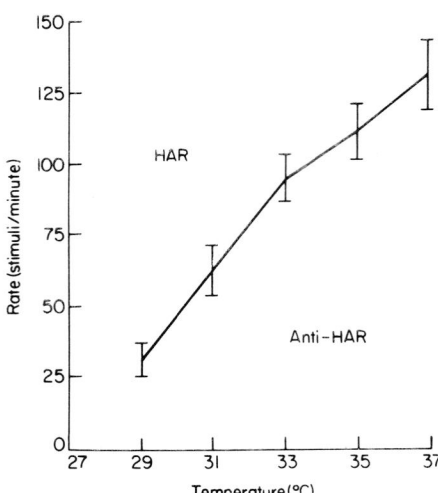

FIG. 5.11b. Locus of iso-HAR points in rate-temperature plane. At rates and temperatures. to the left and above the line, HAR is obtained. Below and to the right anti HAR is found. From Donald *et al.* (1976).

increase in load causes a decrease in contractility while in other circumstances it produces an increase in contractility. Since the latter effect was included in Sarnoff's homeometric autoregulation, it is sometimes given this name (HAR for short). Sometimes it is called the Anrep effect after its discoverer. The opposite effect is called anti-HAR by Hefner's group. It should perhaps be called after Parmley, Brutsaert and Sonnenblick who first described it.

The two effects were shown in the same preparation (dog papillary muscle) by Donald and his colleagues (Fig. 5.11a). At any given temperature, there is a stimulation rate at which no effect is seen (Fig. 5.11b). Above this rate HAR is found; below it anti-HAR occurs. At the temperature and heart rate of the intact dog one would not expect much effect—if anything one should obtain anti-HAR and not obtain an Anrep effect.

This is not an easy phenomenon to study in an intact animal because (1) raising aortic pressure stimulates baroreflexes which affect contractility, (2) indices of contraction during ejection are decreased by an increase in pressure because of the pump function relation. One can overcome these problems by using dogs with denervated hearts and following an index of isovolumic contraction—dP/dt max (Chapter 4). Under these circumstances there is either no effect (Fig. 5.12a) or a slight negative (anti-HAR) response. The phenomenon can be studied in the same way in the cat heart preparation of Elzinga. In this case there is no effect (Fig. 5.12b). Other species have not been studied.

The reader is warned that in many studies in which an Anrep effect is described, the preparations undergo changes in the coronary circulation when aortic pressure is raised. An increase in contractility secondary to increased oxygen supply due to improved myocardial perfusion is not homeometric autoregulation as obtained in

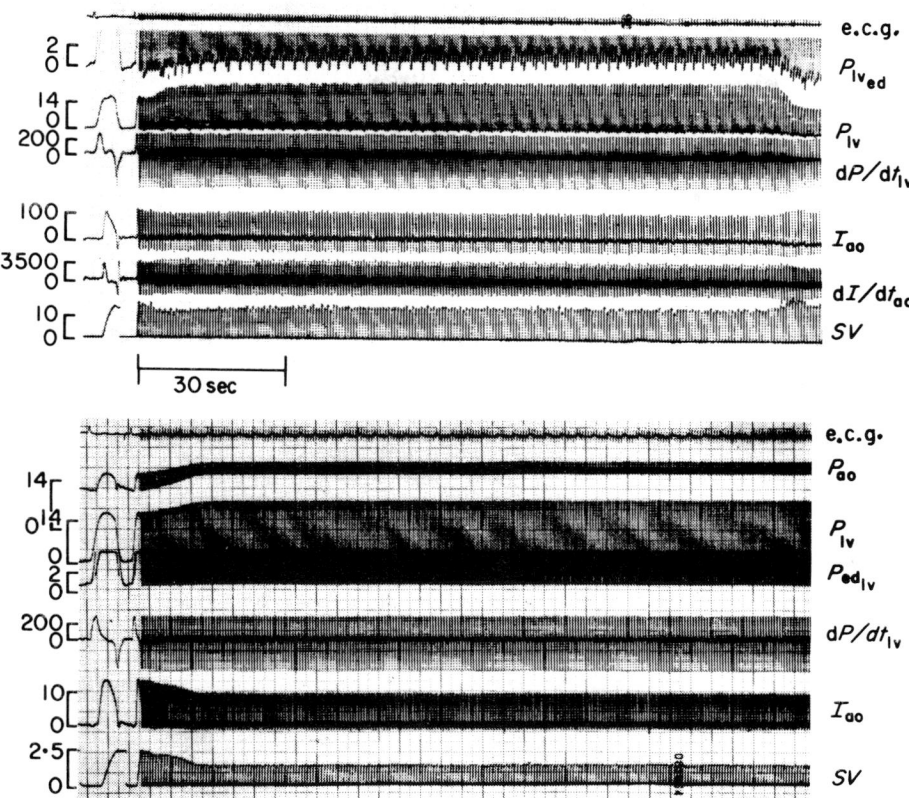

FIG. 5.12. (a) Haemodynamic effects of an occlusion of the thoracic part of the descending aorta in a dog with denervated heart (to remove reflex effects). (b) Haemodynamic effects of an increase in 'peripheral resistance' in the isolated cat heart preparation. P_{lv} = left ventricular (lv) pressure, Ped_{lv} = left ventricular diastolic pressure, dP/dt_{lv} rate of change of P_{lv}. I_{ao} = lv outflow, dI/dt_{ao} = acceleration of blood from the lv. SV = stroke volume. From Elzinga, Noble and Stubbs (1977).

isolated superfused tissue (Fig. 5.11). However it may well be what Anrep and Sarnoff were looking at. It would appear to me to be more important in pathological than in physiological circumstances.

It would appear from the kind of results shown in Fig. 5.11 and 5.12 that homeometric autoregulation has very little effect in physiological circumstances. This is important because of the reliance placed on the pump function and force-velocity curves as basic approaches to the characterisation of contractile performance.

The effect of inotropic influences (altered contractility) on contractile performance

We have already seen that positive inotropic influences like increased Ca^{++} produce an increase in isometric tension development. Therefore they produce similar increases in isovolumic pressure development in the intact heart. One would expect a similar parallel between the increased muscle shortening and increased stroke volume. However, when aortic pressure is normal, no such increase in stroke volume occurs (Fig. 5.13).

It is a common misconception that positive inotropic influences can be studied by giving an intravenous dose of a drug like adrenaline. This is not the case. There are often changes in heart rate which make interpretations very difficult (see Chapter 6). More important, there are large effects on peripheral vessels which have a profound effect on stroke volume through changes in filling and aortic input impedance. In the experiment shown in Fig. 5.13, the intervention was confined to the heart only by close arterial injection of Ca^{++} into the myocardium (through a coronary artery) in a dose insufficient for general effect. Under these circumstances, the indices of speed

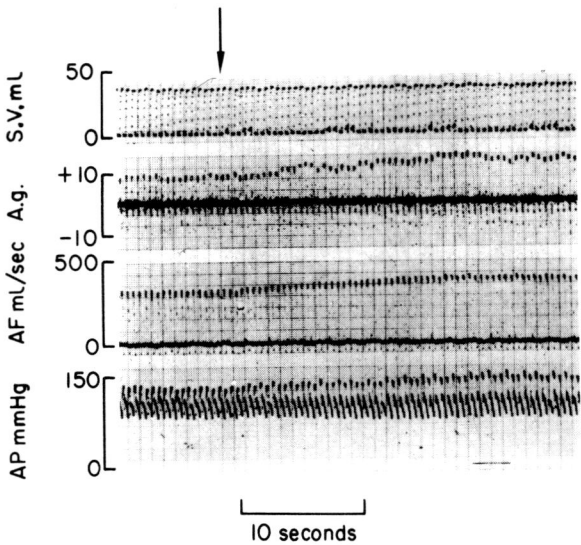

FIG. 5.13. Effect of an injection of 7·5 mg calcium gluconate (arrow) into the anterior descending branch of the left coronary artery. Stroke volume (SV), acceleration (A), aortic flow (AF) and aortic pressure (AP) are shown. From Noble, Trenchard and Guz (1966).

of onset of contraction, maximum acceleration (also dP/dt max not shown), increase greatly but stroke volume is constant.

The reason for this is not clear. It is not due to a simultaneous decrease in end-diastolic volume because the same result is obtained with another positive inotropic intervention, post-extrasystolic potentiation, where the change in contractility occurs between one beat and the next (Fig. 5.14). It is not due to reflex interaction because the same result is obtained with the denervated heart. It appears that there is a limit below which end-systolic volume cannot go unless the pressure against which the ventricle ejects is lowered. Thus when we look at the pump function curves (Fig. 5.15) for normal and increased contractility there is an upward shift which is marked only at the high pressure end of the curve. The heart can generate a considerably higher

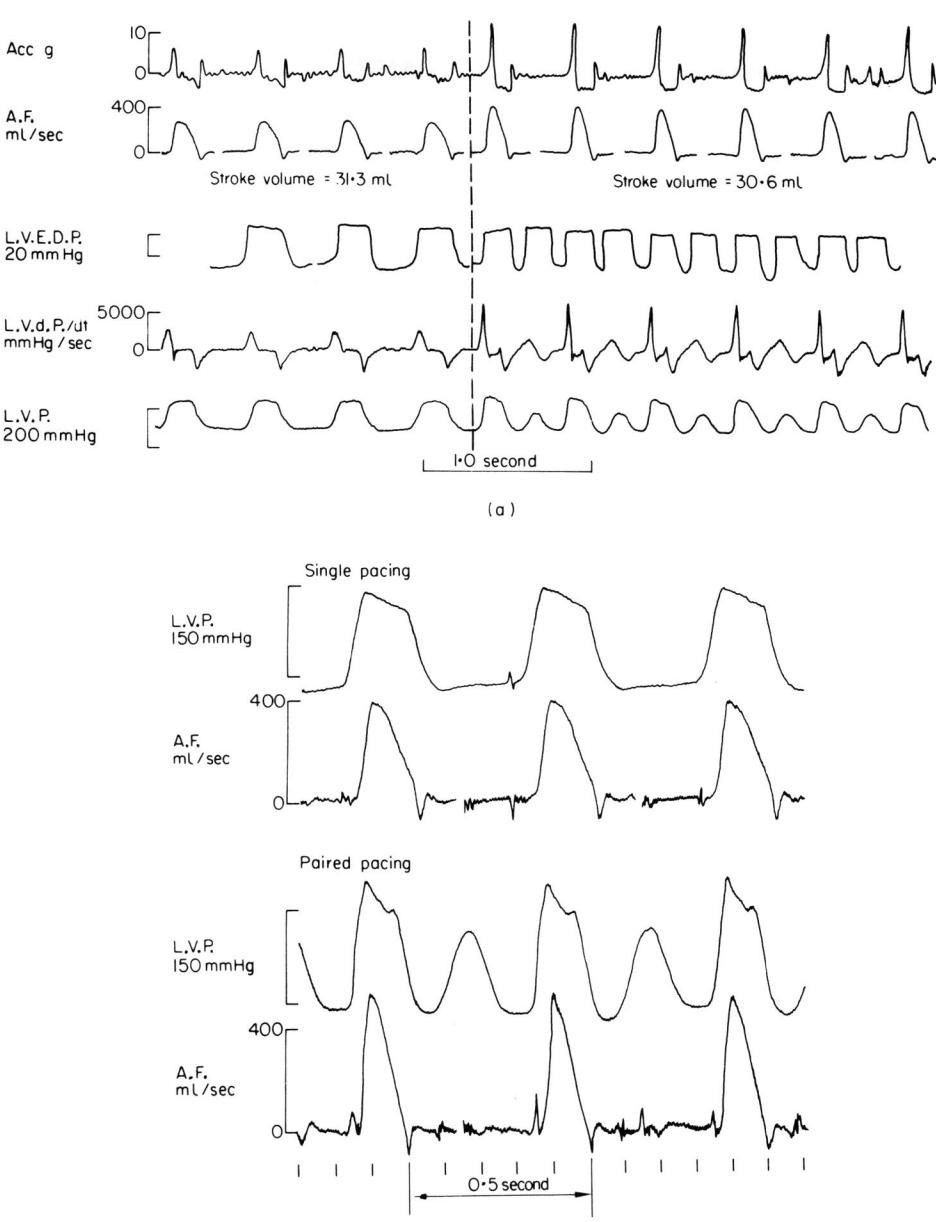

FIG. 5.14. Effect of paired pulse stimulation of the right atrium in a dog with chronic cardiac denervation. (a) Left: single pulse stimulation. Right: paired pulse stimulation at the same basic heart rate but with extrasystoles between each ejecting beat. LVEDP of the ejecting beats is the same. (b) LV pressure and aortic flow (AF) during the same experiment recorded on a high frequency response photographic recorder. From Noble *et al.* (1972).

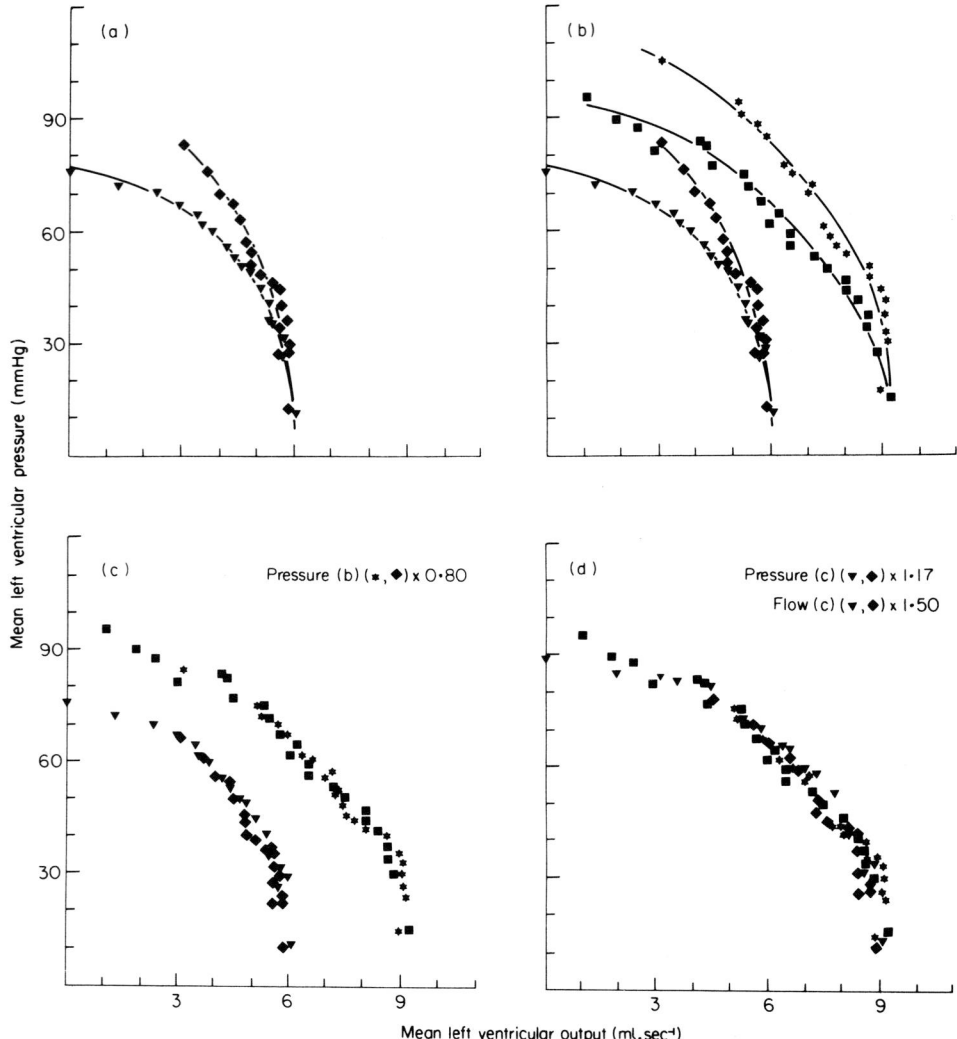

FIG. 5.15. Effect of an increase in contractility on the pump function curve of isolated ejecting cat heart.

(a) ▼ control, ◆ increased contractility by paired pulse stimulation (sustained post-extrasystolic potentiation).

(b)   Data from a run at increased end-diastolic volume (EDV) is added. ▼, ◆ as in (a), ■ control at increased EDV, ★ increased contractility at increased EDV.

(c) At each level of EDV, data superimposes by using a scaling factor (0·80) for the mean left ventricular values only.

(d) Data in (c) superimposes if both mean left ventricular pressure and mean output are multiplied by scaling factors (1·17 for pressure, 1·50 for flow). Compare (c) and (d) with Fig. 5.3. Data from Elzinga G. & Westerhof N. (1979) *Circulation Res.*, **44**, 303.

isovolumic pressure, and increased flow against high pressure. However at normal and low left ventricular pressure, there is only a small increase in mean pressure (see areas under the left ventricular pressure traces in Fig. 5.14) at the same flow.

This result is only obtained if the left ventricle is normal in the control situation. This is often not the case with other preparations. Depression of the heart by anaesthesia, hypercapnia, hypoxia etc results in depression of stroke volume and the entire pump function curve. When positive inotropic interventions are then made, stroke volume and the pump function curve are restored toward normal. This is consistent with the fact that the most commonly used positive inotropic drug—digitalis—is ineffective in producing increased stroke volume and cardiac output in normals; increased flow only follows its use in the depressed, failing heart.

Under physiological circumstances, the contractility of the heart is increased by activation of the sympathetic nervous system leading to release of noradrenaline

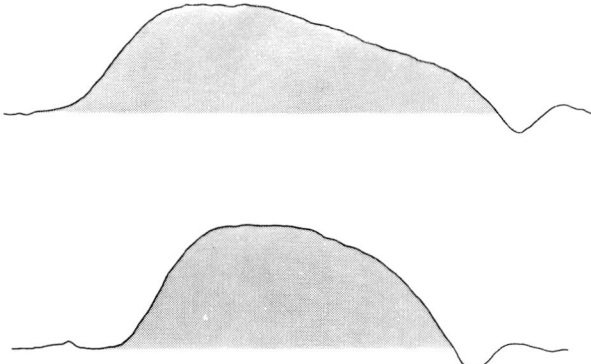

FIG. 5.16.   Left ventricular outflow recorded in the control state (above) and after intracoronary injection of isoprenaline (below). Note shortening of ejection time and decrease in stroke volume (area under the curve, shaded) in spite of greater acceleration and peak outflow.

from nerve terminals in the ventricle, and release of adrenaline into the circulation. These agents, as well as increasing contractility (presumed to be due to increased intracellular Ca^{++}) also lead to an abbreviation of the duration of contraction. This is thought to be due to an acceleration of calcium uptake by the sarcoplasmic reticulum. As a result of this shortening of systole stroke volume falls a little when the drug is confined to the heart (Fig. 5.16) but under the physiological circumstances of general release there is an increase in heart rate due to the effect on the sinus node (Chapter 1). The accelerated relaxation therefore allows greater filling during the abbreviated diastole. This combination, along with changes in the peripheral circulation, result in the increased cardiac output of the adrenergic response.

There are a number of drugs with effects on the contractile state of the myocardium with or without effects on the membrane, action potential, sarcoplasmic reticulum and metabolism. There are also the 'blockers'. This proliferation of drugs makes it necessary to treat cardiac pharmacology as a separate subject which cannot be covered in this text. Similar considerations apply to the more physiologically important subjects of the effects on the heart of ions and hormones.

There is controversy about the question of whether negative inotropic responses mediated by the parasympathetic efferents play a role in physiological responses. Strong electrical stimulation of the vagus nerves is required to show the decrease in contractility of the ventricles; this effect appears to be very small compared with the negative chronotropic effect (slowing of sinus node, bradycardia) and decreased contractility of the atria.

It is doubtful whether the negative inotropic effect of hypercapnia can be considered physiological since the arterial P_{CO_2} is normally controlled within narrow limits. This effect is counteracted by an adrenergic reaction to the hypercapnia which restores the pump function curve and indices of speed of contraction to normal when the high P_{CO_2} is maintained.

Assessment of left ventricular function in patients with heart disease

It is very difficult to attempt to apply any of the approaches described here in the presence of an abnormality of the aortic valve, mitral incompetence or a congenital abnormality involving the left ventricle. Having excluded these conditions, one may then be able to make some progress, e.g. in a case of ischaemic heart disease. Myocardial ischaemia depresses the pump function curve but it is impracticable to measure this in a patient; one cannot change left ventricular pressure over a wide range and one cannot control end-diastolic volume.

The Frank curve is replotted in Fig. 5.17 together with the effect of myocardial disease. In the normal case at normal aortic pressure, the heart contracts isovolumically from A to B and then ejects stroke volume BC. In the diseased case the heart no longer contracts down to the same end-systolic volume. The same stroke volume may be achieved by compensatory dilatation so that now the heart contracts from D to E to F. However, the ratio of stroke volume to end-diastolic volume EF/EX is less than the control value BC/BX. This is called the ejection fraction. It has proved the most useful clinical index of poor left ventricular contraction.

Until recently, the measurement of ejection fraction required cardiac catheterisation, the injection of radiopaque contrast medium into the left ventricle and dynamic radiographic recording of the opacified image in two planes at right angles to one another. The end-diastolic and end-systolic images are selected and the volumes calculated by using some sort of model approximation. Ejection fraction can now be measured without such assumptions or the need for a cardiac catheter by injecting a radioactive indicator intravenously and counting over the precordium with a gamma camera. An alternative approach is to look at left ventricular outflow with a catheter tip velocity probe in the ascending aorta. Peak velocity and acceleration correlate quite well with ejection fraction whereas the correlation between dP/dt max and ejection fraction in these patients is rather poor.

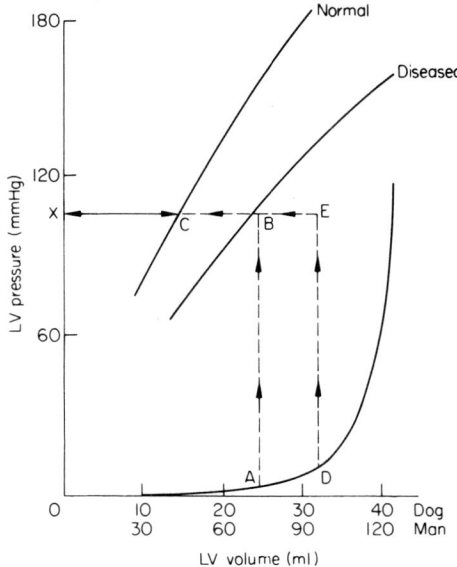

FIG. 5.17. Depression of Frank curve so that ejection can no longer occur from end-diastolic volume *A* at 100 mm Hg. Ventricle distends to volume *D* to compensate, but the new ejection fraction *BE/EX* is reduced compared with control ejection fraction *BC/BX*. From Noble (1978).

Angiography is impractical in acutely ill patients. In these circumstances a soft catheter can be 'floated' into the pulmonary artery. Catheters with a balloon mounted on the end are particularly suitable for this. Inflation of the balloon enables one to record pulmonary capillary 'wedge' pressure which reflects pulmonary venous, left atrial and left ventricular end-diastolic pressures. If thermistors are mounted on the catheter, cardiac output and stroke volume can be measured by thermodilution and points plotted on a graph relating stroke volume to 'wedge' pressure. Such information gives an idea of the position of the heart on the Starling curve and, in particular, whether treatment moves the heart to a higher curve. One has to remember that changes in heart rate and arterial pressure affect the curve and that wedge pressure is not always a reliable reflection of end-diastolic volume.

The difficulties outlined above have created pressure for non-invasive methods of measuring cardiac contraction. These include ballistocardiography, X-ray kymography, systolic time intervals and apex cardiography. The gamma camera method described above is valid and will become the method of choice. Echocardiography is particularly liable to lack of objectivity and to measurement error, particularly when a single beam of ultrasound is used to estimate ventricular diameter. Different parts of the heart move into the line of the beam throughout the cardiac cycle and it is not possible to know the relation between this varying diameter and ventricular volume. The errors can be reduced by obtaining two-dimensional and three-dimensional dynamic ultrasound pictures with arrays of probes or scanning probes.

Blood velocity can also be measured non-invasively by ultrasound using the Doppler principle. Here the problems are the dependence of the signal on the angle between the ultrasound beam and the moving blood, and the fact that signals are picked up from many depths within the body. The latter problem is overcome by using pulsed ultrasound and analysing only those echoes coming from one depth. Angelsen and Brubakk have used this technique to acquire the most promising non-invasive records I have seen (Fig. 5.18). These are records of human ascending aortic velocity obtained from the suprasternal notch. The use of such a technique, combined with improved ways of making dimensional analysis, may make it possible to check many of the mechanisms described in this and the previous chapter, mechanisms which have necessarily been delineated through experience with animal preparations.

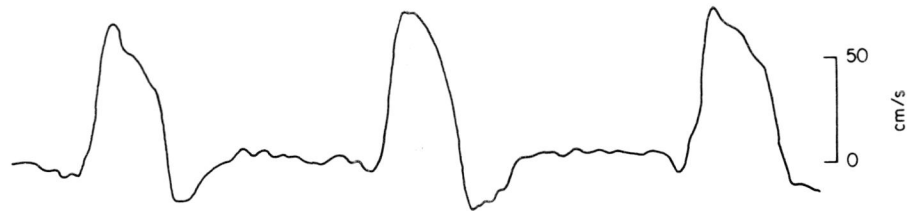

FIG. 5.18.   Record of blood velocity in the human ascending aorta recorded transcutaneously by the gated pulsed Doppler technique by Angelsen and Brubakk (1976).

REFERENCES

ANGELSEN B.A.J. & BRUBAKK A.O. (1976) Transcutaneous measurement of blood flow velocity in the human aorta. *Cardiovasc. Res.*, **10**, 368–379.

BENNETT E.D., ELSE W., MILLER G.A.H., SUTTON G.C., MILLER H.C. & NOBLE M.I.M. (1974) Maximum acceleration of blood from the left ventricle in patients with ischaemic heart disease. *Clin. Sci. Molec. Med.*, **46**, 49–59.

BOM N., LANCER C.T., HONKOOP J. & HUGENHOLTZ P.G. (1971) Ultrasonic viewer for cross-sectional analysis of moving cardiac structures. *Biomed. Eng.*, **6**, 500–503.

Ciba Foundation Symposium: *The Physiological Basis of Starlings Law of the Heart* (1974) Excerpta Medica, Amsterdam.

DONALD T.C., PETERSON D.M., WALKER A.A. & HEFNER L.L. (1976) Afterload-induced homeometric autoregulation in isolated cardiac muscle. *Am. J. Physiol.*, **231**, 545–550.

ELZINGA G., NOBLE M.I.M. & STUBBS J. (1977) The effect of an increase in aortic pressure upon the inotropic state of cat and dog left ventricles. *J. Physiol.*, **273**, 597–616.

ELZINGA G. & WESTERHOF N. (1976) The pumping ability of the left heart and the effect of coronary occlusion. *Circulation Res.*, **38**, 297–302.

ELZINGA G. & WESTERHOF N. (1977) How does a change in end-diastolic volume alter pumping ability of the left heart ? *J. Physiol.*, **266**, 46P.

ELZINGA G. & WESTERHOF N. (1979) How to quantify pump function of the heart. The value of variables derived from measurements on isolated muscle. *Circulation Res.*, **44**, 303–308.

ELZINGA G. & WESTERHOF N. (1978) The effect of an increase in inotropic state and end-diastolic volume on the pumping ability of the feline left heart. *Circulation Res.*, **42**, 620–628.

FABIATO A. & FABIATO F. (1975) Dependence of the contractile activation of skinned cardiac muscle cells on sarcomere length. *Nature*, **256**, 54–56.

FRANK O. (1895) Zur Dynamik des Herzmuskels. *Z. Biol.* **32**, 370. Translated by Chapman C.B. & Wasserman E. (1959) *Am. Heart J.*, **58**, 282 & 467.

FRANKLIN D.L., VAN CITTERS R.L. & RUSHMER R.F. (1962) Left ventricular function described in physical terms. *Circulation Res.*, **11**, 702–711.

FURNIVAL C.M., LINDEN R.J. & SNOW H.M. (1970) Inotropic changes in the left ventricle: the effect of changes in heart rate, aortic pressure and end-diastolic pressure. *J. Physiol.*, **211**, 359–387.

GLEASON W.L. & BRAUNWALD E. (1962) Studies on the first derivative of the left ventricular pressure pulse in man. *J. Clin. Invest.*, **41**, 80–91.

HEFNER L.L., SHEFFIELD L.T., COBBS G.C. & KLIP W. (1962) Relation between mural force and pressure in the left ventricle of the dog. *Circulation Res.*, **11**, 654–663.

HOLT J.P. (1957) Regulation of the degree of emptying of the left ventricle by the force of ventricular contraction. *Circulation Res.*, **5**, 281.

JEWELL B.R. (1977) A re-examination of the influence of muscle length on myocardial performance. *Circulation Res.*, **40**, 221–230.

JEWELL B.R. & ROVELL J.M. (1973) Influence of previous mechanical events on the contractility of isolated cat papillary muscle. *J. Physiol.*, **235**, 715–740.

JULIAN F.J., SOLLINS M.R. & MOSS R.L. (1976) Absence of a plateau in the length-tension relationship of rabbit papillary muscle when internal shortening is prevented. *Nature*, **260**, 340–342.

LAKATTA E.G. & JEWELL B.R. (1977) Length dependent activation: its effect on the length-tension relation in cat ventricular muscle. *Circulation Res.*, **40**, 251–257.

NOBLE M.I.M. (1978) The Frank-Starling curve. *Clin. Sci. Molec. Med.*, **54**, 1–7.

NOBLE M.I.M., STUBBS J., TRENCHARD D., ELSE W., EISELE J.H. & GUZ A. (1972) Left ventricular performance in the conscious dog with chronically denervated heart. *Cardiovasc. Res.*, **6**, 457–477.

NOBLE M.I.M., TRENCHARD D. & GUZ A. (1966) Left ventricular ejection in conscious dogs. II. Determinants of stroke volume. *Circulation Res.*, **19**, 148–152.

NOBLE M.I.M., TRENCHARD D. & GUZ A. (1967) Effect of changes of $PaCO_2$ and PaO_2 on cardiac performance in conscious dogs. *J. Appl. Physiol.*, **22**, 147–152.

PARMLEY W.W., DIAMOND G., TOMODA H. FORRESTER J.S. & SWAN H.J.C. (1972) Clinical evaluation of left ventricular pressures in myocardial infarction. *Circulation*, **45**, 358–366.

PARMLEY W.W., BRUTSAERT D.L. & SONNENBLICK E.H. (1969) Effects of altered loading on contractile events in isolated cat papillary muscle. *Circulation Res.*, **24**, 521–532.

PATTERSON S.W., PIPER H. & STARLING E.H. (1914) The regulation of the heart beat. *J. Physiol.*, **48**, 465.

PERONNEAU P.A., BOURNAT J.-P., BUGNON A., BARBET A. & XHAARD M. (1974). Theoretical & practical aspects of pulsed Doppler flowmetry: real time application to the measure of instantaneous velocity profiles *in vitro* & *in vivo*. In *Cardiovascular Applications of Ultrasound*. R.S. Reneman, Ed. North Holland, Amsterdam.

POLLACK G.H. & KREUGER J.W. (1976) Sarcomere dynamics in intact cardiac muscle. *Europ. J. Cardiol.*, **4**, 53–65.

REEVES T.J., HEFNER L.L., JONES W.B., COGHLAN C, PRIETO G. & CARROLL J. (1960) The hemodynamic determinants of the rate of change in pressure in the left ventricle. *Am. Heart J.*, **60**, 745–761.

SARNOFF S.J. & BERGLUND E. (1954) Ventricular function. I. Starlings law of the heart studied by simultaneous right and left ventricular function curves. *Circulation*, **9**, 706–718.

SARNOFF S.J. & MITCHELL J.H. (1962) The control of the function of the heart. *Handbook of Physiology*, Sec. 2. Circulation 1, 489.

SUGA H., SAGAWA K. & SHOUKAS A.A. (1973) Load independence of the instantaneous pressure-volume ratio of the canine left ventricle and effects of epinephrine and heart rate on the ratio. *Circulation Res.*, **32**, 314–322.

TAYLOR S.R., RUDEL R. & BLINKS J.R. (1975) Calcium transients in amphibian muscle. *Fed. Proc.*, **34**, 1379–1381.

VAN DEN BOS G.C., ELZINGA G., WESTERHOF N. & NOBLE M.I.M. (1973) Problems in the use of indices of myocardial contractility. *Cardiovasc. Res.*, **7**, 834–848.

WEBER K.T., JANICKI J.S. & HEFNER L.L. (1976) Left ventricular force-length relations of isovolumic and ejecting contractions *Am. J. Physiol.*, **231**, 337–343.

WEBER K.T., JANICKI J.S., REEVES R.C., HEFNER L.L. & REEVES T.J. (1974) Determinants of stroke volume in the isolated canine heart. *J. Appl. Physiol.*, **37**, 742–747.

WIGGERS C.J. (1914) Some factors controlling the shape of the pressure curve in the right ventricle. *Am. J. Physiol.*, **33**, 382–396.

WIGGERS C.J. (1926) Studies on the cardiodynamic actions of drugs. II. The mechanism of cardiac stimulation by epinephrine. *J. Pharmac. Exp. Ther.*, **30**, 233–250.

WOHLFART B., GRIMM A.F. & EDMAN K.A.P. (1977) Relationship between sarcomere length and active force in rabbit papillary muscle. *Acta Physiol.*, *Scand.*, **101**, 155–164.

CHAPTER 6

THE DIASTOLIC INTERVAL

Two problems will be discussed. (1) In the preceding two chapters, the ways of characterising cardiac contraction were explored on the basis of a constant heart rate. What are the consequences of a shortening of the diastolic interval so that heart rate increases? (2) In Chapter 5 it was assumed that diastolic pressure was a function of diastolic volume. What other factors may influence diastolic pressure and what are the consequences of a change in diastolic pressure-volume relationships?

THE CONSEQUENCES OF A CHANGE IN HEART RATE

In Chapter 2, the relationship between the force of contraction of heart muscle and the frequency of contraction was explained in detail. The relevant details as regards intact dog and cat hearts are summarised in Fig. 6.1. Human data is still not available.

As the duration of a test interval is increased, force of contraction increases to a maximum (called optimal contractile response) and then declines. In the isolated cat heart of Elzinga, isovolumic pressure of occluded beats is plotted instead of force. In the intact anaesthetised dog LV dP/dt max is used (Fig. 6.1b) which in this situation is independent of changes in end-diastolic volume (see Chapter 5).

When the relationship to test interval is explored at higher basic control steady state heart rates, the entire curve shifts upwards in parallel fashion (Fig. 6.1c). On each curve there is one point corresponding to the steady state interval. The relationship between steady state contractile performance and interval between beats (R-R interval) is given by joining these points and is seen to be quite flat. The relationship between performance and heart rate in the steady state is given by plotting against the reciprocal of these intervals (Fig. 6.1d).

A further illustration of this mechanism in the intact dog is given in Fig. 6.2 where the effect of a sudden step increase in heart rate produced by right atrial pacing is shown. On the first beat after the change a smaller dP/dt max is obtained because of the shorter interval; one has moved to the left along one of the curves shown in Fig. 6.1c. dP/dt max then increases to reach a new level which is similar to the control; one has moved from a lower to a higher curve in Fig. 6.1c. As dP/dt max increases from the first beat after the change to the steady state level, calcium is accumulating in the intracellular compartments (see Chapter 2).

Although it is always possible for the inotropic effect of increased heart rate to be either positive or negative, this effect is small because of the considerations outlined above. I therefore intend to ignore it in the remainder of this chapter. However, all the responses described have been checked in experiments in which steady state *LV*

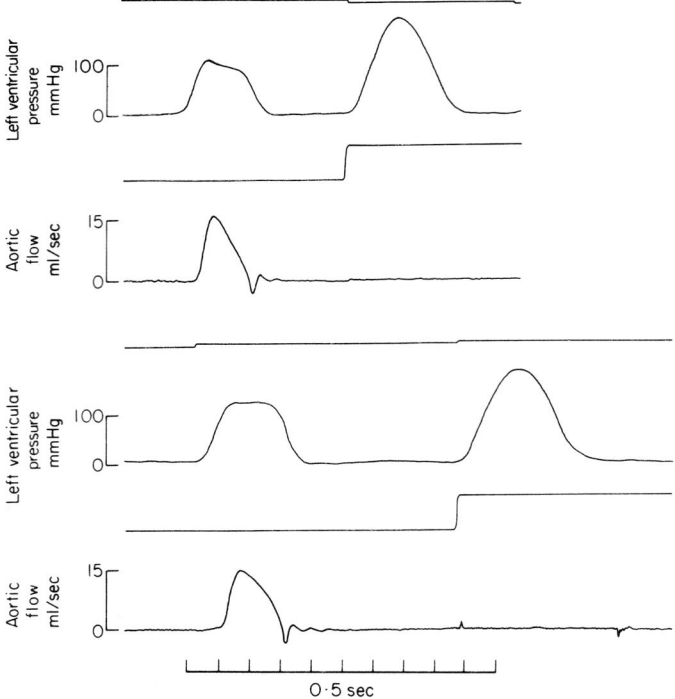

FIG. 6.1a. Left ventricular pressure and outflow from an isolated ejecting cat heart. The second beat in each record is isovolumic. Two different heart rates are compared at the same end-diastolic pressure. Note that there is little difference in the peak systolic isovolumetric pressure at the two heart rates, 218/min above and 138/min below. Tracings kindly provided by Gijs Elzinga.

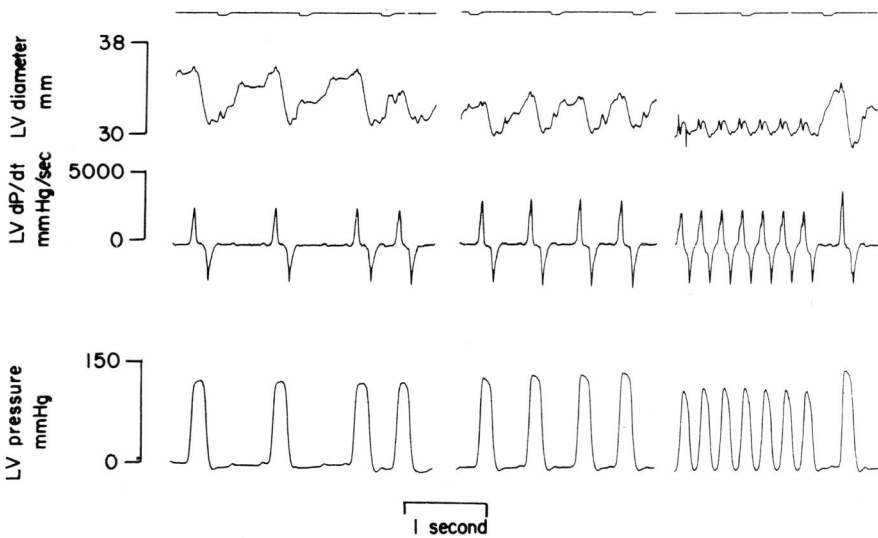

FIG. 6.1b. Dog with heart block. Upper trace—left ventricular (LV) diameter (ultrasonic crystals). Lower trace—LV pressure. Middle trace—rate of change of LV pressure. The last beat in each panel occurs after an optimum test pulse interval. Previous beats—steady state at increasing frequencies from left to right. Note increase in strength (LV dP/dt max) of test pulse (optimum contractile response) with increase in steady state frequency. From a study by Pidgeon et al. to be published.

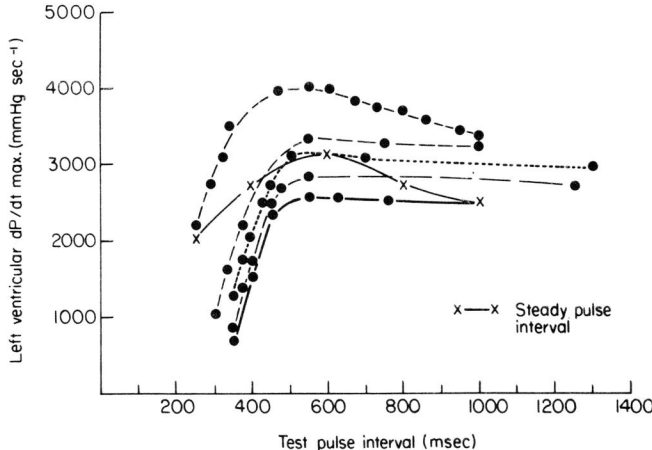

FIG. 6.1C. Each discontinuous line connects test pulse responses for an individual steady state frequency. The interval of the steady state frequencies are indicated by an *X*. Note that the entire test pulse interval curve moves up with increasing steady state frequency and that the steady state response (continuous line) rises and then falls with increasing frequency (shorter interval). From a study by Pidgeon *et al.* to be published.

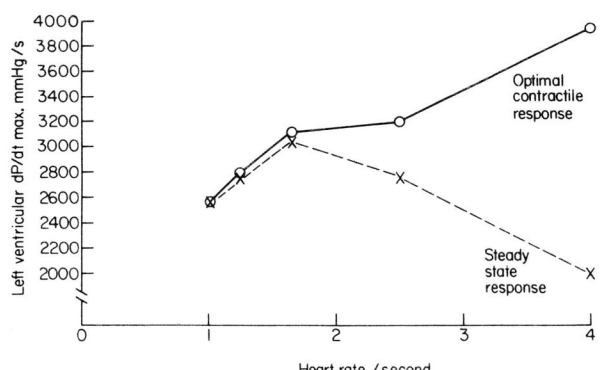

FIG. 6.1d. Relationship of optimal contractile response and steady state response to increasing steady state frequency (heart rate). From a study by Pidgeon *et al.* to be published.

dP/dt max was nearly constant. The results are similar to experiments in which there are small changes in LV *dP/dt* max.

Heart rate, diastolic interval and end-diastolic volume

When the time for diastole is reduced by an increase in heart rate, less blood enters the left ventricle from the left atrium. Therefore there is a reduction in end-diastolic volume. This occurs even in the isolated heart with constant left atrial filling pressure. It is difficult to measure ventricular volume in the intact heart and impossible to measure it precisely. I used a laborious radiological technique involving implantation of radiopaque markers on the cavity walls and frame by frame analysis of synchronised

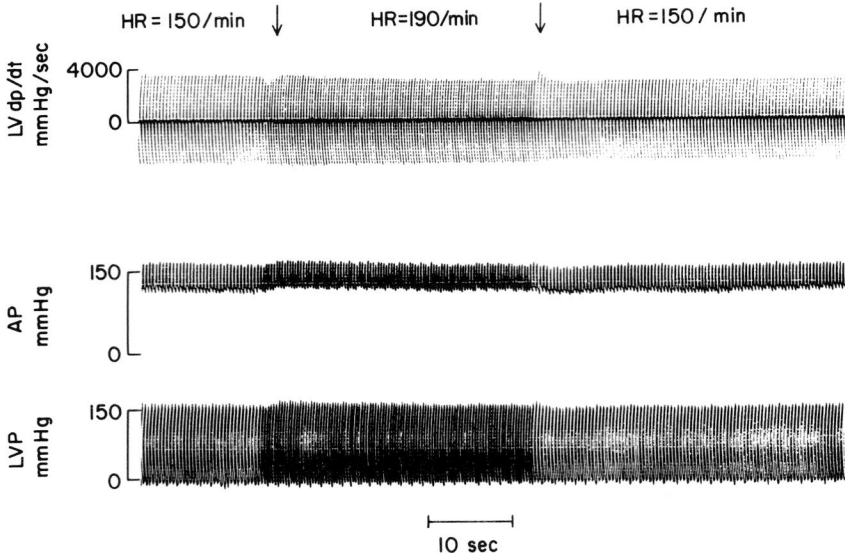

FIG. 6.2. Effect of a sudden step increase (first arrow) and decrease (second arrow) on contractile response as indicated by maximum rate of rise of left ventricular pressure (LV *dp/dt*).
AP—aortic pressure, LVP—left ventricular pressure. From Noble *et al.* (1969).

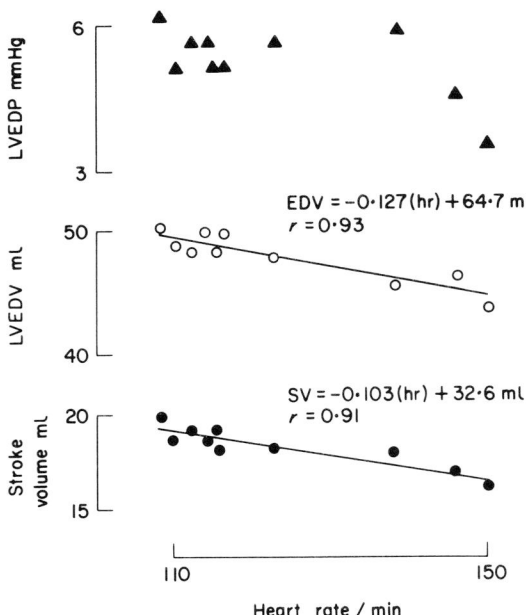

FIG. 6.3. Relationship of stroke volume, left ventricular (LV) end-diastolic volume (LVEDV), and LV end-diastolic pressure (LVEDP) to increasing heart rate in the steady state. From Noble *et al.* (1969).

biplane cineradiographs. This yielded data like that shown in Fig. 6.3 where heart rate was altered by electrical pacing of the right atrium. It appears that the decrease in end-diastolic volume with increasing heart rate is sufficiently linear to give a good fit in a linear regression. The linear equation used is an approximation. There is nothing intrinsically linear about the relationship and it may well not be linear over a wide range of heart rate. However, the *use* of the linear equation has great advantage in developing the consequences of the dependence of end-diastolic volume on heart rate. I draw particular attention to the slope of the line − 0·127 in the case of Fig. 6.3; this means a 0·127 ml fall in end-diastolic volume per beat/min increase in heart rate.

Since stroke volume is dependent on end-diastolic volume (Chapter 5) one would expect stroke volume also to fall, as indeed it does. However, the question arises 'is the end-diastolic volume the only factor controlling stroke volume?' We know from the Weber-Janicki-Hefner curve (Chapter 5) that stroke volume is a function of left ventricular systolic pressure; this remains reasonably constant when one changes heart rate by right atrial pacing (Fig. 6.2). Changes in left ventricular systolic pressure will therefore have only small effects on stroke volume. When describing the relationship between stroke volume and end-diastolic volume (Chapter 5), I pointed out that this was determined by the fact that the left ventricle contracts down to the same end-systolic volume from different end-diastolic volumes. Therefore, the increase in stroke volume consequent upon an increase in end-diastolic volume is identical to the increase in end-diastolic volume. The Starling curve (Fig. 5.2b) has a slope of 1·0. If the left ventricle contrives to eject down to the same end-systolic volume during changes in heart rate, the fall in stroke volume with increasing heart rate will be identical to the fall in end-diastolic volume. The relationship between stroke volume and heart rate is also shown in Fig. 6.3; this is also approximately linear over the range explored. The slope of the line is − 0·103; this means a 0·103 ml fall in stroke volume per beat/min increase in heart rate. This is close to but not identical with the slope of the end-diastolic volume/heart rate line. However, this is an individual experiment. When it is repeated, one finds that the stroke volume slope is sometimes greater and sometimes smaller than the end-diastolic volume slope. The difference in Fig. 6.3 is attributed statistically to experimental error. This is probably due to the errors in the end-diastolic volume measurement which is crude compared with the electromagnetic flowmeter measurement of stroke volume. Therefore one can reasonably conclude (1) that the slopes of the two lines are identical (2) that the ventricle does continue to eject down to the same end-systolic volume (3) that the fall in stroke volume is entirely due to the fall in end-diastolic volume acting through the Starling relationship.

Heart rate and cardiac output

As seen above, stroke volume (SV) decreases almost linearly with increasing heart rate (HR) according to the equation:

$$SV = -a(HR) + b$$

where $-a$ is the slope of the line and b the intercept on the stroke volume axis. This has the form shown in Fig. 6.4a. Cardiac output is the stroke volume multiplied by heart rate, i.e.

$$CO = SV \times HR = -a(HR)^2 + b(HR)$$

This has the form shown in Fig. 6.4b. This is really a mathematical abstraction but the cardiac output/heart rate curve (Fig 6.4b) does fit actual data from dog and man quite well. There is a small rise in cardiac output at rates from 70/min to about 100/min. Cardiac output then remains fairly constant up to about 170/min and then falls off. Cardiac output drops considerably at very low and very high heart rates.

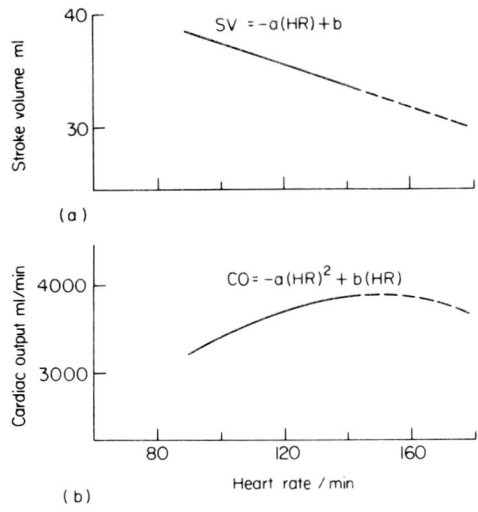

FIG. 6.4.   (a) Inverse linear relationship between stroke volume (SV) and heart rate (HR). (b) If such linear relationship is assumed (a), the relationship between cardiac output (CO) and heart rate will have the form shown. From Noble *et al.* (1966).

Heart rate, the pump function curve and the Weber-Janicki-Hefner curve

Up to this point I have used the pump function curve only at constant heart rate. A change in heart rate, however, raises problems in its use. The mean flow changes are the same as the cardiac output changes (above) but the mean pressure is considerably increased because of the greater number of beats occurring in a given time (Fig. 6.2). Therefore a plot of mean pressure against mean flow would reveal an apparent upward shift of the curve resulting from increased heart rate. However, this is not what would have occurred if the end-diastolic volume had not decreased. In that case the stroke volume is the same and mean flow (cardiac output) increases in proportion to heart rate. A plot of mean pressure against mean flow now reveals an upward and outward shift of the curve.

Similar considerations apply to the mean force—mean velocity curve of a papillary muscle (Chapter 4). The upward and outward shift of that curve consequent upon an increase in contraction frequency does not betoken a fundamental increase in the contractile capabilities of the myocardium; it merely means that the myocardium is being made to contract more often. By the same token, although the increase in the mean pressure/mean flow curve informs the engineer of the increased pumping potential for delivery of blood to the peripheral circulation, it does not mean a fundamental increase in the contractile properties of the myocardium.

The Weber-Janicki-Hefner curve does not suffer from this ambiguity. An increase in heart rate decreases the stroke volume and has no effect on left ventricular systolic pressure (Figs 6.2 and 6.3). The plot of stroke volume against left ventricular systolic pressure is depressed by an increase in heart rate. However, this is entirely due to the fall in end-diastolic volume. If the end-diastolic volume is restored to the control level, exactly the same curve is obtained. This confirms that the ability of the ventricle to generate a given single contraction is the same.

These considerations give rise to thoughts about whether one can combine the advantages and remove the disadvantages of each curve by combining them in some way. The use of a single beat in the Weber-Janicki-Hefner curve removes the sensitivity to heart rate changes. The use of mean left ventricular pressure in the pump function curve removes the sensitivity to aortic input impedance. Mean pressure is the area under the left ventricular pressure divided by the R-R interval between beats (Fig. 6.5).* (This is equivalent to Sarnoff's tension time index per minute). The mean flow is the area under the left ventricular flow curve (stroke volume) divided by the R-R interval between beats (Fig. 6.5). I propose that the division by R-R interval between beats be omitted and a pump function curve be constructed plotting the area under the left ventricular pressure (equivalent to Sarnoff's tension time index per beat) against stroke volume.

This curve will behave in the same way as the Weber-Janicki-Hefner curve under circumstances of changing heart rate (see above). It will also behave as the mean pressure/mean flow curve in that (1) it is not required that the aorta be connected to a Starling resistor, (2) it is not required that the left ventricular pressure remain relatively constant during ejection, (3) it is insensitive to a change in the nature of the aortic input impedance such as might be produced by stiffer arteries (see Chapter 4, Fig. 4.7).

It might be objected that the adoption of such a compromise transgresses the principles of analysis in the frequency domain (Chapter 4). There are two aspects to this: analysis in the frequency domain requires in theory that the system being oscillated be in a steady state, i.e. oscillation at a constant frequency for sufficient length of time to establish absolute constancy of all wave forms from beat to beat. This is impractical in the cardiovascular system, so one needs to know how far away from the steady state one can go and still use the analysis. In the case of the left ventricle, this was checked by Elzinga and Westerhof by interposing single beats of

---

* One can debate the pros and cons of using total pressure (Fig. 6.5a) or developed pressure (Fig. 6.5b) on the basis of muscle models, etc (see page 151, Fig. 6.8). However, developed pressure can be measured correctly, giving it a practical advantage.

higher or lower left ventricular pressure and comparing the results with those obtained at these pressures during a steady state. The mean pressure/mean flow points obtained in the two cases were identical. Therefore in the case of the left ventricle the analysis can be applied to single beats as long as they do not occur after some gross instability such as transient cardiac arrest.

The other aspect of analysis in the frequency domain is the question of higher frequencies. The mean term is merely the first (zero frequency) value in a series pertaining to higher and higher frequencies. Use of 'integrated pressure' and 'integrated flow' (stroke volume) apparently removes time and frequency from the dimensions. However, one can also derive the fundamental sine wave for left ventricular pressure and outflow (1st harmonic) and the higher harmonics over one systole and diastole. This results in a series of values for each harmonic as for aortic input impedance (see Chapter 7). The usefulness of such an exercise has not yet been explored but the use of pressure and flow 'meaned for one beat' (integrated pressure and stroke volume) does not seem to be a serious obstacle.

Heart rate, work and efficiency

In view of the facts that increasing heart rate (1) does not change systolic left ventricular pressure, and (2) produces a fall in stroke volume and that (3) stroke work is stroke volume multiplied by pressure, it is not surprising that stroke work decreases with increasing heart rate in the same, almost linear, manner as stroke volume. The stroke work (SW)/heart rate (HR) relationship is governed by a similar equation:

$$SW = -c(HR) + d$$

where $-c$ is the slope of the line and d the stroke work intercept. The line has the same form as Fig. 6.4a. The value for c in the experiment shown in Fig. 6.3 is 0·177, i.e. stroke work declines by 0·177 Joules per beat/min increase in heart rate.

The work done by the heart in one minute (minute work, MW) is stroke work multiplied by heart rate, i.e.

$$MW = SW \times HR = -c(HR)^2 + d(HR)$$

This has the same form as the curve for cardiac output (Fig. 6.4b). Measured changes in minute work show almost the same changes with increasing heart rate as those of cardiac output.

The oxygen consumption of the left ventricle is determined principally by pressure sustained by it, i.e. the mean left ventricular pressure. This increases almost in proportion to the increase in heart rate (see above) because of the greater number of beats/min. Therefore, over a wide range of heart rate the work done does not change while the oxygen consumed by the heart increases. Thus the ratio minute work/oxygen consumption declines. There are powerful objections to expressing efficiency in this way. Nevertheless, it expresses an important practical consideration—the myocardium does indeed require a greater oxygen supply (causing angina in patients with limited coronary arterial inflow) while no extra blood is supplied to the periphery.

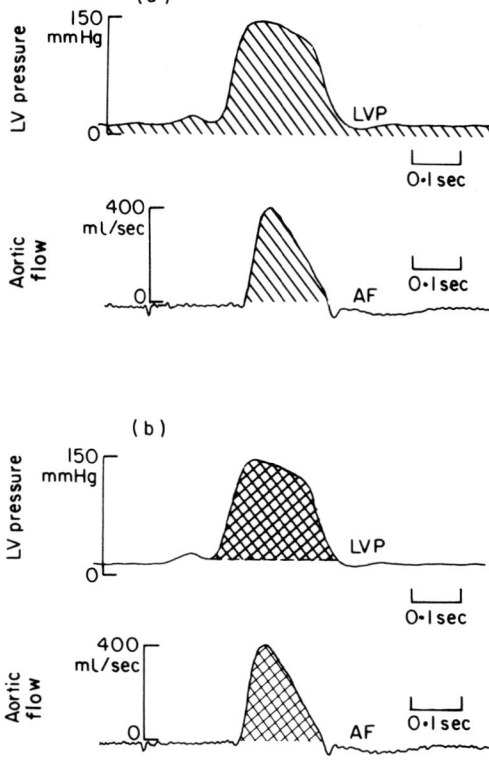

FIG. 6.5.   Left ventricular pressure (LVP) recorded by SF-1 catheter tip manometer and aortic flow (AF) recorded by electromagnetic flowmeter on the ascending aorta in a conscious dog. Hatched areas indicate mean pressure and stroke volume. (a) Total pressure is used. (b) Pressure above the end-diastolic value is used.

Heart rate, blood pressure and peripheral resistance

When one is on the 'ascending limb' of the cardiac output/heart rate relationship (Fig. 6.4b) one also finds a rise in mean arterial pressure (Fig. 6.6). This is associated with a rising diastolic and constant systolic pressure. In some experiments, such as that depicted in Fig. 6.6, there is no detectable change in the ratio mean arterial pressure/cardiac output (peripheral resistance). However, sometimes a plot of mean arterial pressure against cardiac output yields results as shown in Fig. 6.7. The peripheral resistance is the slope of the line connecting the origin of the graph to the data. This slope is steeper at the low cardiac output end of the data than at the high cardiac output end. Does the peripheral vasculature actually open up? This would be expected from stimulation of baroreceptors. The efferent side of the baroreflex is half removed because bradycardia cannot occur (because of the electrical pacing of the right atrium). The fact that the line relating mean arterial pressure to cardiac output (dashed line in Fig. 6.7) has a much lower slope than the peripheral resistance lines

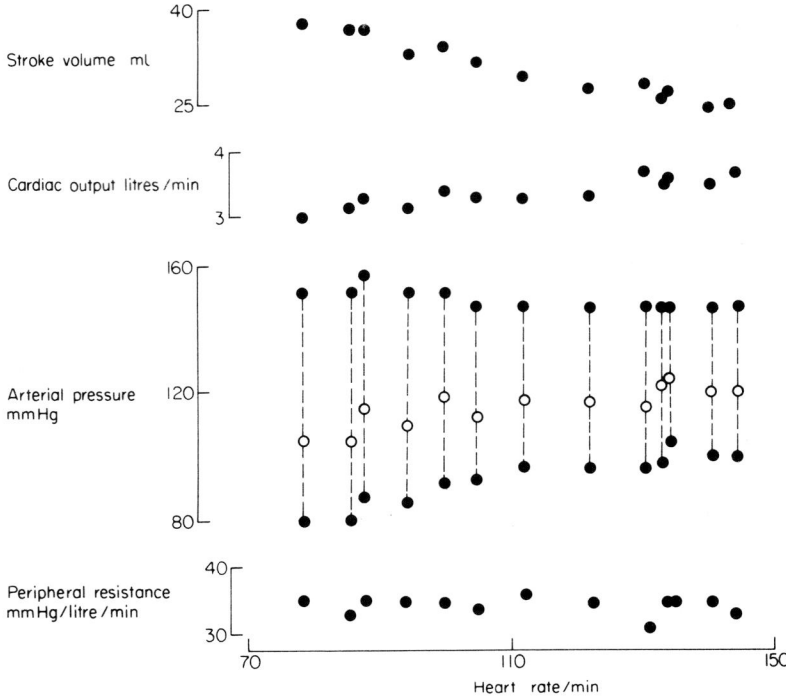

FIG. 6.6.   Effect of heart rate in one dog on stroke volume, cardiac output, arterial pressure and peripheral resistance (mean arterial pressure divided by cardiac output). Open circles in arterial pressure indicate mean values. From Noble *et al.* (1966).

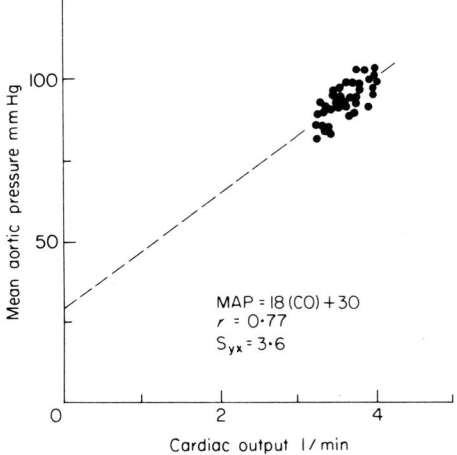

FIG. 6.7.   Relationship between mean arterial pressure (MAP) and cardiac output (CO) in a different dog from that illustrated in Fig. 6.6. A linear regression gave the result shown with a positive intercept on the pressure axis indicating that the slope of the regression line slopes significantly away from a line to the origin. From Noble *et al.* (1966).

raises the question 'Is the pressure-flow diagram of the systemic circulation linear through the origin?' This question will be taken up in the next chapter.

DIASTOLIC FILLING OF THE LEFT VENTRICLE AND VENTRICULAR DIASTOLIC PRESSURE VOLUME RELATIONS

Apart from the pericardium, there are no external constraints on left ventricular filling during the diastolic interval. The stiffness of the myocardium itself prevents overdistension. The mechanical properties of resting diastolic myocardium therefore deserve detailed examination.

The diastolic mechanical properties of isolated papillary muscle

When resting cardiac muscle strips are stretched they develop tension resulting in the resting length tension curve (Fig. 5.1b). This is elastic behaviour but the tissue does not obey Hooke's Law which requires a linear relationship between length and tension with constant slope (tension/length change = stiffness. Length change/tension = compliance). The curve found in cardiac muscle approximates an exponential curve and such curves are usually fitted to length-tension data when convenient mathematical manipulation is required (Hefner & Bowen 1967). However, there is nothing fundamentally exponential about the relationship. It is natural to wonder what structures or mechanisms are responsible for resting tension. This question is tied up with the question of muscle models. There are several possible sources of resting tension: (1) residual contractile activity due to failure of the sarcoplasmic reticulum to lower Ca^{++} concentration below that at which there is no longer any tension produced by the contractile proteins; (2) stretching of the sarcolemma; (3) connective tissue. Since there are also sources of series elasticity both within the sarcomeres and in the elastic ends of the muscle, a model which attempts to include all these factors is too complicated to use (Fig. 6.8c). Most workers have tried to reduce this to the Maxwell (Fig. 6.8a) or Voigt (Fig. 6.8b) models.

Choice between the Maxwell and Voigt models is difficult and the arguments for and against each are inconclusive, probably because both are oversimplifications. On the one hand, Hefner and Bowen showed that the Voigt model has an impossibly

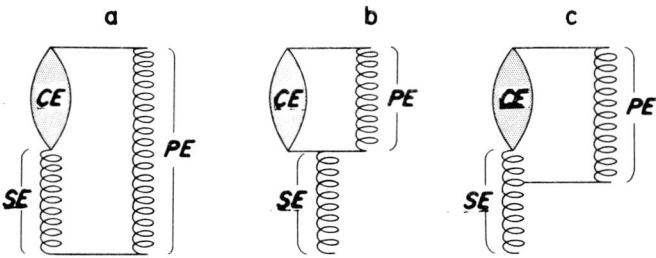

FIG. 6.8. Analogue models of cardiac muscle. (a) Maxwell model. No series elastic element (SE) in series with PE. (b) Voigt model. All SE in series with PE. (c) Part of SE in series with PE.

stiff parallel elastic element while on the other hand Brutsaert showed that contracting muscle performance is determined only by total load as if all resting force was taken up by the contractile element (as would occur in the Voigt model). The argument is not perhaps of much interest or importance to the non-specialist except in that it poses a problem as to whether resting force should be subtracted from total force in order to determine the developed contractile force. This is the usual practice and involves an implicit assumption of the Maxwell model. In the Voigt model, only a small part of the resting tension can be so subtracted. Therefore, if the Voigt model is more correct, the conventional calculation of developed contractile force is incorrect.

In isolated muscle strips it is certain that there is some truth in the Voigt model because recent measurements of sarcomere length show considerable internal shortening of central sarcomeres at the expense of those at the ends of the preparation. In those experiments, it is possible to subtract the correct resting tension corresponding to the sarcomere length during contraction. (This was done in Chapter 5.) The same correction cannot be applied to intact heart where such 'damaged ends' do not occur. The whole question therefore remains unresolved.

The elastic properties of resting myocardium can also be demonstrated by oscillating the length of the muscle sinusoidally. Sinusoidal oscillations of tension then occur. The ratio of the amplitude of the tension to that of the length oscillations is a measure of the stiffness of the myocardium. However, if the frequency of the oscillations is increased, the stiffness apparently increases. This is because the muscle has viscous properties as well as elastic (see below). The stiffness also increases if the overall muscle length is increased. This is because of the steepening of the resting length/tension curve. The large increase in stiffness during contraction is due to the addition of series elasticity (active stiffness).

The elastic properties can also be shown by releasing the end of the muscle so that there is a quick release. There is an accompanying rapid fall in tension. The stiffness is the fall in tension divided by the decrease in length. However, there is also a slower change in tension following the quick release (Fig. 6.9). This is due to stress-relaxation. Stress relaxation can also be shown by slowly stretching the muscle and then relaxing it. The tension for any given length during relaxation falls below that for the same length during stretching; this produces a hysteresis loop (Fig. 6.10).

Viscous resistance to stretch is most simply demonstrated by stretching muscle at different speeds. If the muscle is purely elastic the length-tension curve will be unaffected by speed of stretch. In fact above speeds of stretch of 1–2 muscle lengths/sec, tension for any given length increases (Fig. 6.11).

When a papillary muscle contracts against a higher force in systole, the tension for a given diastolic length is sometimes reduced. This has been attributed to some structure in series with both contractile and parallel elastic elements 'giving' during systole when subjected to the higher force. As a result, this 'series viscous element' is longer and the parallel elastic element shorter during the next diastole. The shorter parallel elastic element carries less force according to its length-tension relationship. Such a change in diastolic tension is not accompanied by any obvious change in

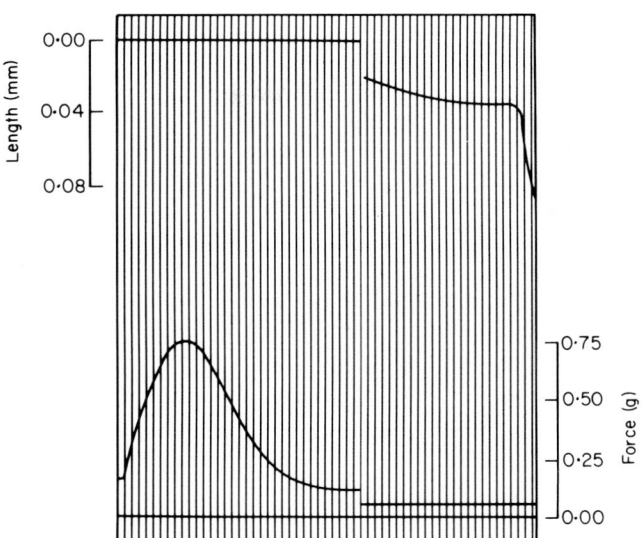

FIG. 6.9. Quick release of resting cardiac muscle produces a sudden drop in tension due to elastic recoil and a slower change due to stress relaxation. From Hefner and Bowen (1967).

viscous resistance to stretch, so presumably this property does not reside in the series viscous element. One would expect all the elements in the muscle (Fig. 6.8) to be viscoelastic rather than purely elastic in common with other biological material. Viscous resistance to stretch is always present to some extent but series viscous behaviour is variable.

There has been much controversy over the question of whether inotropic interventions also change diastolic mechanical properties. While most workers have failed to find such alterations in diastolic properties, there is some evidence to suggest that part at least of the resting tension is determined by an active process or residual

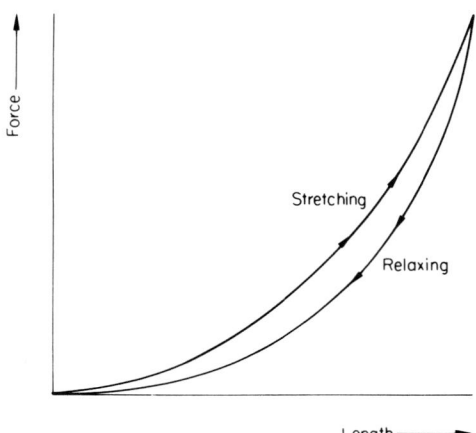

FIG. 6.10. Tension on stretching resting cardiac muscle exceeds that on returning it to original length. Hysteresis.

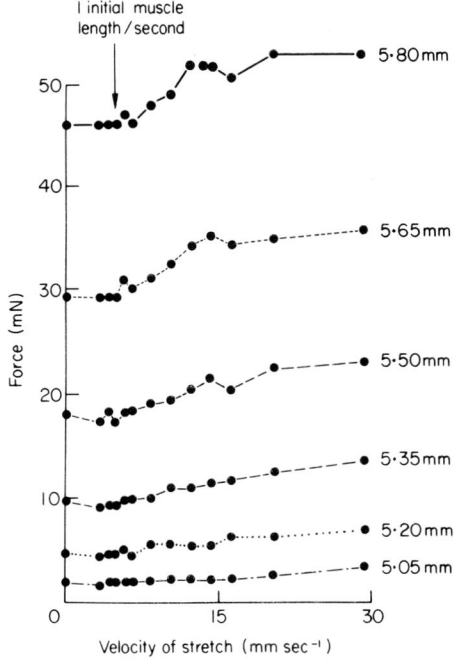

FIG. 6.11. Force at 6 muscle lengths in a cat papillary muscle (ordinate) plotted against velocity of stretch (abscissa). There is increasing viscous resistance to stretch with muscle length. The points on the Y axis are the 'static' forces with increasing length during diastole. From Noble (1977).

activity of the contractile proteins. Hypoxia of papillary muscle certainly leads to a rise in resting tension which could be attributed to failure of the sarcoplasmic reticulum to reduce intracellular Ca^{++} concentration to as low a level as was present in the fully oxygenated muscle.

The diastolic mechanical properties of the intact heart

It is much more difficult to explore the phenomena described above in the intact animal. It is important to look for them because of the consequences of a changing pressure-volume relation (see below). It would not be surprising if some of the effects found in papillary muscle are due to its unphysiological condition (not perfused, low temperature, etc). Additional phenomena are possible in the intact heart: (1) acceleration of a mass of blood into the ventricle may induce inertial effects; (2) changes in coronary perfusion pressure could change the mechanical behaviour of the myocardial vasculature; (3) changes of pressure in the right heart could influence the left ventricle; (4) the pericardium can have an influence; (5) dilatation and hypertrophy can occur over long periods; (6) the left ventricle can 'suck' blood by expanding elastically from its contracted state.

The corresponding relationship to the diastolic length/tension curve in the intact

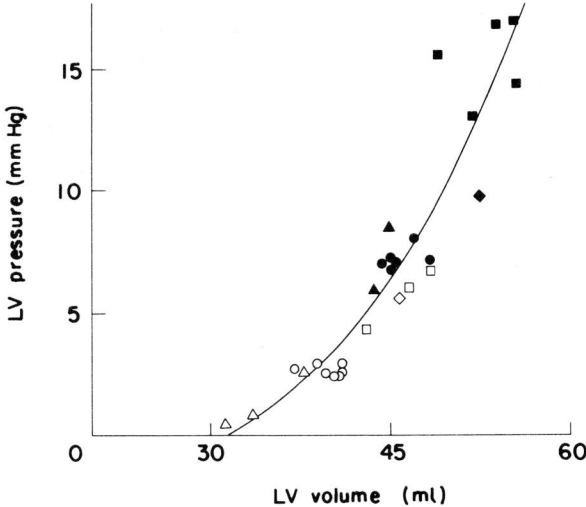

FIG. 6.12. Relationship between left ventricular pressure and volume during diastole. The range of the solid symbols was explored by means of a saline infusion to distend the ventricle. From Noble *et al.* (1969).

heart is the diastolic pressure/volume curve. This is a non-linear relationship. Using the radiopaque marker technique I found that pressure increased ever more steeply with increasing volume (Fig. 6.12). This curve approximates an exponential reasonably well and I used an exponential line fitted to the data by the least squares method as a convenient way of summarising the data. However, this is just as arbitrary as expressing the stroke volume/heart rate relationship by a straight line. There is nothing fundamentally exponential about the pressure/volume relationship. Suppose that the length/tension curve of the muscle fibres is exponential and given by Hefner and Bowen's equation:-

$$F = a(e^{b(l - l_0)} - l)$$

(F = force, l = length, l_0 = unstretched length, a and b are constants). It can readily be shown that if pressure is derived from force by Hefner's equation and volume from length using a cylindrical or spherical model (Chapter 4), the resulting pressure/volume curve cannot possibly be an exponential of the form I used:-

$$P = a + be^{cV}$$

where P = pressure, V = volume and a, b and c are constants. The length/tension curve and pressure/volume cannot both be exponential. It is likely that the length/tension curve fits an exponential most closely over a wide range of stretch. Pressure/volume data may fit an exponential reasonably well over the small range which can be explored in an intact animal but probably departs considerably from it over a wider range.

For this reason I consider the use of the exponential pressure/volume equation for analytical purposes as dangerous. This is especially true when incorrect abbreviation of the formula is used to give an 'index of ventricular compliance' like $dp/dV/P$ which is the stiffness (tangent to the pressure/volume curve) divided by the pressure at which it was measured. This ratio is not constant and one cannot therefore regard changes in it as changes in stiffness. Another dubious practice is to plot the end-systolic and end-diastolic pressure/volume points on semilogarithmic paper and to join them with a straight line.

An additional reason for avoiding this last method is that the end-systolic and end-diastolic points are the least reliable. This is because the filling of the ventricle does not occur at a steady rate throughout diastole. In Fig. 6.13a the filling pattern is shown from radiographic data. This gives only discontinuous points for volume involving scatter. However, the pattern is confirmed by continuous traces of ventricular diameter measured ultrasonically (Fig. 6.13b). What is not in doubt is that there is an early diastolic filling phase which is very rapid. One can see that this is the most rapid event in the cardiac cycle when watching cineradiographs. This early filling phase is followed by a period when the heart is almost stationary. Further filling occurs with atrial systole.

Ideally, elastic properties should be studied when the length of the muscle is not changing because, otherwise, viscous effects may interfere. Thus in the intact heart one should make measurements of the elastic properties during the mid-diastolic quiescent period (diastasis). However, the most common practice is to make measurements at end-systole and end-diastole, times when the ventricle is filling most rapidly. Therefore compliance estimates based on these measurements are unreliable.

The presence of viscous resistance to stretch can be confirmed by the fact that excess diastolic pressure is found when the rate of filling of the ventricle is sufficiently increased, e.g. by infusion of isoproterenol. This has been elegantly shown by Horwitz and Bishop using ultrasonic crystals to monitor the increasing ventricular size in diastole. The filling rate necessary appears to be reasonably consistent with the value of 1–2 muscle lengths/sec found for isolated myocardium if one makes reasonable assumptions about ventricular geometry. Excess pressure from this cause is probably minimal or absent under quiet resting conditions and may not become apparent with slowing or mild quickening of the filling rate from such a control state.

The oscillation technique for studying myocardial mechanical properties has also been applied to the intact heart by Templeton and his colleagues. Instead of applying sinusoidal length changes to a papillary muscle, sinusoidal volume changes were applied to an externally perfused left ventricle. The amplitude of the pressure oscillations divided by the amplitude of the volume changes—$\delta P/\delta V$ behaved in a similar manner to $\delta F/\delta L$ for the papillary muscle. Viscous effects were shown by the increase in $\delta P/\delta V$ with a higher frequency of oscillation. This method is particularly valuable for exploring the effect of changes in the coronary vessels. Increase in coronary perfusion pressure and coronary vasodilation by glyceryl trinitrate failed to produce changes in the diastolic mechanical properties.

In the intact animal no obvious changes in diastolic pressure can be detected at

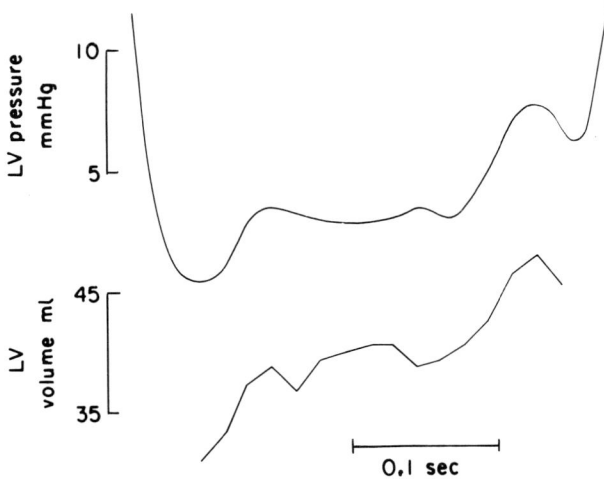

FIG. 6.13a.   Changes in left ventricular pressure and volume during one diastole in a quietly resting dog. From Noble *et al.* (1969).

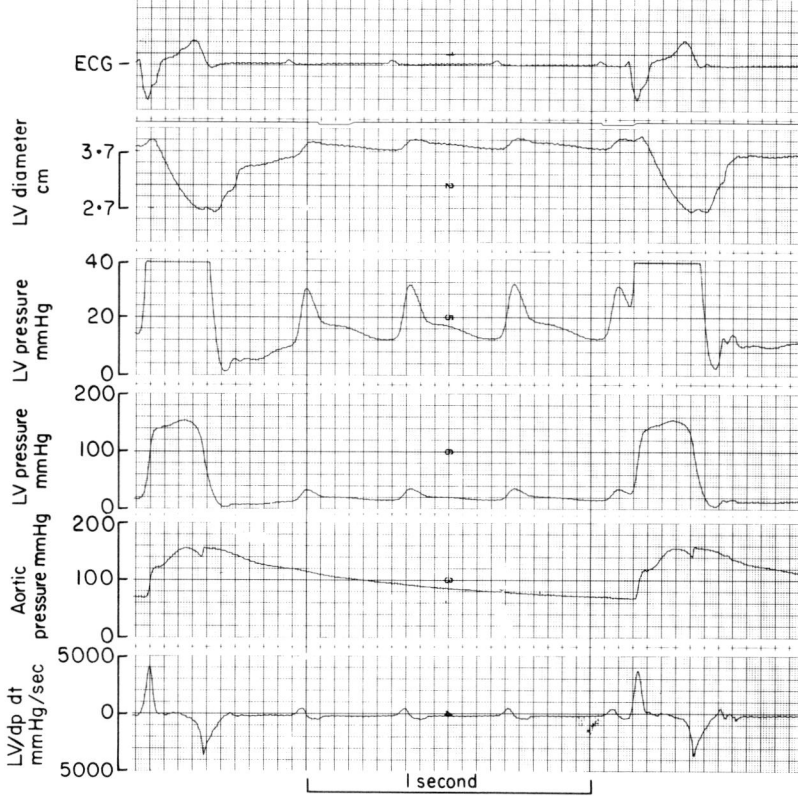

FIG. 6.13b.   Changes in left ventricular pressure and diameter in an anaesthetised dog with heart block. Aortic pressure and *dP/dt* also shown. The contribution to filling of atrial contraction is illustrated here. Atrial systoles produce an increase in diameter which is not sustained when the ventricle is distended.

times of greatest acceleration and deceleration of blood flowing into the left ventricle. Inertial forces seem to be too small to be detectable under normal circumstances. The effect attributed to a 'series viscous element' (see above) is also too small to be detected—no change in the mid-diastolic pressure/volume relation occurs acutely in response to an increase in left ventricular systolic pressure. In such acute experiments it is also not possible to detect stress relaxation although this phenomenon may play a role in long term ventricular dilatation (see below).

Changes in the right ventricle do affect the left ventricular diastolic pressure/ volume relation. This can be easily shown in excised hearts in which different right ventricular volumes produce different left ventricular pressure/volume curves by changing the stresses in the intraventricular septum. This effect is more difficult to show in the intact heart. Elzinga, in an even more sophisticated version of his isolated cat heart preparation, connected the pulmonary artery to a hydraulic model of the pulmonary arterial input impedance. Unfortunately ventricular dimensions were not measured. However, it was possible to show an influence of right ventricular pressure on left ventricular pressure. Elzinga's preparation has an intact pericardium. Removal of the pericardium showed that the influence of right on left ventricular pressure was very much reduced. Thus, quite apart from any direct influence of the pericardium *per se* on diastole, it increases the interventricular 'cross-talk'. The direct influence of the pericardium was shown in the classic study of Hefner and colleagues who related left ventricular pressure and external circumference. Pericardectomy caused flattening of the pressure/circumference curve at pressures above 10 mm Hg (Fig. 6.14). This study embodies a definitive exposition of the principles governing ventricular compliance. However, limitation in available methods led to the use of external circumference as an index of ventricular size. This is affected by changes in ventricular

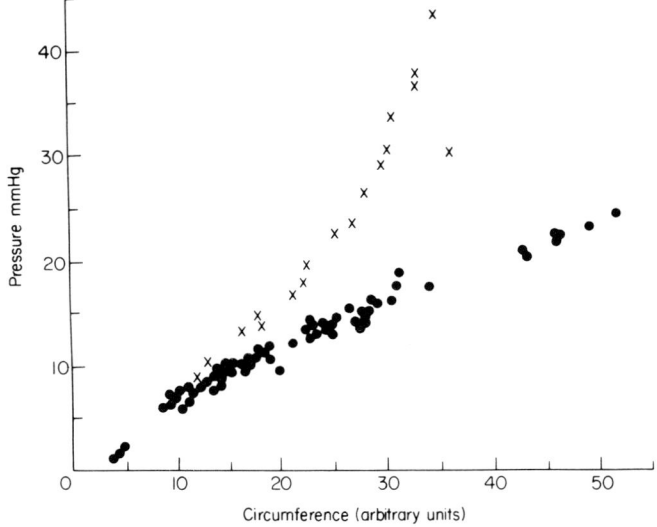

FIG. 6.14. Relationship between left ventricular pressure (ordinate) and external circumference (abscissa) with pericardium closed (×) and open (●). From Hefner *et al.* (1961).

wall thickness and these may have caused the apparent change in ventricular distensibility accompanying a positive inotropic intervention. Ultrasonic and radiographic estimates of internal dimensions do not confirm this.

Left ventricular 'suction' certainly occurs in an excised heart placed in a bath of saline. Such a heart fills and expels fluid thus propelling itself around the bath. In order to do this the ventricle has to empty to a much lower end-systolic volume than ever occurs against a normal end-systolic pressure according to the Frank curve. In order to demonstrate it in an intact animal one would have to show a downward inflection of the quasi-exponential pressure/volume curve downward to the left of that normally measured (Fig. 6.12) with negative transmural pressures. Such a result has not been shown convincingly at normal arterial pressure. However, it is likely that filling by 'suction' can occur at very low arterial pressure.

The majority of papers dealing with ventricular compliance deal with changes induced by disease. Myocardial ischaemia affects a region of the ventricle and it is necessary to measure changes in force and dimension of the ischaemic segment rather than overall pressure and volume. The question whether there is a change in compliance of the ischaemic muscle is unresolved. Undoubtedly resolving infarcts and post-infarction scars and aneurisms are stiffer than normal myocardium as one would expect from replacement by fibrous tissue. Thus the diastolic pressure/volume curve of such hearts may be shifted to the left.

In generalised left ventricular disease, dilatation may occur causing a shift of the entire pressure/volume curve to the right. Hypertrophy, by making the ventricular wall thicker and therefore stiffer, shifts the entire pressure/volume curve to the left. Combinations of dilatation and hypertrophy occur as in experimental 'volume over-

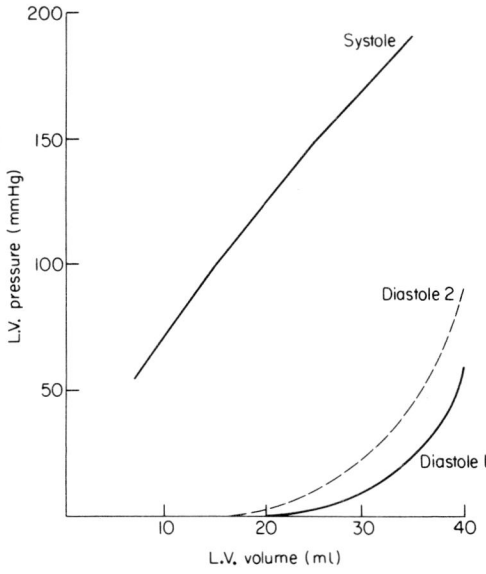

FIG. 6.15a. Left ventricular pressure-volume (Frank) curves for systole and two diastoles with different resting compliance, the stiffer case being represented by the dashed line.

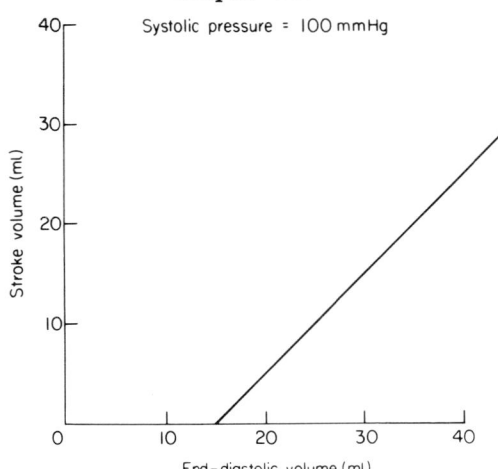

FIG. 6.15b.   Stroke volume/end-diastolic volume (Starling) curve for the two circumstances in (a) are identical.

load'. For instance, anastomosis of the aorta to the inferior vena cava produces chronic distension of the ventricle, the pressure/volume curve first shifts to the right and then moves to the left. In the presence of hypertrophy and/or dilatation it is virtually impossible to determine whether the muscle itself is of normal compliance.

Consequences of a change in the diastolic pressure/volume relationship

In Fig. 6.15a the Frank curve is plotted together with two diastolic pressure/volume curves. From any given end-diastolic volume, the ventricle ejects the same stroke volume, so that the Starling curve is the same for both cases (Fig. 6.15b). However, if stroke volume (or stroke work) is plotted against end-diastolic pressure (Fig. 6.15c)

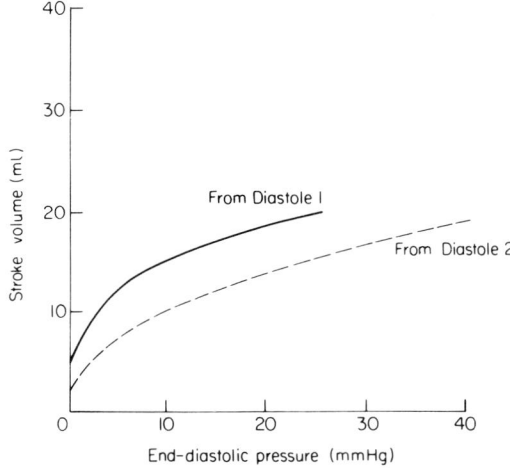

FIG. 6.15c.   Stroke volume/end-diastolic pressure curves for the two circumstances in (a) are different.

completely different curves are obtained. Therefore, if stroke volume (or work) against end-diastolic pressure is used as a 'ventricular function curve' it becomes a function of the diastolic pressure/volume relation as well as the contractile properties. The rate of filling of the ventricle, myocardial infarction, dilatation, hypertrophy etc will all influence this sort of ventricular function curve. This makes the interpretation of changes in these curves extremely difficult.

REFERENCES

ALEXANDER R.S. (1962) Viscoelastic determinants of muscle contractility and 'cardiac tone'. *Fed. Proc.*, **21**, 1001.

BERGLUND E., BORST H.G., DUFF F. & SCHREINER G.L. (1958) Effect of heart rate on cardiac work, myocardial oxygen consumption and coronary flow in the dog. *Acta Physiol., Scand.*, **42**, 185.

BRAUNWALD E., FRYE R.L. & ROSS J. (1960) Studies on Starling's law of the heart. Determinants of the relationship between left ventricular end-diastolic pressure and circumference. *Circulation Res.*, **8**, 1254.

BRECHER G.A. & KISSEN A.T. (1957) Relation of negative intraventricular pressure to ventricular volume. *Circulation Res.*, **5**, 157.

BRECHER G.A., KOLDER H. & HORRER A.D. (1966) Ventricular volume of non-beating excised dog hearts in the state of elastic equilibrium. *Circulation Res.*, **19**, 1080.

EDMAN K.A.P. & JOHANNSSON M. (1976) The contractile state of rabbit papillary muscle in relation to stimulation frequency. *J. Physiol.*, **254**, 565–581.

ELZINGA G. (1972) Crosstalk between left and right heart: PhD Thesis, Free Univ. Amsterdam.

ELZINGA G. & WESTERHOF N. (1979) How does a change in heart rate affect pump function of the left heart ? *J. Physiol.* In Press.

GLANTZ S.A. & KERNOFF R.S. (1975) Muscle stiffness determined from canine left ventricular pressure-volume curves. *Circulation Res.*, **37**, 787–794.

HAWTHORNE E.W. (1961) Instantaneous dimensional changes of the left ventricle in dogs. *Circulation Res.*, **9**, 110.

HEFNER L.L. & BOWEN T.E. (1967) Elastic components of cat papillary muscle. *Am. J. Physiol.*, **212**, 1221.

HEFNER L.L., COGHLAN H.C., JONES W.B. & REEVES T.J. (1962) Distensibility of the dog left ventricle. *Am. J. Physiol.*, **201**, 97–101.

HOFFMAN B.F., BASSETT A.L. & BARTELSTONE H.J. (1968) Some mechanical properties of isolated mammalian cardiac muscle. *Circulation Res.*, **23**, 219–312.

HORWITZ L.D. & BISHOP V.S. (1972) Left ventricular pressure-dimension relationships in the conscious dog. *Cardiovasc. Res.*, **6**, 163–171.

KOCH-WESER J. & BLINKS J.R. (1963) Influence of the interval between beats on myocardial contractility. *Parmacol. Rev.*, **15**, 601.

LEACH J.K. & ALEXANDER R.S. (1965) Effect of epinephrine on stress relaxation and distensibility of the isolated heart. *Am. J. Physiol.*, **209**, 935–940.

LINDEN R.J. & MITCHELL J.H. (1960) Relation between left ventricular diastolic pressure and myocardial segment length and observations on the contribution of atrial systole. *Circulation Res.*, **8**, 1092.

LITTLE R.C. & WEAD W.B. (1971) Diastolic viscoelastic properties of active and quiescent cardiac muscle. *Am. J. Physiol.*, **221**, 1120–1125.

LOEFFLER L. & SAGAWA K. (1975) A one dimensional viscoelastic model of cat heart muscle studied by small length perturbations during isometric contraction. *Circulation Res.*, **36**, 498–512.

LUNDIN G. (1944) Mechanical properties of cardiac muscle. *Acta Physiol., Scand.*, **7** (suppl. 20) 1–85.

MILLER D.E., GLEASON W.L., WHALEN R.E., MORRIS J.J. & McINTOSH H.D. (1962) Effect of ventricular rate on the cardiac output in the dog with chronic heart block. *Circulation Res.*, **10**, 658.

MITCHELL J.H., LINDEN R.J. & SARNOFF S.J. (1960) Influence of cardiac sympathetic and vagal nerve stimulation on the relation between left ventricular diastolic pressure and myocardial segment length. *Circulation Res.*, **8**, 1100.

MITCHELL J.H., WALLACE A.G. & SKINNER N.S. (1963) Intrinsic effects of heart rate on left ventricular performance. *Am. J. Physiol.*, **205**, 41.

MONROE R.G. & FRENCH G.N. (1961) Left ventricular pressure-volume relationships and myocardial oxygen consumption in the isolated heart. *Circulation Res.*, **9**, 362.

NINOMIYA I. & WILSON M.F. (1965) Analysis of ventricular dimension in the unanaesthetized dog. *Circulation Res.*, **16**, 249.

NOBLE M.I.M. (1977) Diastolic viscous properties of cat papillary muscle. *Circulation Res.*, **40**, 287–292.

NOBLE M.I.M., MILNE E.N.C., GOERKE R.J., CARLSSON E., DOMENECH R.J., SAUNDERS K.B. & HOFFMAN J.I.E. (1969) Left ventricular filling and diastolic pressure-volume relations in the conscious dog. *Circulation Res.*, **24**, 269–283.

NOBLE M.I.M., TRENCHARD D. & GUZ A. (1966) Effect of changing heart rate on cardiovascular function in the conscious dog. *Circulation Res.*, **19**, 206.

NOBLE M.I.M., WYLER J., MILNE E.N.C., TRENCHARD D. & GUZ A. (1969) Effect of changes in heart rate on left ventricular performance in conscious dogs. *Circulation Res.*, **24**, 285–295.

PIDGEON J., LAB M.J., SEED W.A., ELZINGA G., PAPADOYANNIS D. & NOBLE M.I.M. (1979) The contractile state of cat and dog heart in relation to stimulation frequency. (Submitted for publication.)

PINTO J.G. & FUNG Y.C. (1973) Mechanical properties of the heart muscle in the passive state. *J. Biomech.*, **6**, 597–616.

RUSHMER R.F. & CRYSTAL D.K. (1951) Changes in configuration of the ventricular chambers during the cardiac cycle. *Circulation*, **4**, 211.

RUSHMER R.F., CRYSTAL D.K., WAGNER C., ELLIS R.M. & NASH A.A. (1954) Continuous measurement of left ventricular dimensions in intact anaesthetized dogs. *Circulation Res.* **2**, 14.

SONNENBLICK E.H., ROSS J., COVELL J.W. & BRAUNWALD E. (1966) Alterations in resting length-tension relations of cardiac muscle induced by changes in contractile force. *Circulation Res.*, **19**, 980–988.

TEMPLETON G.H., DONALD T.C., MITCHELL J.H. & HEFNER L.L. (1973) Dynamic stiffness of papillary muscle during contraction and relaxation. *Am. J. Physiol.*, **224**, 692–698.

WALKER S.M. (1960) Potentiation and hysteresis induced by stretch and subsequent release of papillary muscle. *Am. J. Physiol.*, **198**, 519–522.

WARNER H.E. & TORONTO A.F. (1960) Regulation of cardiac output through stroke volume. *Circulation Res.*, **8**, 549.

CHAPTER 7

THE LOAD SYSTEM—AORTIC INPUT IMPEDANCE

The left ventricle ejects into a complex system of branching tubes. It is common to evaluate it by dividing mean aortic pressure by cardiac output and to regard this as the peripheral resistance. The justification for using mean values has already been discussed in the introductory section of Chapter 4. However, further questions arise: (1) What does the ratio mean pressure/mean flow for the systemic arterial system mean? (2) Are there reactive elements in the system and how can they be characterised? (3) Are there reflections of the pressure-flow pulse? (4) Is the loading system optimised for the left ventricle in any way?

Peripheral resistance

A straightforward resistance can be evaluated by dividing mean pressure drop by mean flow. In electrical analogy we say that the resistance obeys Ohm's law, i.e. the relationship between voltage (or pressure difference) and current (or flow) is a straight line extending from zero with a positive slope (Fig. 7.1a). If this is not the case, difficulties arise. For instance, a number of peripheral vascular beds have a relationship like that in Fig. 7.1b where there is an intercept on the pressure axis, i.e. a certain pressure is required before any flow can occur at all. This is called the critical opening pressure. Another problem is alinearity of the pressure/flow line as occurs in the pulmonary bed (Fig. 7.1c). In either of these situations (Figs. 7.1b and c) pressure/flow is different at every point on the line and cannot therefore be used directly to evaluate the resistance of the bed. The equation for the line must be used instead.

It is not unreasonable to expect the systemic arterial system to behave like Fig. 7.1b because (1) a number of peripheral beds have critical opening pressures, so why not the whole arterial bed? (2) in pacing experiments a rise of cardiac output was accompanied by a smaller percentage rise in mean arterial pressure (Fig. 6.7).

If this is the case, the consequences illustrated in Fig. 7.2 would result. The thick line AB represents the mean pressure/mean flow relationship of the arterial system. At the lowest values of pressure and flow the conventional peripheral resistance is the slope of the dashed line OA. At the highest values of pressure and flow it is given by the slope of the dotted line OB. This slope is considerably less, yet the vascular bed has not changed; there has been no change in the calibre of any constituent vessels. Clearly it is erroneous to say the peripheral resistance has fallen even if the pressure/flow ratio is less.

The result found in the pacing experiment (Chapter 6) could have resulted from

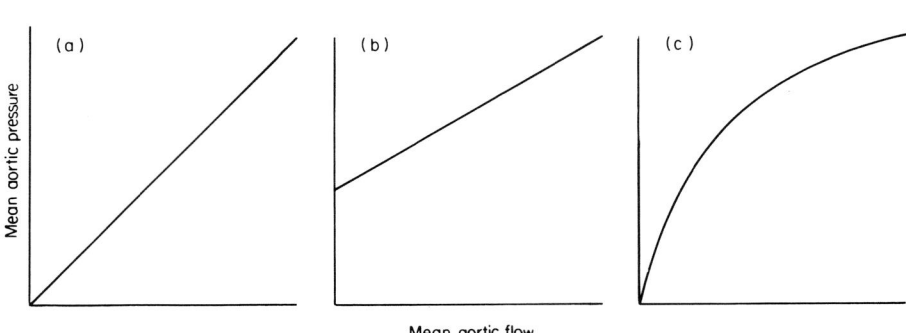

FIG. 7.1. Pressure-flow diagrams for vascular beds. (a) Linear through the origin. (b) Linear with pressure intercept (critical closing pressure). (c) Non-linear.

the baroreflexes responding to a rise in arterial pressure to produce peripheral vaso-dilation. To test whether the peripheral vascular bed is really like Fig. 7.2 it would be necessary to change cardiac output and follow arterial pressure after blockade of nervous reflexes and possibly also catecholamine release. It is surprising that this experiment has only recently been done by Sagawa and Eisner. They interposed a pump between the vena cavae and the right atrium so that the flow through the right ventricle, pulmonary circulation and left heart was controlled by the pump setting. The pressure-flow relationship found was similar to that obtained in the pacing experiment (Fig. 6.7). They then removed the baroflexes by (1) destroying the vagus and carotid sinus nerves, or (2) producing generalised autonomic ganglionic blockade with hexamethonium. The latter intervention causes hypotension so that the pre-hexamethonium level of pressure had to be resored with a noradrenaline infusion.

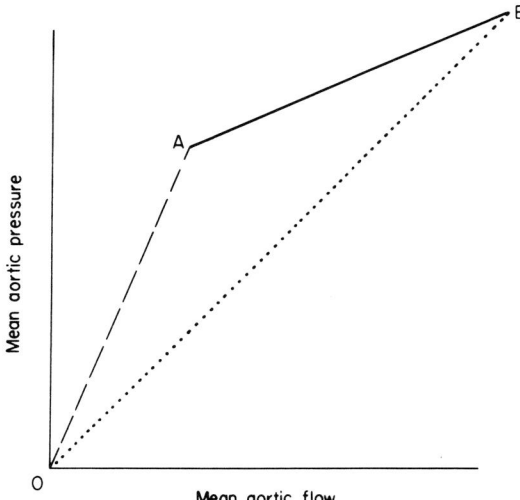

FIG. 7.2. Consequences of vascular bed of type shown in Fig. 7.1b. 'Peripheral resistance', i.e. pressure/flow, at *A* is the slope of the dashed line. At *B* this has declined to the value of the slope of the dotted line.

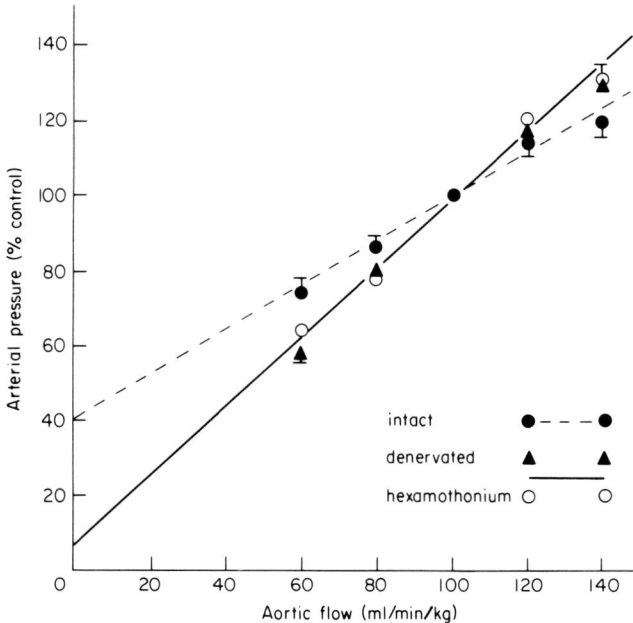

FIG. 7.3. Pressure flow diagrams obtained in dogs for the entire systemic bed. The results in the control state (dashed line) are similar to those shown in Figs. 6.7. and 7.2. Removal of the baroreflexes causes the relationship to pass through the origin as in Fig. 7.1a (continuous line). From Sagawa and Eisner (1975).

The results are shown in Fig. 7.3. The control dashed line shows a pressure/flow line angled away from the origin with an apparent pressure intercept of about 40 mm Hg. The continuous line is fitted to the data after denervation and pharmacological blockade. All three sets of data are reasonably linear. The pressure intercept after baroreflex removal is 3 mm Hg which is not significantly different from zero. Sagawa and Eisner therefore conclude that 'the conventional practice of calculating total peripheral resistance as pressure/flow and evaluating reflex control of it in terms of the changes in that value involves only a small error in the moderately sub- and supranormal flow range'. Thus, the change in the pressure/flow ratio with increasing flow in Fig. 7.2 and Fig. 7.3 dashed line does indeed indicate a true fall in resistance and opening and/or widening of peripheral vascular channels.

Dynamic resistance

In view of the importance of the conclusion of Sagawa and Eisner (above), the experiment deserves to be repeated and confirmed. The possibility of a slope to the pressure/flow line which is less than the peripheral resistance (Fig. 7.2) leads to other thoughts. Could it be that if one produced very slow excursions of pressure and flow through the systemic vascular bed, say sinusoidal variations at a fifth of cycle/sec (e.g. with breathing), the ratio of the amplitudes of the pressure and flow waves in the physiological range might be different from the mean pressure/flow ratio or peripheral resistance. Such very slow oscillations would be too slow to produce much in the way of reactive (capacitative and inductive) effects and the pressure/flow ratio can be considered as a 'dynamic resistance'. If Sagawa and Eisner are correct, dynamic resistance is a function of baroreflex sensitivity. A lower 'resistance' to changing flow than to steady flow might be of some advantage to the heart. The heart produces intermittent pulses of flow, the periphery requires a reasonably constant flow so that potentially one might think the oscillatory pump was a bad design, wasting energy. The question 'how does the arterial system match the pulsating pump to the peripheral resistance?' will be a recurring one in this chapter. One contribution to the solution of the problem could be by having a lower resistance to slow flow oscillations (dynamic resistance) than to steady flow (peripheral resistance).

The experiment of passing very slow sine waves of flow through the systemic arterial tree is impractical. An alternative way of obtaining similar information is to pace the heart in a random fashion. With random flow and pressure signals it is possible to calculate mathematically the pressure/flow ratio at frequencies far below

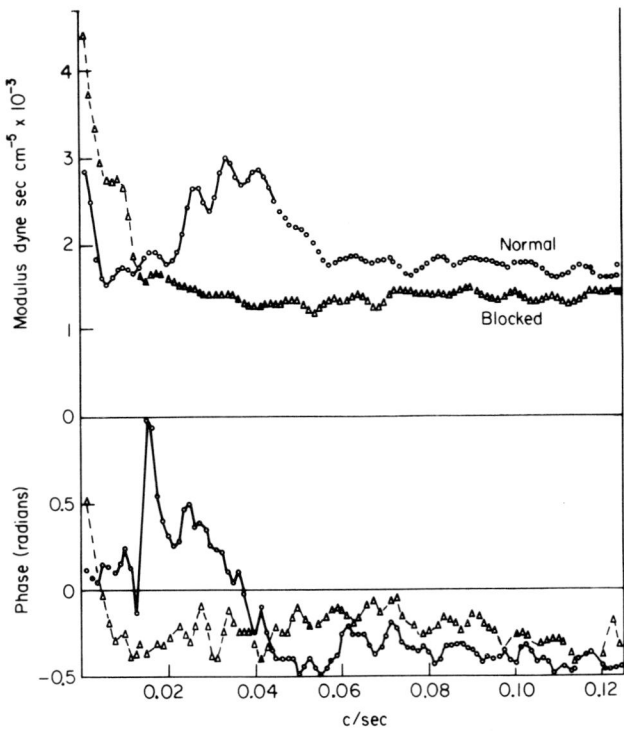

FIG. 7.4. Aortic impedance at very low frequencies before and after ganglionic blockade (blocked). The modulus of impedance (pressure/flow) in the blocked case approaches a value of 5000 dyne sec cm^{-5}, a value of the same order of magnitude as I would expect for the peripheral resistance of a dog (actual value not given). With baroreflexes intact the modulus approaches a lower value as one would expect from the lower slope of the unblocked pressure flow diagram in Fig. 7.3. From Taylor (1966).

the natural heart rate frequency. This was done by Taylor (Fig. 7.4) whose data indicate that the pressure/flow ratio is less than the peripheral resistance. This was probably not the case after pharmacological reflex blockade (Fig. 7.4) suggesting that this phenomenon is due to baroreflexes. The factors influencing impedance at frequencies below 0·5 cycles/sec will be considered in Chapter 9.

Aortic input impedance

If the arterial system was a pure resistance, aortic pressure would have the same wave shape as aortic flow and would drop to zero in diastole as does aortic flow. However, aortic pressure has a different wave form and remains high in diastole—an important feature for the maintenance of tissue perfusion particularly in the coronary bed. Hales was the first to measure arterial pressure directly by cannulation of an artery. He thought the arteries must act as a compression chamber, damping the flow oscillations and providing a steady pressure head as is the case in old fashioned fire engines. This idea later became known as the Windkessel theory. It will become evident in this and subsequent chapters that the arterial system is more complicated than this. However, an important function of the arterial system is to act as a Windkessel thus helping again to match the oscillating pump to the peripheral resistance. Moreover, the input impedance of the aorta (below), i.e. the arterial system as the left ventricle 'sees' it, can be closely simulated by a hydraulic Windkessel model (see below).

In order for the waveforms of aortic flow and pressure to be different there must be reactive (capacitative and/or inductive) components to the system. The Windkessel is a simple capacitance. Therefore, in order to characterize the system we cannot just consider the mean pressure and flow terms; we must know about higher frequencies or harmonics, i.e. more of the frequency domain.

Imagine that one disconnected the left ventricle from the aorta and substituted a mechanical pump which pushed sine waves of pressure and flow into the arterial system. If the impedance to flow is high there will be large fluctuations of pressure. The magnitude of the impedance is given by the amplitude of the pressure sine wave divided by the amplitude of the flow sine wave; this ratio is called the 'modulus of impedance'.

In the arterial system we find that the pressure and flow sine waves are not in phase. In Fig. 7.5 is illustrated a case where flow peaks before pressure, in fact it peaks as pressure is crossing zero on the upstroke. The time that flow is in advance is one quarter of a complete cycle which is measured as 360°. Thus the flow is 90° ahead of pressure; this is called (by convention) a phase angle of −90°, and occurs when the impedance is a pure capacitance. If the impedance is a pure resistance, pressure and flow are in phase and the phase angle is zero. If the impedance is a pure inductance (inertance), pressure will be 90° ahead of flow and the phase angle is +90°. Thus the phase angle of aortic input impedance can be between −90° and +90°. The whole impedance is characterized by the modulus and phase angle together.

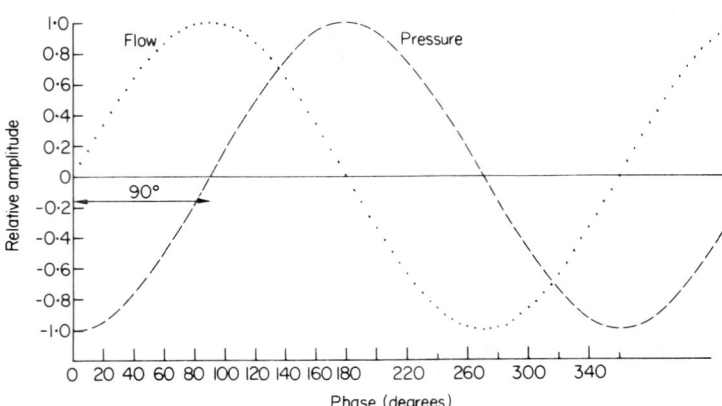

FIG. 7.5.   Diagram of sine waves of flow and pressure with flow leading pressure in phase by 90°.

When one examines the arterial system in this way, one finds that the values for the modulus and phase of impedance vary with the frequency of the sine waves of pressure and flow with which one oscillates the system. Thus the complete aortic input impedance consists of a plot of modulus and phase of impedance against frequency. This analysis as a function of frequency will be called 'analysis in the frequency domain'. It is a difficult concept to grasp when looking at naturally occurring pressure and flow signals which change as functions of time. However, impedance as a function of time is difficult to evaluate in the 'time domain' (see below).

If one did actually replace the left ventricle by a sinusoidal pump it would be very impractical to make measurements of impedance. The arterial bed would also change as a result of the procedure. This difficulty is circumvented by use of Fourier analysis. Any repetitive waveform can be synthesised by adding together a sine wave of the same frequency as the waveform (e.g. flow and pressure), a sine wave of twice the frequency, one of three times the frequency and so on until one reaches a total sum which reproduces the waveform exactly. All these sine waves have different amplitude and phase angle. The sine wave of the same frequency as the waveform (in our case equal to heart rate) is called the fundamental or first harmonic. The sine wave of twice this frequency is called the second harmonic and so on for the other frequencies. There is also a 'zero frequency' term, sometimes called the 'zeroth harmonic'. This is merely the mean value used in the calculation of peripheral resistance (above), i.e. mean arterial pressure in the case of aortic pressure and cardiac output of aortic flow. Thus a complete description of aortic input impedance consists of the peripheral resistance (mean aortic pressure/mean aortic flow) plus a series of values at heart rate frequency, twice heart rate frequency, etc for modulus of impedance (amplitude of pressure harmonic/amplitude of flow harmonic) and phase angle of impedance (phase angle of pressure harmonic minus phase angle of flow harmonic) (Fig. 7.6). The reader might be daunted by the prospect of the mathematical calculations involved in deriving all the pressure and flow harmonics from his measurements of

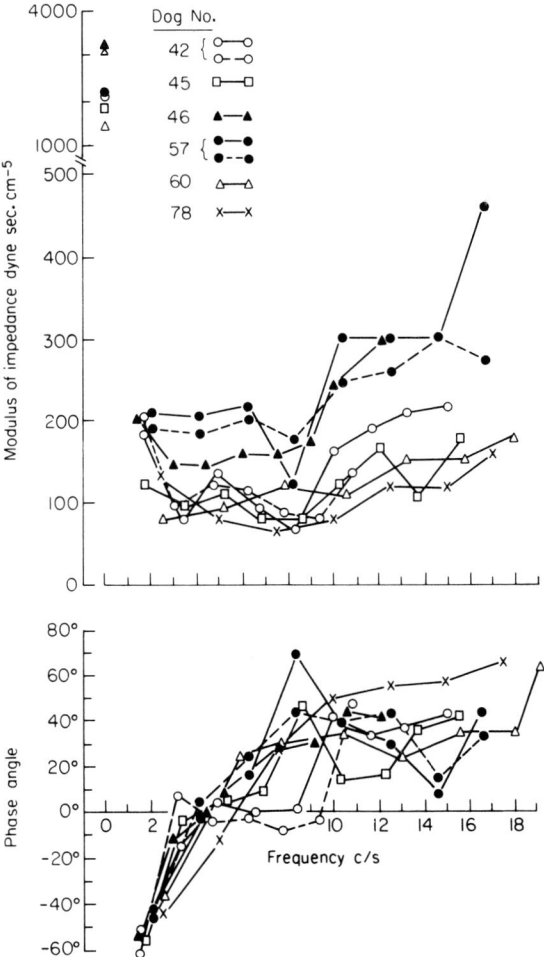

F IG. 7.6. Aortic input impedance in dogs. The points at zero frequency represent peripheral resistance. From Noble *et al.* (1967).

the aortic pressure and flow waveforms. In fact the calculations are readily available in modern computer 'packages'. In order to check that the computer has produced the correct answers it should be asked to add up all the pressure harmonics to check that the resultant waveform is the same as the original aortic pressure waveform and likewise for flow. Care is required with phase measurements to exclude two common sources of error: (1) electromagnetic flowmeters have greater electronic delays than pressure amplifiers leading to an instrumental cause of more positive phase angles of impedance. (2) Pressure and flow must be measured at the same point. If pressure is measured proximal to flow, phase angles of impedance will be too positive; if pressure is measured distal to flow the reverse is the case.

A much more serious worry arises in the use of this method of calculation of aortic input impedance. If the plot shown in Fig. 7.6 truly characterises the arterial system above, it must be the same regardless of the nature of the pressure and flow pulses put into the arterial system by the heart. The test usually applied to check this point is to pace the heart at different frequencies, with results similar to those shown in Fig. 7.7. Here we see that the impedance plots for different heart rates are all very close together. However, this is not a fair test. As we saw in Chapter 6, increasing heart rate by pacing can raise the arterial pressure and lead to baroreflex vasodilation. This is indicated in Fig. 7.7 by the fall in the value of the 'zero frequency term', i.e. the peripheral resistance, with increasing heart rate. One requires to change the input to the system without changing it by the intervention. This is achieved in Fig. 7.8a by giving intracoronary injections of calcium ion or catecholamine to make the heart put out a more rapidly rising flow curve with a higher peak flow and shorter duration. A different series of sine waves (harmonics) is required to synthesise the flow and pressure waveforms resulting from this intervention. However, the impedance plot calculated from these different pressure and flow harmonics is the same (Fig. 7.8b). This confirms that the input impedance plot describes the arterial system.

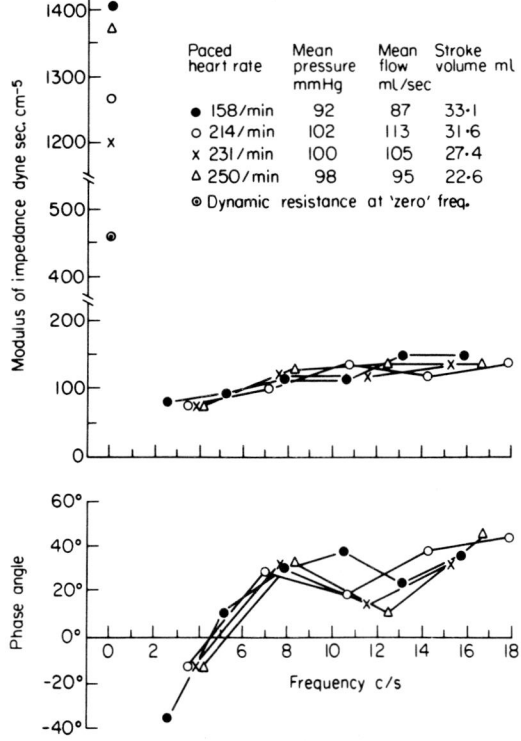

FIG. 7.7. Aortic input impedance at four different heart rates achieved by electrical pacing of the right atrium over a period of 20 sec. Points at zero frequency represent peripheral resistance, except ○, the 'dynamic resistance at zero frequency' obtained from the slope of the regression line between mean pressure and mean flow (Fig. 6.7). Note superposition of impedance values. From Noble *et al.* (1967).

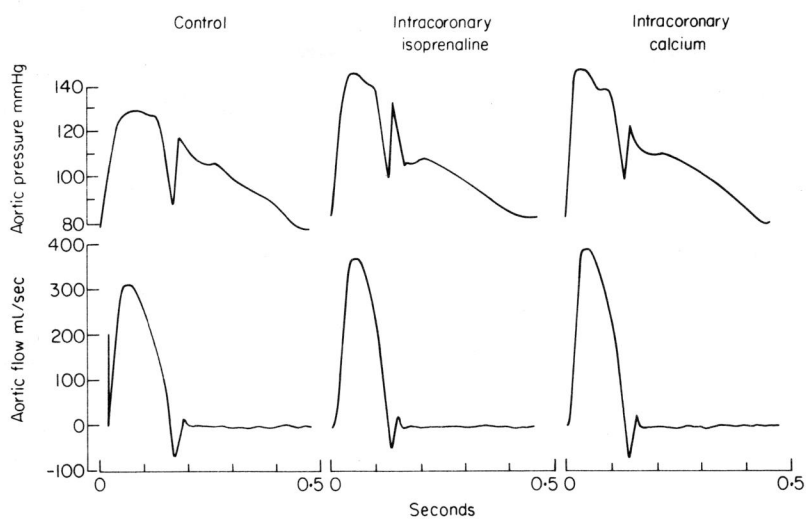

FIG. 7.8a.   Aortic input impedances during a control period and following intracoronary injection of isoprenaline and calcium gluconate. From Noble *et al.* (1967).

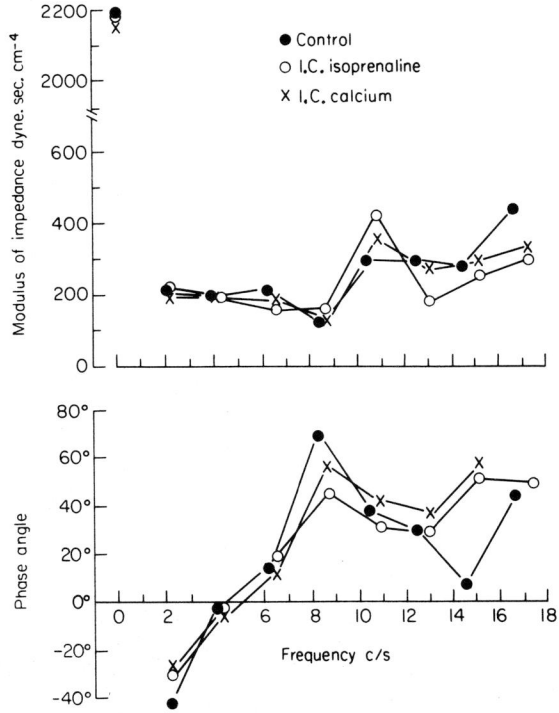

FIG. 7.8b.   Aortic pressure and flow waveforms during a control period and after intracoronary injection of isoprenaline and calcium. Note that impedances in (*b*) are superimposed in spite of the different wave shapes (*a*) used in their calculation. From Noble *et al.* (1967).

Having gone to all this trouble to obtain aortic input impedance one might well wonder whether it has any use. Fig. 7.7 shows that peripheral vasodilatation causes a fall in the peripheral resistance (zero frequency term) but little change in any other aspect of impedance. This indicates that impedance at higher frequencies is rather insensitive to changes in the peripheral vascular bed; this impression is confirmed by experiments with vasoconstricting and vasodilating drugs. The impedance at higher frequencies is changed more by alterations in the compliance of the arterial walls, e.g. stiff arteries give higher moduli and more positive phase angles. However, again impedance is not particularly sensitive to such changes which can be detected just as easily by finding increased pulse pressure for the same output.

The usefulness of input impedance is therefore not as a practical sensitive measure of changes in the arterial system. It is rather to understand the system and how it is adapted to its function of converting a totally pulsatile aortic inflow to a reasonably steady pressure head for perfusion of peripheral vascular beds. An examination of this function will be carried out in subsequent sections of this book. Before embarking on this it should be pointed out that the magnitude of the impedance (Fig. 7.6) (expressed as moduli) is very low compared with peripheral resistance. This is of great practical importance in regard to the work done by the heart. It means that although the output of the heart is totally *pulsatile*, nearly all the mechanical energy is dissipated in the production of *steady* flow through the peripheral vascular bed. Less than 10% of the mechanical energy is wasted in overcoming frequency dependent impedance to flow, at least under normal resting conditions.

The Windkessel

Earlier mention was made of this idea of the arterial system as a compression chamber. The model has fallen into disfavour because it was realised that there are pressure waves which travel along the elastic tubes (arteries). Wave travel does not occur in a Windkessel. However recent studies have reinstated the value of the Windkessel. Westerhof, Elzinga and Sipkema built a hydraulic model which is illustrated in Fig. 7.9 and is a modified Windkessel. There is an inlet tube with resistance similar to the characteristic impedance of the aorta, there is an air filled chamber (c) which is the Windkessel itself, there is a 'peripheral resistance' consisting of a number of parallel capillary tubes.

The important point is that this simple model with rigid walls which do not allow wave travel has the same input impedance as the arterial system (Fig. 7.10). Thus when a real heart is attached to this model, the resulting flow and pressure waveforms are also like those in an intact animal (Fig. 7.11). Thus when the heart 'looks into' the aortic input impedance it 'sees' a load which is almost indistinguishable from a Windkessel.

The flow delivered through the capillary tubes of the peripheral resistance has little pulsatility because of the damping effect of the air chamber (c). The perfusion

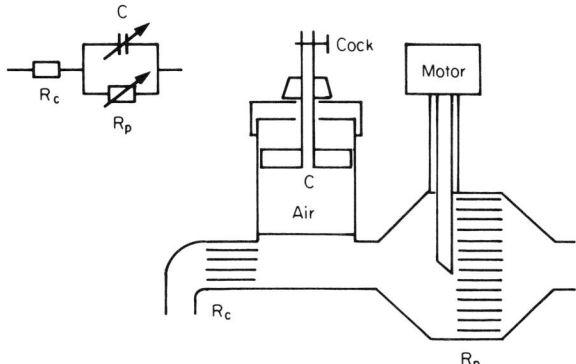

FIG. 7.9. Hydraulic model of the systemic arterial system R_c = aortic characteristic impedance (impedance of proximal aorta alone), C = compliance (Windkessel) controlled by amount of air allowed via cock, R_p = peripheral resistance controlled by motor operated sliding shutter. Electrical analogue equivalent inset. From Westerhof *et al.* (1977).

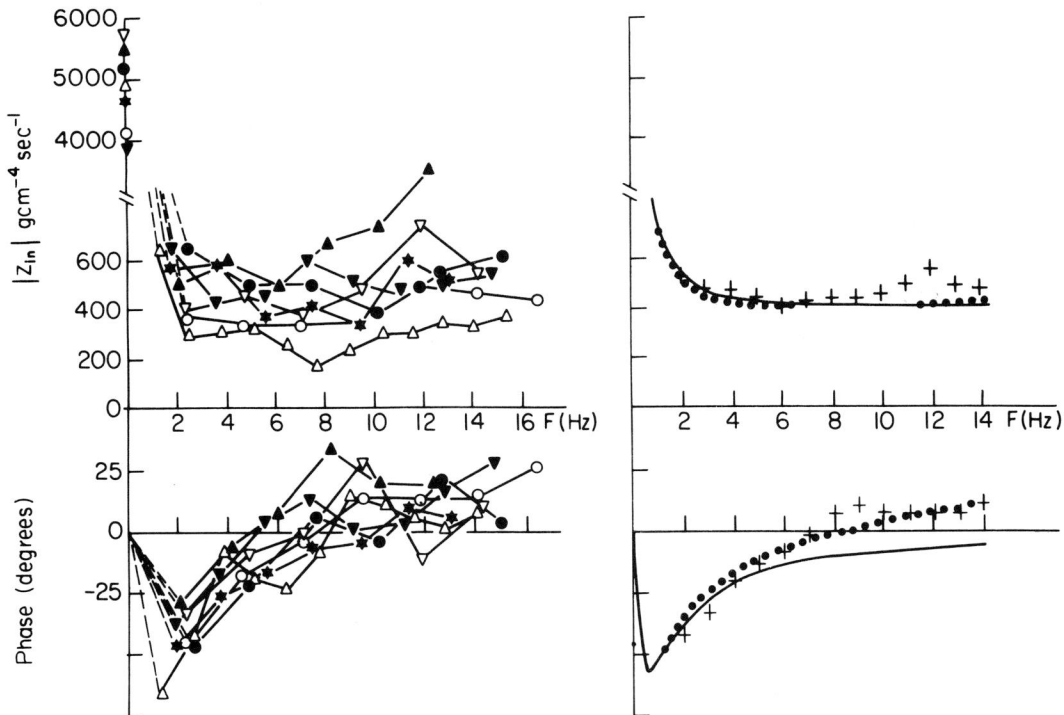

FIG. 7.10. Left: modulus and phase of the hydraulic input impedance in seven dogs. Pressure and flow were measured in the ascending aorta. Right: Plusses, average impedance values of seven dogs are determined by averaging the interpolated data (left) at integer values of frequency. Fully drawn line: impedance of the three element Windkessel model (Fig. 7.9.). Dotted line: Impedance of the same Windkessel but with an inertia element in series with R_c. From Westerhof *et al.* (1977).

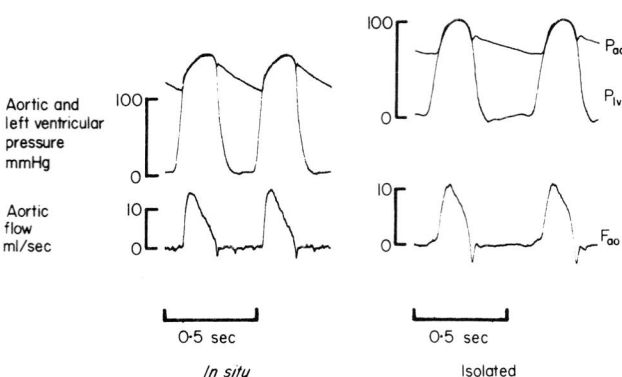

Aortic and left ventricular pressure mmHg

Aortic flow ml/sec

In situ   Isolated

FIG. 7.11.   Left ventricular (P_{lv}) and aortic (P_{ao}) pressures and aortic flow (F_{ao}) as measured (left), in the open thorax of a cat and (right) when an isolated cat heart pumps into the hydraulic model in Fig. 7.9. Pressures in mm Hg, flows in ml/sec.

pressure of this resistance, 'arterial pressure' has much less pulsatility than the aortic inflow pulse. Therefore, this simulated arterial system functions very like a Windkessel.

As we shall see later the real arterial system is very different from a Windkessel because of the features necessary to distribute blood, i.e. branching tubes traversing the various distances from the heart to different organs. However, the experiments of Westerhof do highlight the fact that this arterial system fulfills with remarkable accuracy the *functions* of a Windkessel.

The elastic tube

The simplest way to simulate the arterial system might be to use a long piece of rubber tube closed off at the end. This was done by Taylor. He showed that in such a tube pressure and flow waves travelled down to the end of the tube and were reflected back from the end. They then travelled back towards the entrance and interacted with new forward going waves. The input impedance of this model has a number of high peaks and troughs (Fig. 7.12). If the length of the tube is such that it is a multiple of half a wave length, maxima are obtained as forward and reflected waves summate. Minima occur half way between so that the first minimum is obtained at one quarter wave length. For a tube of given length, the impedance at the inlet changes with frequency from maxima to minima and back every time the length of the tube is a multiple of a quarter of a wave length. (Wave length = velocity of wave travel down the tube (see Chapter 9) divided by frequency.) The phase angle of impedance crosses zero (changes sign) at the same frequency as the maxima and minima.

It is very clear that the input impedance of this tube is very different from that of the aorta (Fig. 7.6); the tube simulates aortic input impedance much less well than does a Windkessel (Fig. 7.10). Nevertheless, because it is more like an arterial system than is an air chamber, many authors have tried to interpret the aortic input impedance in terms of Taylor's model. This leads to the conclusion that the frequency at which the

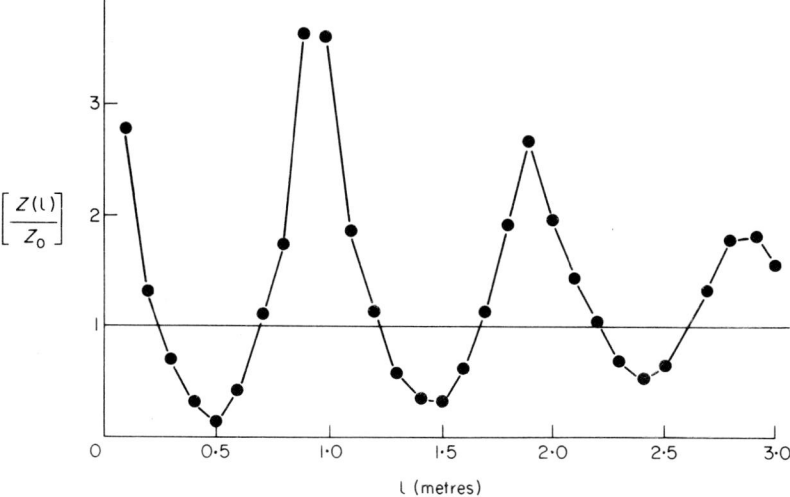

FIG. 7.12. The input impedance of a rubber tube with closed end, plotted with distance from the inlet (left) to which the oscillations were applied. The frequency used was 7 Hz, wave length 2·0 metres. The deviation of the nodes and antinodes diminished progressively with distance from the pump due to damping. From Taylor (1957).

phase angle reaches zero (5–10 Hz) is accompanied by a minimum in the impedance moduli! This then leads to the conclusion that, for a wave velocity of 5 m/sec, the end of the tube (the so-called 'major reflecting site') is 12–25 cm from the aortic valve. In order to examine this problem it is necessary to look at reflections in the arterial system in a simpler fashion.

The forward and backward pressure and flow waves in the aorta

When pressure and flow waves are reflected and travel backwards towards the entrance of the tube, the backward pressure wave is added to the forward going pressure wave; the measured wave is the sum of the two. The backward flow wave is subtracted from the forward going flow wave; the measured wave is the difference between the two. It is therefore possible for each pair of pressure and flow harmonics, with knowledge of the proportion of the wave reflected (the reflection coefficient, a function of impedance), to calculate the forward and backward components of each pressure and flow harmonic. We can then add the forward components of the pressure and flow harmonics to obtain the forward pressure and flow waveforms, add the backward components of the pressure and flow harmonics to obtain the backward pressure and flow waveforms. New equations by Westerhof *et al.* (1978) indicate that these waveforms can be obtained more simply and directly by addition and subtraction in the time domain.*

* If P_m and F_m = measured pressure and flow, P_f and F_f = forward pressure and flow, P_b and F_b = backward pressure and flow, and Z_c = characteristic impedance of aorta, then: P_f and $F_f \times Z_c$ both equal $\frac{1}{2}(P_m + F_m \times Z_c)$; P_b and $-F_b \times Z_c$ both equal $\frac{1}{2}(P_m - F_m \times Z_c)$.

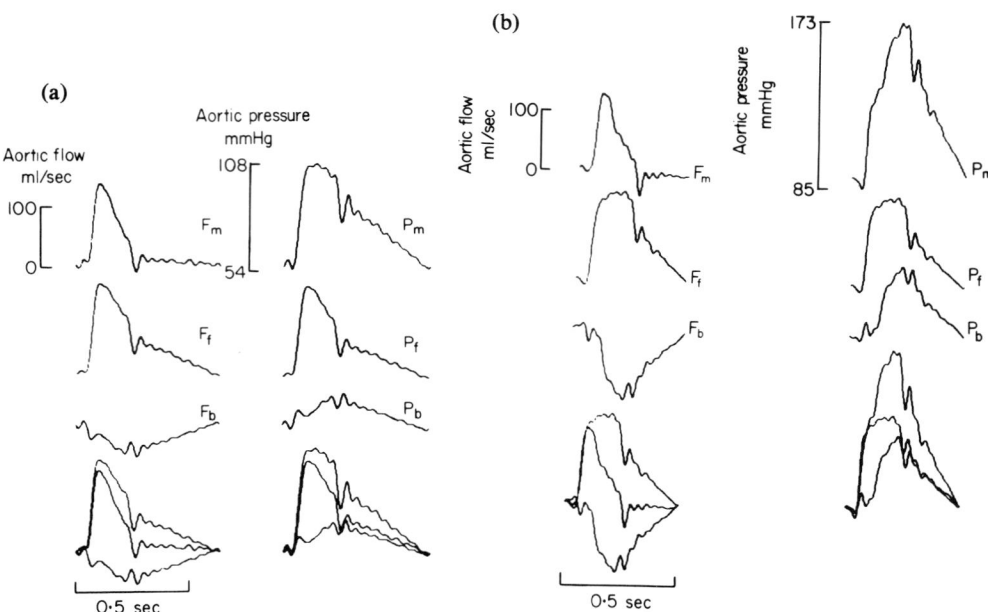

FIG. 7.13.   Relation between measured (F_m, P_m), forward (F_f, P_f) and reflected (F_b, P_b) flow (F) and pressure (P). The lower part of each panel shows how summation of forward and reflected waves gives the measured flow or pressure. (a) control traces. (b) Occlusion of the descending aorta to give a larger reflected component. From Van den Bos *et al.* (1976).

An example of such waveforms is shown in Fig. 7.13a. It is possible for the physiologist unfamiliar with Fourier analysis to check that the computations are correct because with reflected waves the forward pressure and flow waveforms are identical; this is indeed the case (Fig. 7.13). The backward pressure and flow waveforms are also identical but because reflected flow subtracts from forward flow it is presented upside down (Fig. 7.13). It is clear that these forward and backward waves are the only ones which, when added together, give the measured pressure waveform and when subtracted give the flow waveform.

It is apparent that the reflected waves F_b and P_b in Fig. 7.13a are small and diffusely spread out in time. This is unlike the result to be expected from a major reflecting site which would give a distinct peak in the reflected wave. That this would be the case can be shown by introducing a major reflecting site artificially by blowing up a balloon in the descending aorta (Fig. 7.13b). We now see steeply rising reflected waves occurring after time has elapsed for them to travel from the aortic valve to the balloon and back. It can also be seen from Fig. 7.13b that the large reflected wave causes a much higher pressure (reflected pressure adds) and lower flow (reflected flow subtracts).

The important consequence of this is that major reflections increase the pressure load on the heart which would be disadvantageous. In reality, the arterial system seems to be adapted in such a way that this disadvantage (seen in its most extreme form in Taylor's model, Fig. 7.12) is avoided. The way in which the amount of reflected pressure reaching the heart is minimised is an important feature of the function of the arterial system (Chapter 9). The important point in the present context, i.e. the aortic input impedance 'as the heart sees it' is that this reflected pressure is small in magnitude and diffused in time (Fig. 7.13a). It is also clear that the zero phase angle of impedance at 5–10 Hz (Fig. 7.6) is not indicative of a major reflecting site but merely reflects the change from predominantly capacitative properties at low frequency (negative phase angle, flow leading pressure in time) to a dynamic resistance at 5–10 Hz (flow and pressure in phase). At higher frequencies, positive phase angles may be obtained due to the dominance of blood mass inertia in the proximal aorta (Chapter 8).

The unit impulse response of the arterial system

Mention has already been made of the conceptual difficulties experienced by the cardiovascular physiologist confronted with the need to think of impedance as a function of frequency. He feels a need to express impedance as a function of time which has more realism and this leads to erroneous calculations of 'instantaneous impedance' from instantaneous values of pressure and flow.

One of the virtues of the forward and reflected wave analysis (above) is that these waves can be reconverted to the 'time domain' (Fig. 7.13). However, the actual waves produced still depend, of course, on the contraction of the heart. Different waveforms will be produced if the heart is stimulated, e.g. by intracoronary calcium (Fig. 7.8a). In order to determine the characteristics of the arterial system alone one needs to remove this dependence on left ventricular ejection.

The difficulties of such analysis are very great. The most successful attempt is that of Laxminarayan *et al.* who used mathematical processes even more complicated than Fourier analysis. If it were possible to derive impedance plots which are continuous functions of frequency, i.e. defined at all frequencies not just harmonics, and for a frequency range to infinitely high frequencies, then the impedance could be easily converted into the time domain. A difficulty arises, however, in that one can only obtain the impedance function up to some maximum frequency in the range 20–30 Hz where the pressure and flow components become very small. Then the derived time domain function shows large oscillations with that arbitrary cut off frequency. Laxminarayan *et al.* dealt with this problem by adding a filter to remove this frequency from the time domain function.

The time domain function is called 'the unit impulse response' (Fig. 7.14). The reader has to imagine that the heart is removed and a very large, brief, square wave of flow is forced into the arterial system. This input spike is called a 'unit impulse'. The resulting pressure, the response to the unit impulse; is solely determined by physical characteristics of the arterial system. The pressure also rises rapidly to a peak as one would expect, but the slow decay is due to the damping (capacitative) properties of the system. This is what one would expect from a Windkessel.

In a pure Windkessel, the pressure would decay steadily to zero. In an elastic

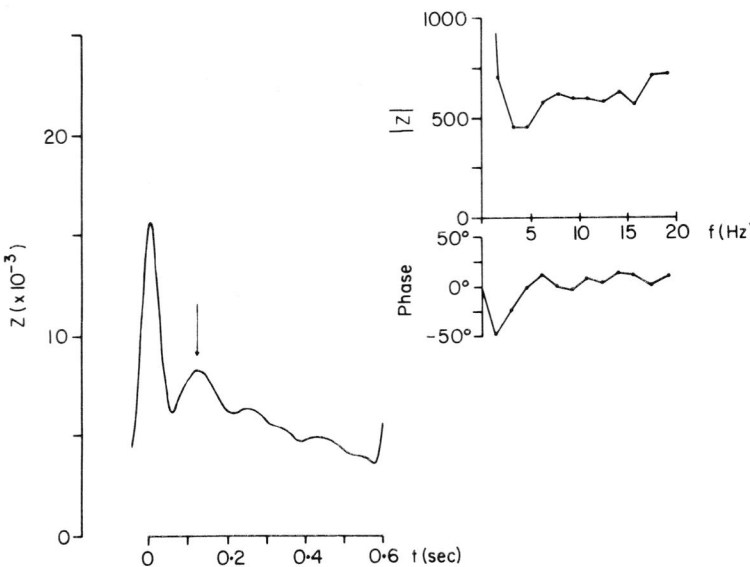

FIG. 7.14. Unit impulse response of dog systemic arterial system. Units are g cm^{-4} sec^{-2}. Arrow denotes reflected wave. To the right is shown the simultaneously calculated impedance as a function of frequency. Units are g cm^{-4} sec^{-1}. From Laxminarayan *et al.* (1977).

tube the steep pressure would travel to the end and back again and produce a sharp second peak in the unit impulse response. That this is not found in the arterial system (Fig. 7.14) is entirely consistent with the flat impedance as a function of frequency (Fig. 7.6) and the lack of a sharp peaked reflected wave (Fig. 7.13a). The unit impulse response does not decay smoothly to zero as a single function (Fig. 7.14). There is a small amplitude diffuse secondary pressure wave. This is consistent with the small diffuse reflected waves obtained with a physiological flow pulse (Fig. 7.13a) instead of a unit impulse.

REFERENCES

ATTINGER E.O. (Ed.) (1964) *Pulsatile Blood Flow.* McGraw-Hill, New York.

ATTINGER E.O., ANNE A. & McDONALD D.A. (1966) Use of Fourier series for the analysis of biophysical systems. *Biophys. J.*, **6**, 291–304.

BERGEL D.H. (Ed.) (1972) *Cardiovascular Fluid Dynamics.* Academic Press, London and New York.

CARO C.G., PEDLEY T.J., SCHROTER R.C. & SEED W.A. (1978) *The Mechanics of the Circulation.* Oxford Univ. Press.

ELZINGA G. & WESTERHOF N. (1973) Pressure and flow generated by the left ventricle against different impedances. *Circulation Res.*, **32**, 178–186.

FRANK O. (1899) Die Grundform des Arteriellen Puls. *Z. Biol.*, **437**, 483–526.

FRANK O. (1905) Der Puls in den Arterien. *Z. Biol.*, **46**, 441–553.

GABE I.T., KARNELE J., PORJE G. & RUDEWALD B. (1964) The measurement of input impedance and apparent phase velocity in the human aorta. *Acta Physiol.*, *Scand.*, **61**, 76–85.

HALES S. (1769) *Haemostatics.* Statical Essays, London.

JAGER G.N., WESTERHOF N. & NOORDERGRAAF A. (1965) Oscillatory flow impedance in electrical analog of arterial system. *Circulation Res.*, **16**, 121–133.

LAXMINARAYAN S., SIPKEMA P. & WESTERHOF N. (1977) Characterization of the arterial system in the time domain. *I.E.E.E. Trans, Bio-Med. Eng.*

MILLS C.J., GABE I.T., GAULT J.H., MASON D.J., ROSS J., BRAUNWALD E. & SHILLINGFORD J.P. (1970) Pressure-flow relationships and vascular impedance in man. *Cardiovasc. Res.*, **4**, 405–417.

MILNOR W.R. (1975) Arterial impedance as ventricular afterload. *Circulation Res.*, **36**, 565–570.

MCDONALD D.A. (1974) *Blood Flow in Arteries*. Edward Arnold, London.

MCDONALD D.A. & TAYLOR M.G. (1959) The hydrodynamics of the arterial circulation. *Progress Biophys. and Biophys. Chem.* Vol. 9. J.A.V. Butler and B. Katz Eds. Pergamon Press, Oxford.

NICHOLS W.W., CONTI R., WALKER W.E. & MILNOR W.R. (1977) Input impedance of the systemic circulation in man. *Circulation Res.*, **40**, 451–458.

NOBLE M.I.M., GABE I.T., TRENCHARD D. & GUZ A. (1967) Blood pressure and flow in the ascending aorta of conscious dogs. *Cardiovasc. Res.*, **1**, 9–20.

NOBLE M.I.M., TRENCHARD D. & GUZ A. (1966) Effect of changing heart rate on cardiovascular function in the conscious dog. *Circulation Res.*, **19**, 206–213.

O'ROURKE M.F. (1967) Steady and pulsatile energy losses in the systemic circulation under normal conditions and in simulated arterial disease. *Cardiovasc. Res.*, **1**, 313–326.

O'ROURKE M.F. & TAYLOR M.G. (1967) Input impedance of the systemic circulation. *Circulation Res.*, **20**, 365–380.

PATEL D.J., DE FREITAS F.M. & FRY D.L. (1963) Hydraulic input impedance to aorta and pulmonary artery in dogs. *J. Appl. Physiol.*, **18**, 134–140.

PATEL D.J., MASON D.T., ROSS J. & BRAUNWALD E. (1965) Harmonic analysis of pressure pulses obtained from the heart and great vessels of man. *Am. Heart J.*, **69**, 785–794.

PETERSON L.H. (1954) The dynamics of pulsatile blood flow. *Circulation Res.*, **2**, 127–139.

SAGAWA K. & EISNER A. (1975) Static pressure-flow relation in the total systemic vascular bed of the dog and its modification by the baroreceptor reflex. *Circulation Res.*, **36**, 406–413.

SPENCER M.P., JOHNSTON F.R. & DENISON A.B. (1958) Dynamics of the normal aorta, 'Inertance' and compliance of the arterial system which transforms the cardiac ejection pulse. *Circulation Res.*, **6**, 491–500.

TAYLOR M.G. (1957) An approach to an analysis of the arterial pulse wave. *Phys. Med. Biol.*, **1**, 258–321.

TAYLOR M.G. (1969) Use of random excitation and spectral analysis in the study of frequency dependent parameters of the cardiovascular system. *Circulation Res.*, **18**, 585–595.

TAYLOR M.G., (1966) The input impedance of an assembly of randomly-branching elastic tubes. *Biophys. J.*, **6**, 29–46.

VAN DEN BOS G.C., WESTERHOF N., ELZINGA G. & SIPKEMA P. (1976) Reflection in the systemic arterial system: effects of aortic and carotid occlusions. *Cardiovasc. Res.*, **10**, 565–573.

WESTERHOF N. (1968) *Analog studies of human systemic arterial hemodynamics*. Ph. D. Thesis, Univ. Pennsylvania.

WESTERHOF N., BOSMAN F., DE VRIES C.J. & NOORDERGRAAF A. (1969) Analog studies of the human systemic arterial tree. *J. Biomed.*, **2**, 121–143.

WESTERHOF N., ELZINGA G. & SIPKEMA P. (1971) Artificial system for pumping hearts. *J. Appl. Physiol.*, **31**, 776–781.

WESTERHOF N., ELZINGA G., SIPKEMA P. & VAN DEN BOS G.C. (1977) Quantitative analysis of the arterial system and heart by means of pressure-flow relations. *Cardiovascular Flow Dynamics and Measurements*. N.H.C. Hwang and N.A. Normann Eds. University Park Press, Baltimore.

WESTERHOF N., ELZINGA G. & VAN DEN BOS G.C. (1973) Influence of central and peripheral changes on the hydraulic input impedance of the systemic arterial tree. *Med. Biol. Engng.*, **11**, 710–723.

WESTERHOF N., SIPKEMA P., VAN DEN BOS G.C. & ELZINGA G. (1972) Forward and backward waves in the arterial system. *Cardiovasc. Res.*, **6**, 648–656.

WESTERHOF N., VAN DEN BOS G.C. & LAXMINARAYAN S. (1978) Arterial reflection. In *International Symposium. Dynamics and regulation of the arterial system. Erlangen.*

WETTERER E. & KENNER TH. (1968) *Die Dynamik des Arterien-pulses.* Springer-Verlag, Heidelberg.

CHAPTER 8
PRESSURE GRADIENT

THE RELATIONSHIP BETWEEN THE PULSATILE PRESSURE GRADIENT ALONG AN ARTERY AND FLOW

We now turn from the entire arterial system as seen from the left ventricle (Chapter 7) to the arteries themselves. What governs the flow of blood through these tubes? It is well recognised that the flow along a tube is determined by the difference in pressure between one end and the other. This derives from Poiseuille's law and equation. It is now necessary to use equations which I have, as far as possible, tried to avoid in this book. I now resort to them because there are too many factors to convert the equations into words.

Poiseuille's equation

There are a number of preconditions which are supposed to be fulfilled before the application of this relationship.

(1) The fluid must be homogeneous—an ideal Newtonian liquid. Blood certainly is not such a liquid because of the presence of red cells.

(2) The flow through the tube must be steady. Obviously this is not true in arteries where we have seen that flow is highly pulsatile.

(3) The flow must be laminar and not turbulent. However there is turbulence in the aorta (Fig. 8.1). Turbulent flow is more likely if the mean velocity of blood flow is high, if the density of the liquid is high, if the viscosity of the liquid is low, if the diameter of the tube is large and if there are projections, roughnesses or irregularities in the tube. Turbulence is energy wasting—a larger pressure gradient is required for turbulent than for laminar flow.

(4) There should be no liquid slip at the liquid-tube wall interface.

(5) The tube must be long compared to the region studied. This is because it takes a considerable distance from the inlet of the tube for the distribution of velocities across the tube to become parabolic (Fig. 8.2). Clearly this does not apply to the arterial system where the aorta is an inlet and where there are many branches.

(6) The tube diameter must be constant. The arteries taper.

Having pointed out these pre-conditions and that they are not satisfied in arteries, we can look at Poiseuille's equation:

$$Q = \frac{(P_1 - P_2)\,\pi r^4}{8L\mu} = \frac{p\,\pi r^4}{8\mu}$$

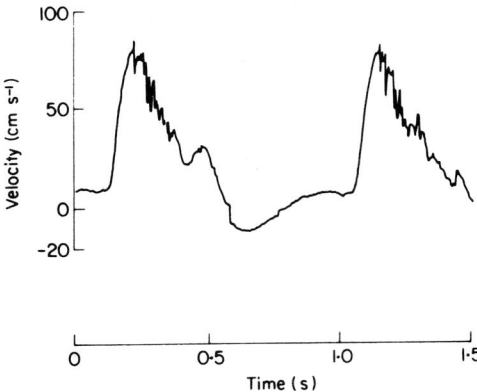

FIG. 8.1.   Record of blood velocity made in the aorta with a hot film anemometer by A. Seed. Note the turbulence during deceleration. From Caro, Pedley, Schroter and Seed (1978).

Q is the flow. P_1 is the pressure at one end of the tube and P_2 at the other end of the tube of length L. This pressure gradient will be abbreviated to $p = [(P_1 - P_2)/L]$, the pressure gradient for unit length. r is the radius of the tube, and μ the viscosity of the liquid. The resistance of the tube (pressure gradient divided by flow) is P/Q which is $8\mu/\pi r^4$, i.e. it increases in proportion to viscosity and decreases in proportion to the fourth power of the radius. For a given tube and liquid this resistance is constant and Q is proportional to p,

$$Q = \frac{p}{\text{resistance}}$$

as in the case of current and voltage with an electrical resistance (Ohm's law). In order to find a modification of Poiseuille's equation which could be applied to arteries, we must turn to Womersley's equation.

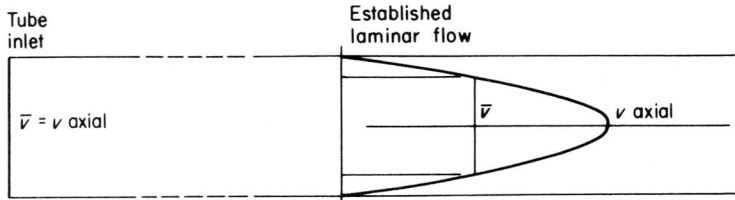

FIG. 8.2.   Velocity of blood flow plotted against distance across the diameter of a tube. At the inlet (left) the velocity is the same across the tube (flat velocity profile) and average velocity ($\bar{v}$) is the same as velocity in the centre (V axial). With established laminar flow (right). The velocity profile is parabolic and average velocity is half axial velocity.

Womersley's equation

Womersley's equation requires all the same preconditions as Poiseuille's except for the second. In place of steady flow through a tube, Womersley considered a sinusoidally oscillating pressure gradient and flow. Here I have to introduce the equation for the sinusoidal pressure gradient (illustrated in Fig. 8.3).

$$p = M \cos (\omega t - \phi)$$

In Fig. 8.3, continuous line, we have the graph of a cosine against angle. At 0° the base equals the hypotenuse and the ratio (cosine) equals 1. In this case it is multiplied by a factor M which is the amplitude of the wave. With increasing angle, the cosine decreases to 0 then goes to $-M$, then back to 0 at 270° and finally reaches $+M$ at 360°. The dashed line shows a cosine wave which is shifted on the angle axis by $\phi°$. Now we need to have time on the angle axis and this is done by multiplying time by the angular frequency ω (cycles/sec $\times$ 360°). The dashed line can now be expressed as:

$$p = M \cos (\omega t - \phi)$$

This is the pressure gradient considered by Womersley.

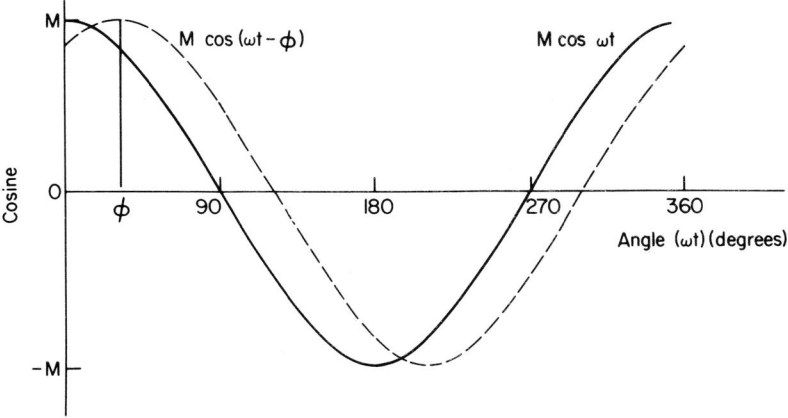

FIG. 8.3.   Diagram of cosine wave with and without phase shift of ϕ degrees.

One can imagine that if a pressure gradient like this was oscillating back and forth slowly in a tube, the flow would follow it quite closely but if the oscillations are faster, the liquid will acquire a momentum during flow in one direction which will make it continue in that direction rather than reverse when the pressure gradient reverses. Therefore, the flow will lag behind the pressure gradient.

One can also imagine that as this tendency increases, the flow will move to and fro less and less until the frequency of oscillation of the pressure gradient is so high that the liquid's inertia holds it virtually stationary. Thus, as frequency increases, flow lags more and more behind pressure gradient, the flow amplitude falls and the velocity profile (Fig. 8.2) becomes flatter. The same tendencies follow from an increase in diameter of the tube because there is a greater mass of fluid with greater inertia. Increased density of liquid will also have the same effect by increasing inertia.

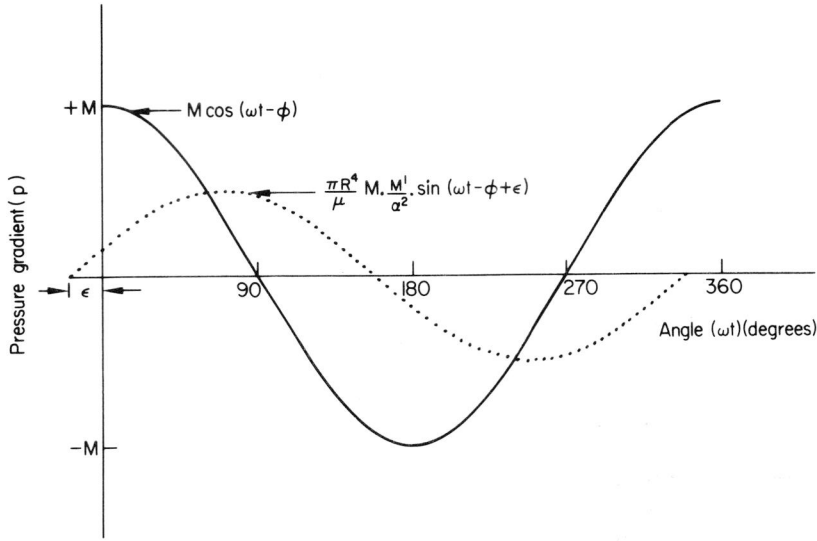

FIG. 8.4.   Diagram of sinusoidal pressure gradient (continuous line) and resultant flow (dotted line).

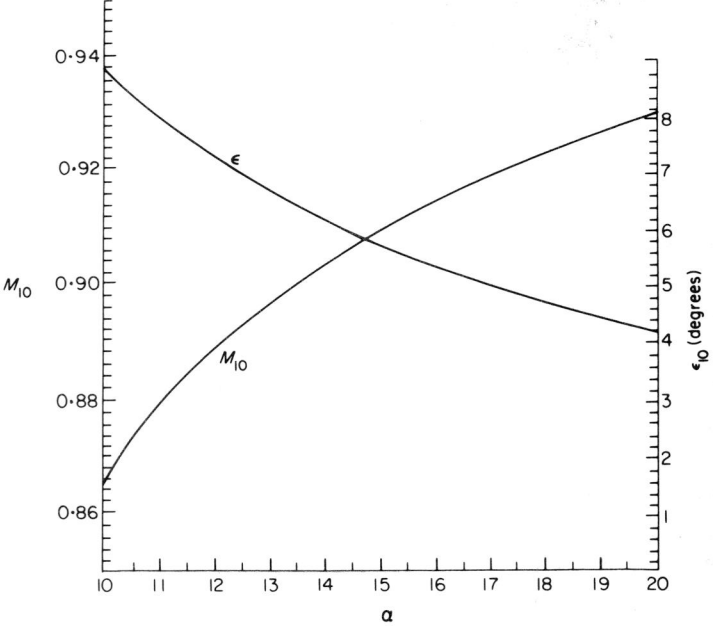

FIG. 8.5.   Relationship between Womersleys factors M^1 and ε and α.

Increased viscosity will counteract these effects. Womersley devised a factor called α to express this tendency:

$$\alpha = R\sqrt{\frac{\omega\rho}{\mu}}$$

where R = radius of tube, ω = angular frequency of oscillation (above), ρ = density of fluid, and μ = viscosity of fluid.

Womersley calculated that the flow resulting from a sinusoidal pressure gradient [$M \cos(\omega t - \phi)$] would also be a sinusoidal wave whose amplitude would be determined by the amplitude of pressure gradient M, the Poiseuille factor $\pi r^4/\mu$ and two other factors M' (a function of α) and $1/\alpha^2$. He also calculated that the lag of flow behind pressure gradient could be expressed by a phase shift $90 - \varepsilon$ (also a function of α).

Thus Womersley's equation states that if $p = M \cos(\omega t - \phi)$

$$Q = \frac{\pi r^4}{\mu} \cdot M \cdot \frac{M^1}{\alpha^2} \sin(\omega t - \phi + \varepsilon)$$

This is illustrated in Fig. 8.4. A sine wave is shifted 90° to the right of a cosine wave, so the phase lag of flow behind pressure gradient is 90° $- \varepsilon$. The details of M' and ε (Fig. 8.5) are not important conceptually but are required if one is to test the correctness of the equation. They are given in tables and can be expressed in formulae for $\alpha > 10$:

$$M' = 1 - \frac{\sqrt{2}}{\alpha} + \frac{1}{\alpha^2}$$

$$\varepsilon = \frac{\sqrt{2}}{\alpha} + \frac{1}{\alpha^2} + \frac{19}{24\sqrt{2}.\alpha^3}$$

It will be noted that Womersley's equation has similar features to Poiseuille's. The amplitude no longer varies linearly with p but is modified by M'/α^2 and lags by 90° $- \varepsilon$. If α is very small, i.e. as α tends towards zero, M'/α^2 tends towards $1/8$ and ε tends towards 90° (Fig. 8.5) when

$$\varepsilon = 90°, \sin(\omega t - \phi + \varepsilon) = \cos(\omega t - \phi).$$

Womersley's equation then becomes

$$Q = \frac{\pi r^4}{\mu} \cdot \frac{1}{8} \cdot M \cos(\omega t - \phi)$$

i.e. $$Q = \frac{\pi r^4}{\mu} \cdot \frac{1}{8} \cdot p$$

which is the same as Poiseuille's equation. It turns out that the difference between Poiseuille's equation and Womersley's equation for values of α of 0·5 or less is negligible.

The importance of this is that in a very small artery, pressure gradient and flow will be in phase and related to one another by the resistance along the vessel. This would also be true if one had a low frequency and high kinematic viscosity (viscosity/density ratio). This does not apply to arterial blood flow but applies to such situations as air flow through a pneumatachograph where flow during breathing is measured by taking the pressure gradient across a small mesh resistance. This linear relation between p and Q breaks down in vessels other than very small arteries and breaks down more and more as α increases, i.e. artery diameter increases.

When one comes to the aorta α is very large and conditions are approaching the limiting conditions of very large α. In this case ε tends towards 0 (Fig. 8.5), the flow tends to lag a complete 90° behind pressure gradient. M'/α^2 tends towards a very low value (Fig. 8.5) so that the amplitude of the flow sine wave is small. This situation is due to the predominance of blood inertia and is analogous to the voltage and current across an electrical inductance.

Application of Womersley's equation to arteries

It will be apparent from this analysis that Womersley's equation only deals with sine waves of pressure gradient and flow and with none of the other preconditions required by Poiseuille's equation. It is therefore necessary to apply it to arterial blood flow to see how well it fits. Since flow in arteries is not sinusoidal, we revert again to Fourier analysis as we did for the calculation of input impedance in Chapter 7.

Thus one takes a measured pressure gradient along an artery.* This is then broken down into a mean term, a fundamental and a series of harmonics. A flow harmonic is derived from each pressure gradient harmonic using Womersley's equation. These flow harmonics including the zeroth harmonic are then added together to obtain the actual predicted flow wave.

One then compares the resulting predicted flow with an actual (measured) flow wave and the correspondence is found to be close (Fig. 8.6a). Thus it seems that the various factors which should have interfered with this result (non-Newtonian fluid, etc) are sufficiently small to be neglected.

Longitudinal impedance

In the case of Poiseuille's equation we were able to relate pressure gradient to flow by the constant ratio of the two, resistance (P/Q). This is not possible with Womersley's equation because there is a combination of inertial and resistive factors along the tube. These can be taken into account by taking the impedance between the two pressure measuring points along the artery—called the longitudinal impedance.

---

* Technically very difficult because of the need to have two exactly matched pressure measuring systems of identical static and dynamic calibration.

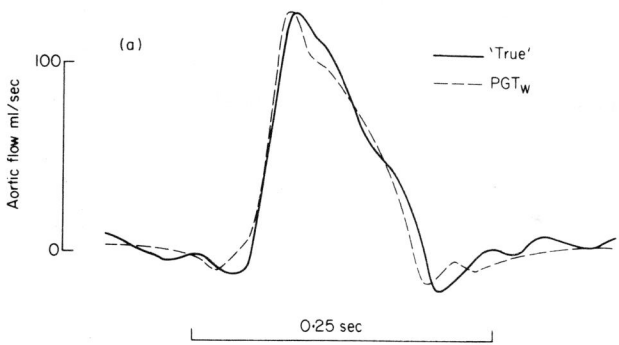

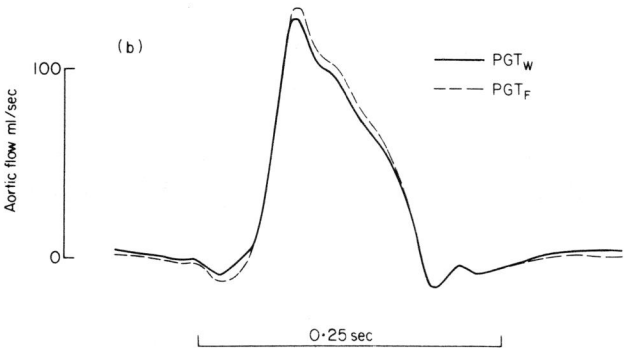

FIG. 8.6. (a) Flow curves measured simultaneously by electro-magnetic flowmeter (continuous line) and by calculation from the pressure gradient using Womersley's equation (dashed line). (b) Comparison of flow calculated from the pressure gradient by Womersley's equation (solid line) and by Fry's method (dashed line).

Since, in this case, capacitance can be ignored, the ratio p/Q or Z (longitudinal impedance) is given by:

$$ Z = \frac{\rho}{\pi r^2} [R(\alpha) + j\omega\lambda(\alpha)] $$

where ρ is the density of blood as before and ω the angular frequency as before ($j = \sqrt{-1}$). However, $R(\alpha)$ and $L(\alpha)$ are functions of $\alpha^\star$ as illustrated in Fig. 8.7. Note that as α gets bigger $R(\alpha)$, the resistance term, gets smaller and $L(\alpha)$ the inertance (inductance) term gets bigger and dominates the impedance.

The situation in the aorta, where there is an inlet, a flat velocity profile and turbulence, is handled by Fry by a much more approximate solution. He assumes here

---

$\star$ $R(\alpha) = (\omega \sin \varepsilon)/M'$ or $(\nu/R^2)\cdot(\alpha^2 \sin \varepsilon)/M'$, $L(\alpha) = (\cos \varepsilon)/M'$. $R(\alpha)$ is not to be confused with the radius of the tube r.

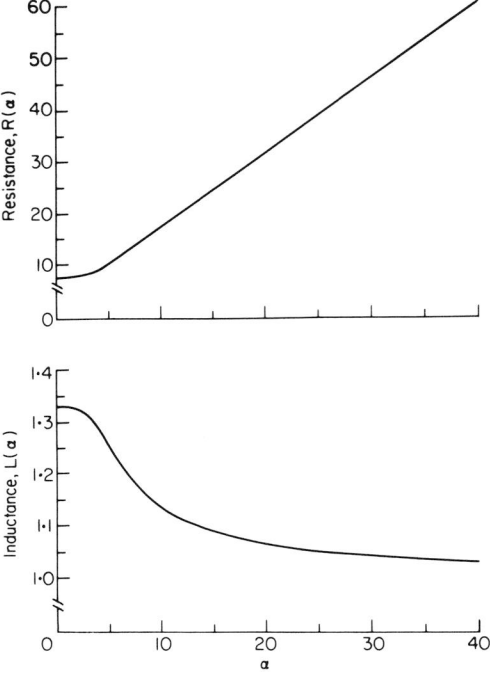

F I G. 8.7.   Relationship between fluid resistance (above) and inductance (below) and α.

that the resistance is so small that it can be regarded as constant. The almost pure inductive conditions result in a situation where pressure gradient is proportional to the acceleration of flow rather than to flow itself. Acceleration is 90° ahead of flow in phase in these conditions. Thus acceleration is in phase with pressure gradient which is also 90° ahead of flow (high α, see above). Thus Fry writes:

$$p = L \cdot \frac{dQ}{dt} + RQ$$

where dQ/dt is the rate of change of flow (acceleration) and Q is the flow. R is a proportionality constant (resistance) between p and Q; this is certainly not correct to use since p is not proportional to Q in this case. However, the term is so small that the correct flow is still predicted quite well by the equation (Fig. 8.6b). It is even simpler and probably more correct to ignore resistance. The pressure gradient has virtually the same waveform as acceleration (Fig. 8.8).

The pressure gradient across the aortic valve

The aortic valve represents a non-linear device in what would otherwise be a large tube (left ventricular outflow tract and ascending aorta) which allows flow in the forward direction only. We have seen (Fig. 8.8) that the pressure gradient in the

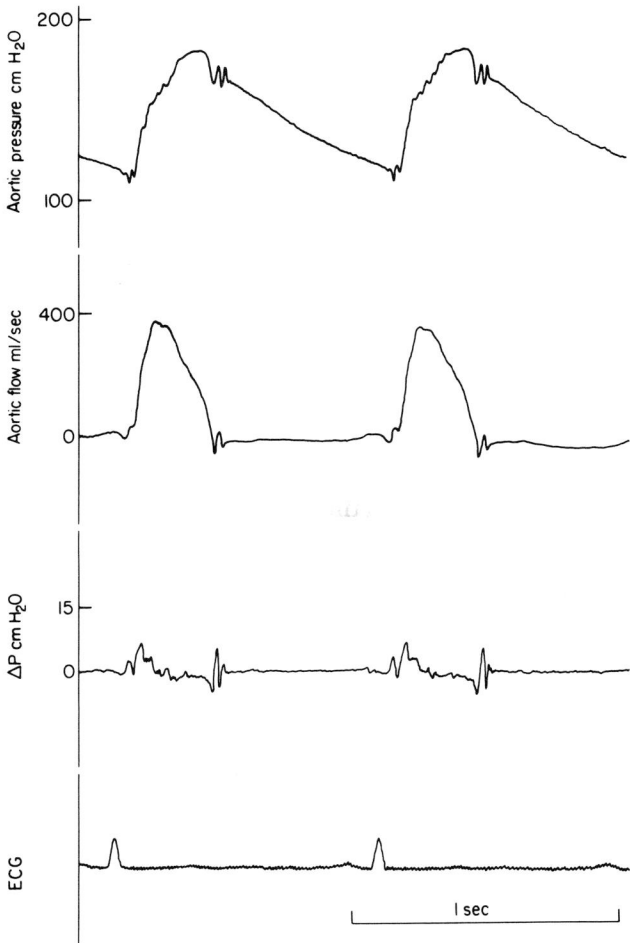

FIG. 8.8. Measurements of instantaneous pressure, flow and pressure gradient (ΔP) made in the ascending aorta of a normal human. In this case flow was obtained by integration of ΔP, the waveform of which is therefore the same as that of acceleration. From Snell *et al.* (1965).

ascending aorta is proportional to and in phase with flow acceleration. This means that there is a positive pressure gradient up to peak flow and subsequently as flow decelerates from its peak value to zero the pressure gradient is negative, i.e. the pressure further along the aorta is higher than the pressure closer to the heart. However, flow is still going forward, in spite of the backward pressure gradient, because of its momentum. If the conditions proximal to the aortic valve, in the left ventricular outflow tract are similar one might also expect to see a positive pressure gradient in early ejection and a negative pressure gradient in late ejection when flow is declining. This is indeed the case (Fig. 8.7).

It must now be apparent that the pressure gradient across the aortic valve during

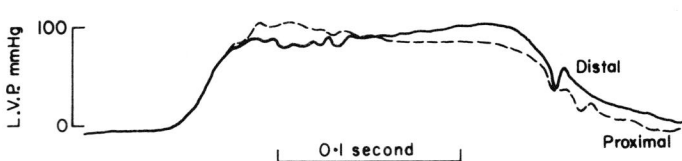

FIG. 8.9. Left ventricular pressure measured simultaneously at two positions in the left ventricular outflow tract with two high fidelity micromanometers at identical gain and zero.

ejection must be similar to that in the aorta distal to it and the left ventricular outflow tract proximal to it. This is also the case (Fig. 8.10). This result has often elicited surprise. How can the pressure in the aorta be higher than that in the left ventricle and outflow still be continuing? This question arises from a misconception about haemodynamics which is similar in a way to the erroneous idea that left ventricular or aortic pressure at any instant in time can be related to flow at that instant to give an instantaneous impedance. In the present case the absurdity of that procedure is more apparent since it would lead to the conclusion that in late systole there is a negative longitudinal impedance.

The occurrence of a negative pressure gradient during deceleration of flow is however a very natural consequence of a longitudinal impedance dominated by inertia because of the high value of α. The broadening of the concept of Poiseuille by Womersley and the consideration of impedance rather than resistance is worthy of attention by cardiologists and cardiac physiologists as well as by bioengineers.

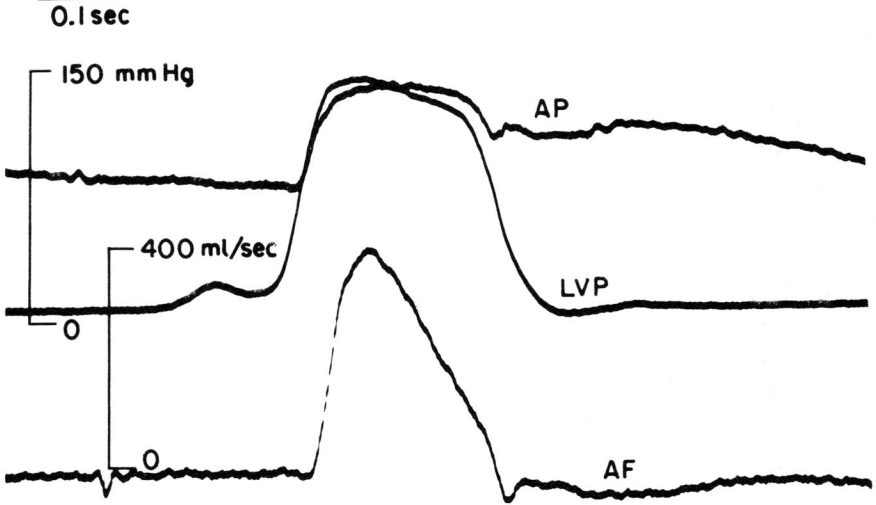

FIG. 8.10. Aortic pressure (AP) and left ventricular pressure (LVP) recorded simultaneously with identical gain and zero with two high fidelity micromanometers. Aortic flow (AF) also measured simultaneously with an electromagnetic flowmeter. From Noble (1968).

The contribution of blood momentum to left ventricular ejection

This was the title of a paper I published in 1968 from which Figs. 8.7 and 8.8 are taken. At that time I was rather taken with a concept of Isaac Starr which is perhaps worth repeating here:

'So many of our colleagues continue to think of the function of the heart as the Greeks thought of motion in general, e.g., the sun is drawn by Apollo's chariot because, like a wagon on earth, if not continually worked upon, its motion would stop. Similarly, many think that the heart must keep pushing out the blood up to the end of ejection. That this is not necessary has been clearly demonstrated by Spencer and Greiss (1962) the data of Rushmer and associates (1964) are also consistent with this view. The blood, once set into motion, will continue in motion because of its inertia until resistance stops it. So, after positive acceleration is over and maximum velocity has been attained, little if any cardiac effect will be required and this effort may cease well before the end of ejection.'

The finding of a negative pressure gradient during late ejection indicating, because of the inductive longitudinal impedance, that flow is maintained by momentum, naturally led one to consider this proposition seriously.

However, the longitudinal impedance is not 'seen' by left ventricle. As was demonstrated in Chapter 7, the left ventricle 'sees' the aortic input impedance which is mainly resistive and capacitative. It is probable that the aortic input impedance phase angles go positive at high frequencies although this is the least accurate part of the input impedance measurement. This conclusion is certainly suggested by the greater initial rise in aortic pressure with increased acceleration (Fig. 8.9). However, the impedance during late ejection is certainly dominated by the low frequency capacitative components.

Nevertheless, momentum must be contributing to flow during deceleration and the backward transmission of pressure from the aorta to the left ventricle must be contributing to the maintenance of left ventricular pressure. Further points in favour of this conclusion are (1) that the pressure response to a unit impulse of flow indicating time dependent impedance (Fig. 7.14) has dropped to about half its peak value by 0.1–0.2 sec, (2) that an increase in aortic pressure due to a large reflected wave when the descending thoracic aorta is occluded causes a marked rise in left ventricular pressure and fall in aortic inflow during late ejection (Fig. 7.13), and (3) that left ventricular pressure drops precipitously when the aorta is occluded during late ejection; this effect can also be explained on the basis of deactivation of the ventricular muscle but it cannot be thus easily deactivated earlier in systole. Thus, although one can reiterate that blood momentum contributes to left ventricular ejection, the magnitude of the contribution remains unknown.

REFERENCES

AMBROSI C. & STARR I. (1965) Incoordination of the cardiac contraction, as judged by the force ballistocardiogram and the carotid pulse derivative. *Am. Heart J.*, **70**, 761.

FRY D.L., MALLOS A.J. & CASPAR A.G.T. (1956) A catheter tip method for measurement of the instantaneous aortic blood velocity. *Circulation Res.*, **4**, 627.

GABE I.T. (1965) Arterial blood flow by analogue solution of the Navier-Stokes equation. *Phys. Med. Biol.*, **10**, 271.

GREENFIELD J.C. & FRY D.L. (1965) Relationship between instantaneous aortic flow and the pressure gradient. *Circulation Res.*, **17**, 340.

HALE J.F., McDONALD D.A. & WOMERSLEY J.R. (1955) Velocity profiles of oscillating arterial flow with some calculations of viscous drag and the Reynolds number. *J. Physiol.*, **28**, 629–640.

HALES S. (1733) *Statistical Essays: Containing Haemastaticks.* Reprinted 1964, No. 22, History of Medicine series, Library of New York Academy of Medicine. Hafner Publishing, New York.

McDONALD D.A. (1955) The relation of pulsatile pressure to flow in arteries. *J. Physiol.*, **127**, 533.

McDONALD D.A. (1974) *Blood Flow in Arteries.* Edward Arnold, London.

NOBLE (1968) The contribution of blood momentum to left ventricular ejection in the dog. *Circulation Res.*, **23**, 663–670.

NOBLE M.I.M., GABE I.T., TRENCHARD D. & GUZ A. (1967) Blood pressure and flow in the ascending aorta of conscious dogs. *Cardiovasc. Res.*, **1**, 9.

PORJÉ I.G. & RUDEWALD B. (1961) Hemodynamic studies with differential pressure technique. *Acta Physiol., Scand.*, **51**, 116.

RUDEWALD B. (1962) Haemodynamics of the human ascending aorta as studied by means of a differential pressure technique. *Acta Physiol., Scand.*, **54**, Suppl. 187.

RUSHMER R.F. (1964) Initial ventricular impulse. A potential key to cardiac evaluation. *Circulation*, **29**, 268.

SNELL R.E., CLEMENTS J.M., PATEL D.J., FRY D.L. & LUCHSINGER P.C. (1965) Instantaneous blood flow in the human aorta. *J. Appl. Physiol.*, **20**, 691.

SPENCER M.P. & GREISS F.C. (1962) Dynamics of ventricular ejection. *Circulation Res.*, **10**, 274.

WOMERSLEY J.R. (1955) Method for the calculation of velocity, rate of flow and viscous drag in arteries when the pressure gradient is known. *J. Physiol.*, **127**, 553.

CHAPTER 9
PULSE TRANSMISSION

In the previous chapter it was assumed that a short length of artery was rigid. This enabled one to obtain a very close correspondence between the pulsatile flow wave derived from the pressure gradient along such a short section and measured flow. Along great lengths of artery such an assumption is untenable, because the length can no longer be regarded as negligible compared to the wavelength. The elasticity of the arterial walls (without which there would be no Windkessel function) causes a number of important effects which must be considered when thinking about the function of the arterial system as a whole.

Elasticity of arteries

Since the arteries have the shape of tubes it is usual to examine the elastic properties of the wall indirectly. This is done by increasing the distending pressure inside the tube and measuring the change in radius. The stress around the circumference of the tube can be calculated from PR/h (where P = pressure, R = radius and h = wall thickness) and related to the increase in radius or circumference.*

If the arterial wall obeyed Hooke's Law (stress proportional to strain), the plot of wall tension against radius would be a straight line but in fact it curves upwards (Fig. 9.1) because the wall gets stiffer as it is distended. This produces difficulty in describing the elasticity quantitatively with Young's modulus. The incremental modulus is the ratio of a change in stress to the corresponding relative change in length, i.e. strain; this increases with strain in the case of a non-linear elastic body of this type (Fig. 9.2). Actual measurements of incremental modulus as a function of radius are shown for a femoral artery in Fig. 9.3. This stiffening of the wall with increasing pressure is important in preventing arteries from bursting.

The arteries are also elastic in the longitudinal direction. The relationship between elongating force and length extension is also alinear (as Fig. 9.1). A further complication is that arteries *in vivo* are tethered by branches and tissues so that longitudinal extension is prevented.

The description of the elasticity above concerns slowly changing or steady values of stress and strain. However, during the cardiac cycle pressure is changing rapidly. If one subjects an artery to a pulsating pressure the artery appears to be stiffer (greater pressure change for the same radius change). This effect can be expressed by the ratio of the pulsatile (dynamic) incremental modulus to the static incremental

---

* The strain is the change in circumference but changes in radius are proportional ($\frac{1}{2}\pi \times$ circumference).

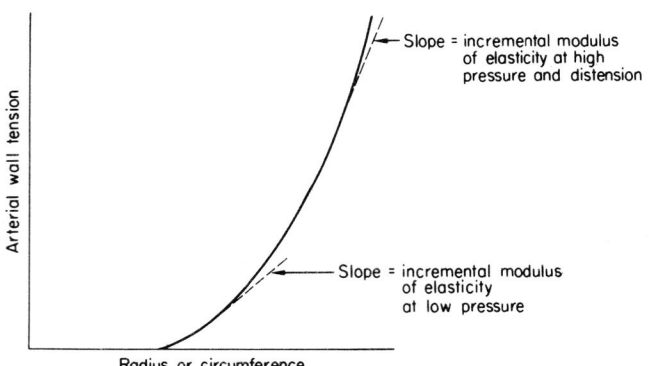

FIG. 9.1.   Relationship between arterial wall tension and artery size showing nature of
non-linearity. Note increase in incremental elastic modulus with increase in pressure and
distension.

modulus. This ratio does not change very much with frequency but varies considerably between arteries (Fig. 9.4). There is also a phase lag between pressure and
radius.

The difference between different arteries (Fig. 9.4) can be accounted for by
differences in the composition of the wall, e.g. there is a greater proportion of elastin
in the thoracic aorta. As one goes to peripheral arteries like the carotid there is also
smooth muscle in the wall, contraction of which will increase its stiffness. The
increasing stiffness of arteries as one goes peripherally from the heart has important
consequences for pulse transmission (see below).

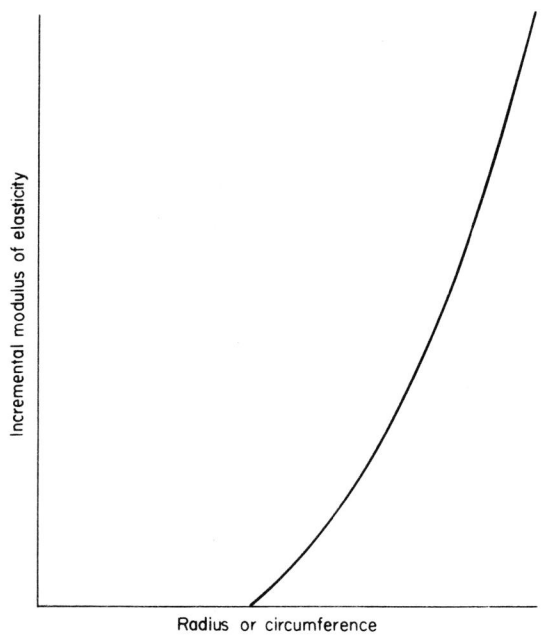

FIG. 9.2.   Non-linear relationship between incremental arterial elastic modulus and artery size.

Wave travel

If the arterial system were rigid, flow and pressure waves would be transmitted without distortion at the speed of sound. The elasticity of the arteries introduces distortion and slows the speed of transmission down. In the aorta where distensibility is greatest, the wave velocity is slowest; it speeds up as one moves out to the stiffer arteries in the

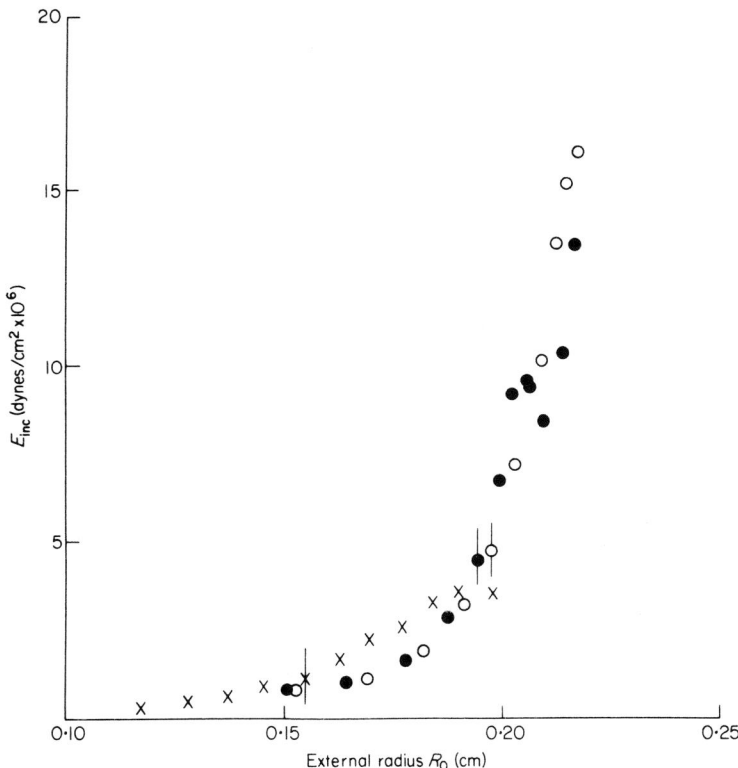

FIG. 9.3. Incremental modulus plotted against radius for three separate runs in one artery. In each case measurements were made when pressure was increasing on the first ($\times$), second ($\bullet$) and third ($\bigcirc$) occasion. Vertical lines indicate points at 100 mm Hg pressure. From Bergel (1971a).

periphery. This relationship between wave velocity and stiffness is expressed by the Moens-Korteweg equation:

$$C_0 = \sqrt{\frac{E \cdot h}{2\,R\rho}}$$

(C_0 = wave velocity, E = elastic modulus, h = wall thickness, R = radius, ρ = density of blood).

Wave velocity can be measured by displaying two pressure or flow pulses together in time (Fig. 9.5). There is a time difference between the systolic upstrokes of the two pulses. The distance between the two sites of measurement along the arterial system divided by this time difference gives the pulse wave velocity. Note that the shapes of the two pulses are different and that the measurement would be different and more difficult using other parts of the pulse waveforms than the upstrokes. This is because different components of the wave travel at different speeds causing distortion. It will be appreciated that a measurement of pulse wave velocity is a useful way of estimating

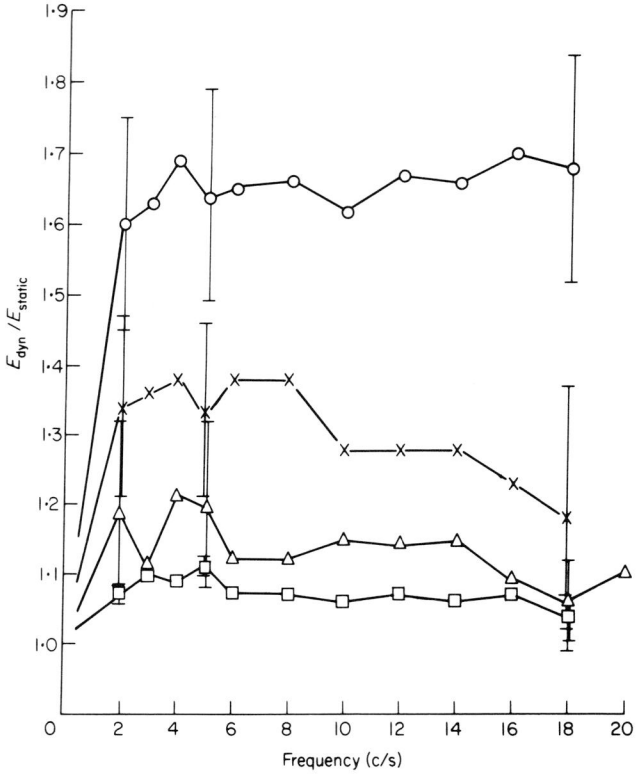

FIG. 9.4.   Elastic modulus measured dynamically (Edyn) as a ratio of the static modulus (*E* static) plotted as a function of the frequency at which the dynamic measurement was made. □ thoracic aorta, △ abdominal aorta, × femoral artery, ○ carotid artery. From Bergel (1971b).

arterial stiffness indirectly. Thus, in man a higher than normal pulse wave velocity indicates stiffened arteries.

   Another feature of the change in the pulse as it travels down the arterial system is that the amplitude of the pressure gets bigger while the amplitude of fluid velocity decreases (Fig. 9.6). This amplification of the pressure pulse is related to reflections and to the increasing stiffness of the arteries as one tracks peripherally. The effect is greater if the arteries as a whole are stiffer than normal. Thus, subjects with stiffened arteries have increased pulse pressure in peripheral arteries.

Phase velocity

In order to sort out what is happening to alter the shape of the pulse waveform (Fig. 9.5), one requires the use of Fourier analysis. If each waveform is broken down into a Fourier series (as for impedance measurements, Chapter 7) it will be found that there is a phase lag between the upstream and downstream first harmonics. The distance between measuring sites divided between this time lag gives the so called apparent wave velocity for the first harmonic. The same procedure for the higher harmonics gives their corresponding apparent wave velocities which can then be plotted against

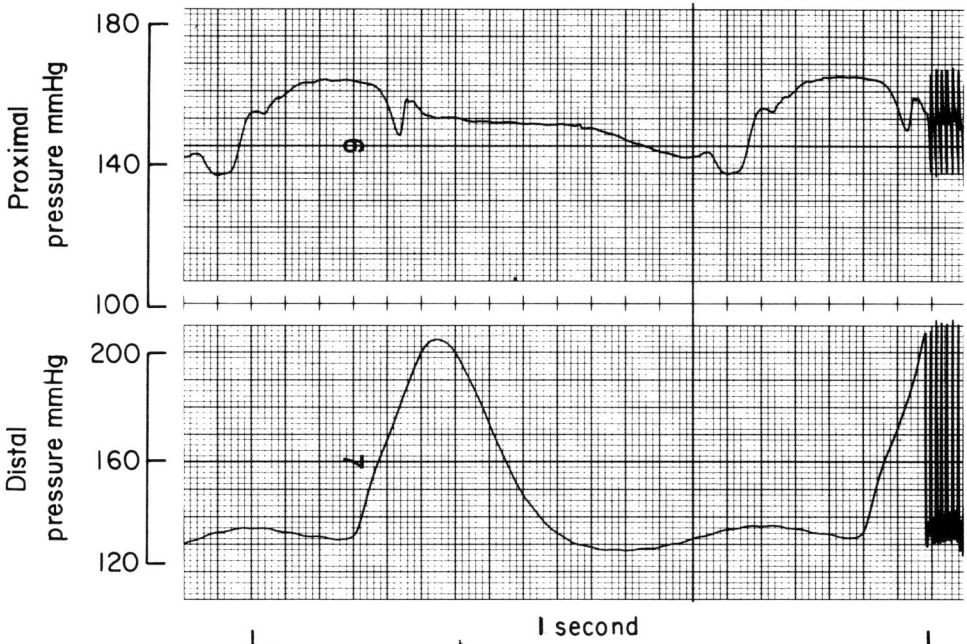

FIG. 9.5. Simultaneous recording of pressure in the ascending aorta and femoral artery. Note the time difference between the initial upstrokes. Pulse wave velocity is the distance between recording sites divided by this time ('foot to foot' velocity).

frequency. It is found that these values vary with frequency in a similar way to input impedance (Fig. 9.7).

The apparent wave velocity is affected by reflections. In Taylor's tube there are peaks at the antinodes and troughs at the nodes (Fig. 9.8). In the absence of such reflections, the tube has a uniform phase velocity along its length, called the true phase velocity. The apparent wave velocity deviates from the true phase velocity depending on the amount of reflection present in the system.

This interference by reflections makes interpretation of data obtained from pressure pulses (e.g. Fig. 9.5) difficult. The effect of reflections can be avoided by

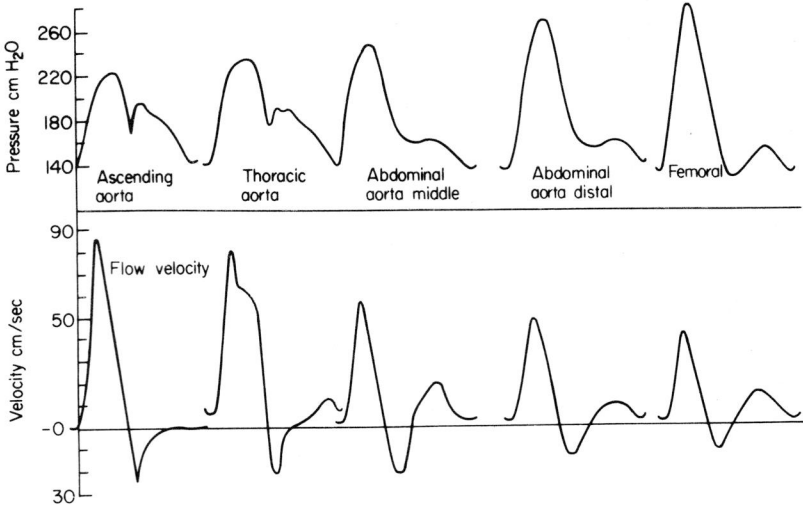

FIG. 9.6.   The pressure pulses and the oscillatory flow velocity curves measured simultaneously at different sites. Pressure oscillations increase with distance from the heart but velocity oscillations show a progressive decrease. This is due to the increase in impedance with increasing distance from the heart. From McDonald (1974).

studying very high frequencies. For this reason Anliker imposed artificial high frequency pulses and measured their speed of transit down the system.

Reflections in the arterial system

As was seen in the case of aortic input impedance (Chapter 7) the fluctuations with frequency of wave velocity and impedance in the aorta are small (Fig. 9.7). This shows that, from the inlet, the system does not appear to be like Taylor's closed tube. It

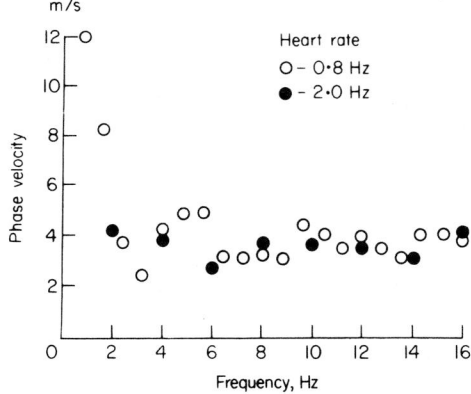

FIG. 9.7.   Average apparent phase velocities in the ascending aorta under control conditions (●) and during vagal stimulation to slow the heart rate (○). From Nichols and McDonald (1972).

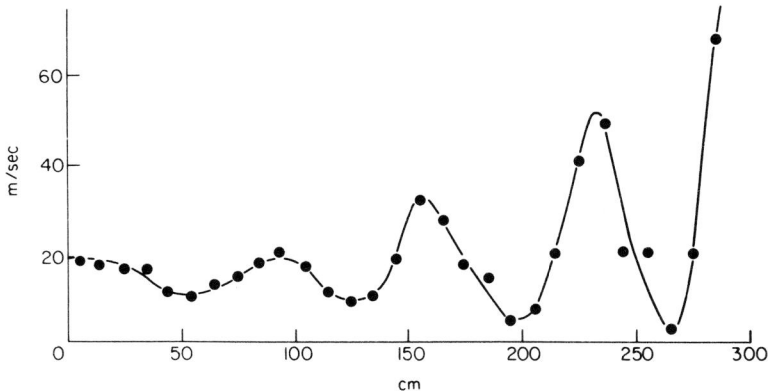

FIG. 9.8(a). The apparent phase velocity in the rubber tube used in Fig. 7.12. Frequency of oscillations 10 Hz. From Taylor (1957).

could be argued that this is because the arterial system consists of two Taylor tubes, one with the inlet at the descending aorta having a different distance from the major reflecting site than the other, with the inlet at the main arteries to the upper body from the arch of the aorta. The reflected waves from these two tubes would cancel out and not appear at the ascending aorta. However, in such a case, as one measured pressure pulses at points progressively further out along the system, one would find fluctuations in amplitude with peaks at nodes where apparent phase velocity is high and troughs at antinodes where apparent phase velocity is low (Fig. 9.8). In fact this is not the case. There is an increase in pressure pulse amplitude (see above) but

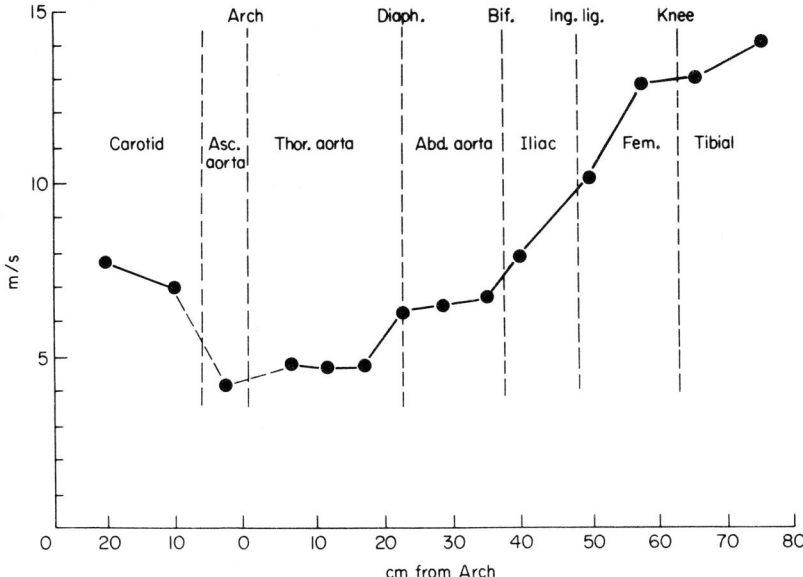

FIG. 9.8(b). Wave front (foot to foot) velocity recorded in a dog in relation to distance from the heart. From Nichols and McDonald (1972).

no fluctuations superimposed (Fig. 9.9). This could be due to the fact that the system is short with respect to the wavelengths.

The analysis in Chapter 7 showed that there are reflections which come back to the ascending aorta but these are spread out to produce a diffuse reflected wave (Fig. 7.13). The smooth increase in pulse pressure with distance from the heart (Fig. 9.9) shows that the same diffuseness of the reflected waves occurs everywhere in the

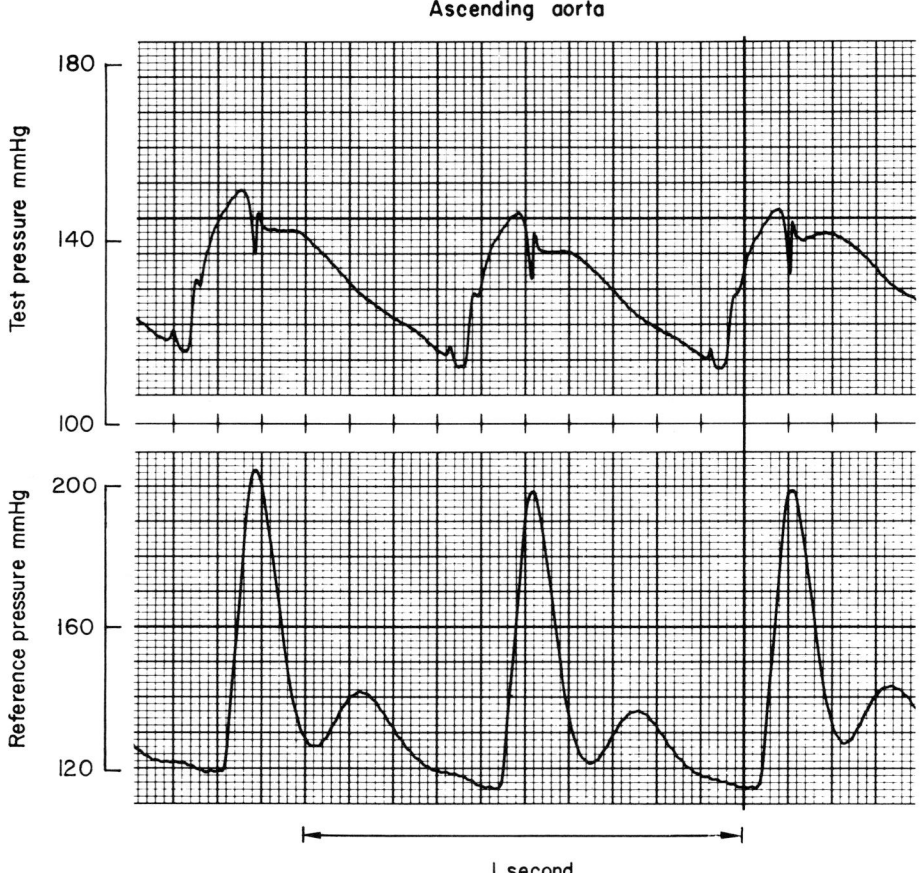

FIG. 9.9a (i)

system. One can list the following characteristics of the arterial system with increasing distance from the heart: (1) increasing stiffness, (2) branching, (3) increasing pulse pressure, (4) increasing wave velocity, (5) increasing impedance (even when normalised for size of bed by taking pressure/velocity), (6) decreasing amplitude of velocity pulse.

The first two of these are causes of reflections. A stiff artery distal to a distensible one implies an increase in characteristic impedance* and such an impedance step will

---

* I.e. impedance of the proximal vessel given by the input impedance at high frequencies.

cause a reflection. Since the stiffness increase is a smooth continuum, not an abrupt step at a particular site, the resulting reflections will be arising from all parts of the system distributed broadly in distance and therefore also in time.

Branches also cause reflections because of the change in characteristic impedance between the mother vessel and daughter vessels causing an impedance mismatch. Each branching produces small reflections but there are many branches along the

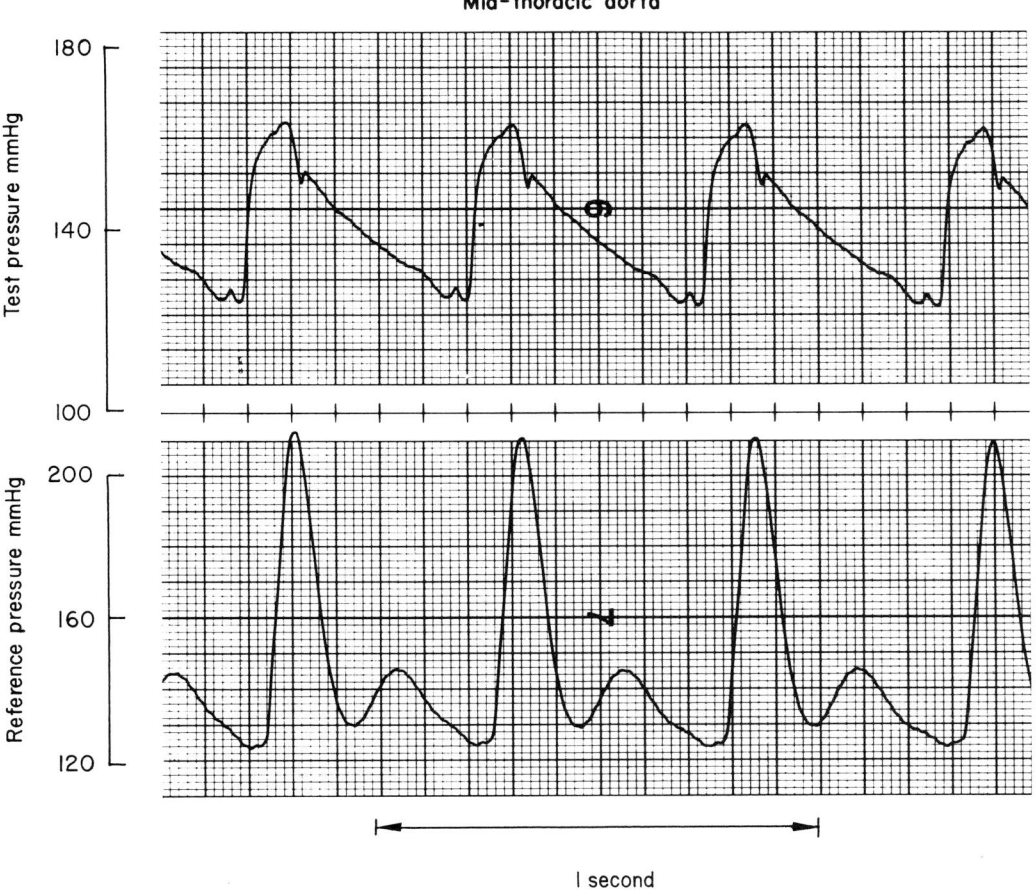

FIG. 9.9a (ii)

system. In this case the reflection sites are discreet but are nevertheless distributed fairly evenly throughout the system.

We may therefore conclude that these reflections are present and will cause amplification of pressure and diminution of velocity pulses, because reflected pressure waves add and reflected flow waves subtract from the forward going waves. These effects and the consequent increase in impedance with increasing distance down the system may thus be attributed to the effects of reflections. However, one may ask why these effects increase with distance down the system. It will be noted from Fig. 9.9

that there is much more pressure amplification, i.e. more reflections in the femoral artery than in the thoracic aorta. There is also much more pressure amplification of the first harmonic than of the fourth harmonic. Why are low frequencies reflected back more than high frequencies? (Remember the low frequency composite reflected wave at the ascending aorta, Chapter 7.)

Westerhof explains what would happen at a branching point (Fig. 9.10). Consider

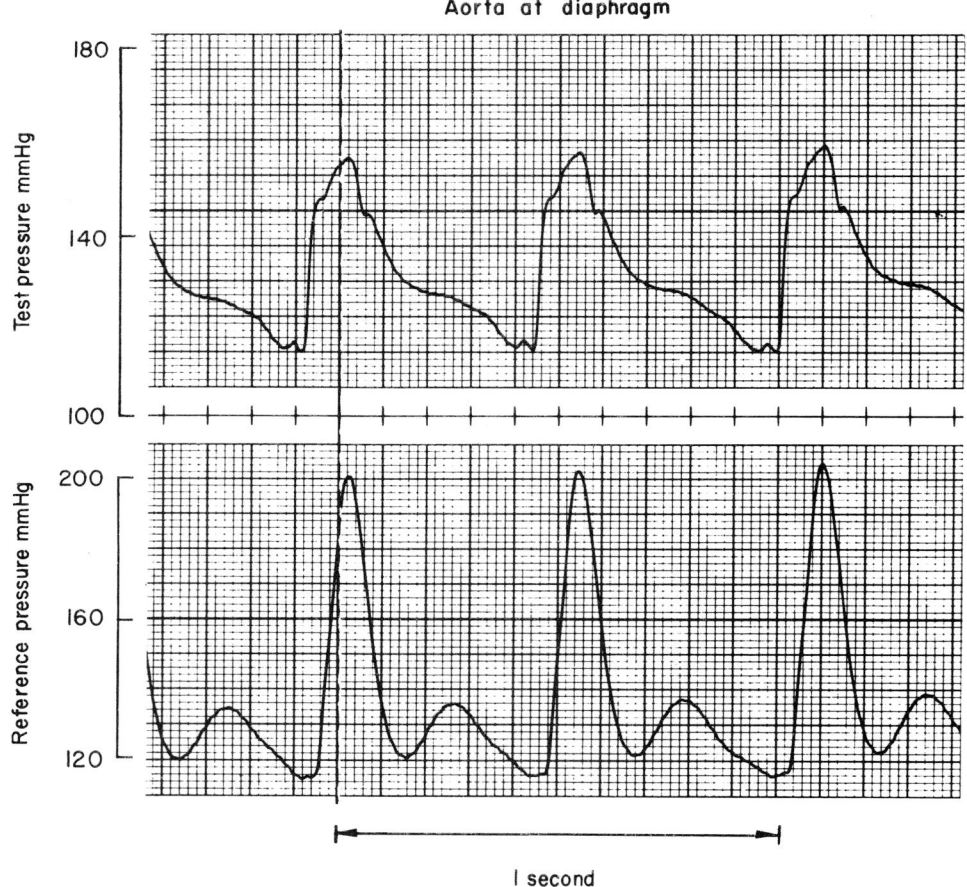

FIG. 9.9a (iii)

a forward going wave. There will be a small reflection set up but since the impedance mismatch is not great, most of the wave is transmitted into the daughter branches. Consider now a reflected wave coming backwards up one of the daughter branches. The impedance mismatch between this daughter branch and the junction between the other branch and the parent vessel is great. Thus most of this backward wave will be reflected back again towards the periphery. The design of the branching system is such as to cause reflected waves to be bottled up in the periphery.

Now consider the effects upon reflected waves of different frequencies. The amount of reflection of waves in tubes depends on how the wave length matches the length between reflecting sites. Low frequency waves have a wave length which is long compared to the distances between two branching points in the periphery. These will therefore tend to pass back through branching points towards the heart. High frequency waves on the other hand have wave lengths which are less than the distances between two branching points in the periphery. These waves, therefore, have

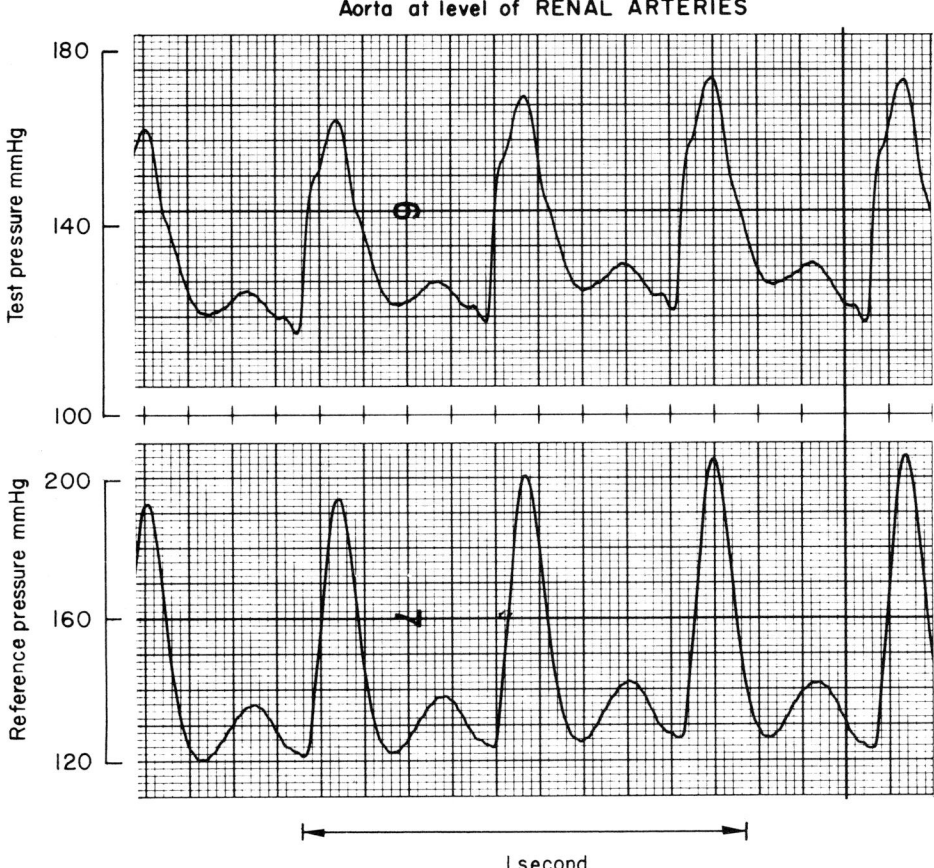

FIG. 9.9a (iv)

a greater chance of being reflected back centrifugally at branching points. High frequency reflected waves are bottled up in the periphery more than low frequency waves.

Design of the arterial system

The process of natural selection appears to have resulted in a design of arterial system which is well suited to its purpose. If the system consisted of simple conduits ending in the high resistance of peripheral vascular beds it would serve well for delivery of steady flow. In the body, there is the disadvantage that the pump has a highly pulsatile output.

When the heart is connected to a tube system, the minimum of extra work resulting from pulsatility is achieved by having a distensible tube with a low wave

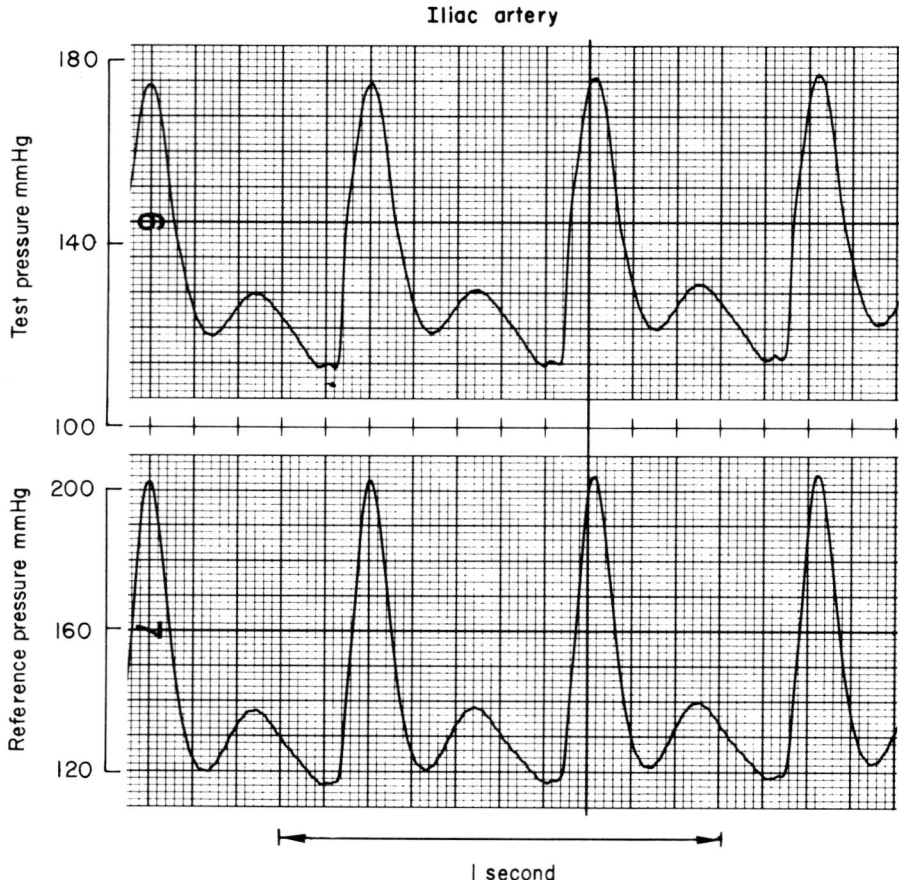

FIG. 9.9a (v)

FIG. 9.9a.   Pressure recorded at locations from ascending aorta to iliac artery (above). Femoral artery pressure is recorded throughout (below). Note increase of amplitude of pressure oscillation (pulse pressure) with distance from the heart.

velocity. These requirements are similar to those of a Windkessel which also minimises cardiac pulsatile work by being distensible. If such distensibility of the walls extended over the entire system, there would be two further disadvantages:
(1) Very distensible arteries cause instability of control of blood volume distribution; large volumes of blood would shift from veins to arteries disturbing the capacitative functions of the venous system.

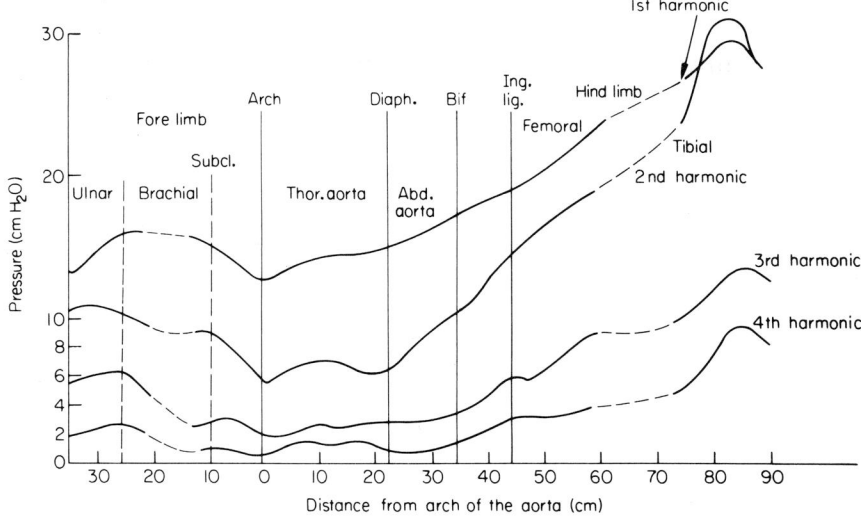

FIG. 9.9b. The first four harmonics of pressure plotted as a function of distance from the heart. Note that the second harmonic increases most and that the first and second harmonics increase more than the third and fourth. From McDonald (1974).

(2) If the distensibility is high and the impedance low, there will be a large step up in impedance when the tubes connect on to the high peripheral resistance. This will lead to large reflected waves which come back to the heart and load it with an impedance with large fluctuations from frequency to frequency; this would demand that the heart only works at the critical frequency at which the impedance is low (at a 'node'). (3) Control of blood pressure would be slow. In order to prevent large reflected waves it is necessary to choose a characteristic impedance for the tubes which matches the peripheral resistance. This means making them very stiff with consequent increase in the input impedance to be similar to peripheral resistance. The required pulsatile cardiac work is then greatly increased, negating one of the desirable functions

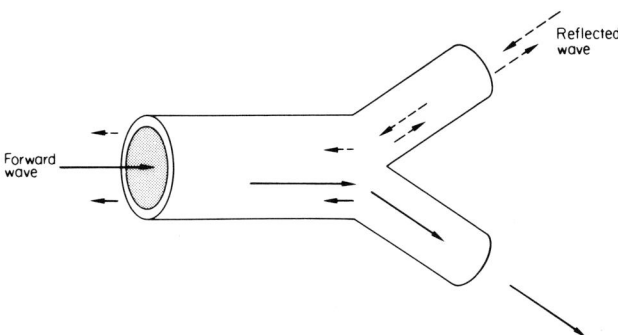

FIG. 9.10. Diagram of arterial bifurcation. Most of the reflected wave is reflected back again at the junction whereas a relatively smaller proportion of the forward wave is reflected.

of the system, the Windkessel function. As Taylor has pointed out this uniform transmission system is a much poorer design for the arteries than a simple Windkessel.

Taylor suggests that the required objectives, (1) low input impedance, (2) low overall distensibility, and (3) matching of characteristic impedance of the terminal part of the system to the peripheral resistance, are achieved by a non-uniform transmission system. In this system the physical properties of the arteries are functions of distance from the heart. The system remains essentially linear with maintenance of super-position (see Chapter 7 for tests of superposition of aortic input impedance). In this particular case, arterial wall stiffness, wave velocity and characteris-

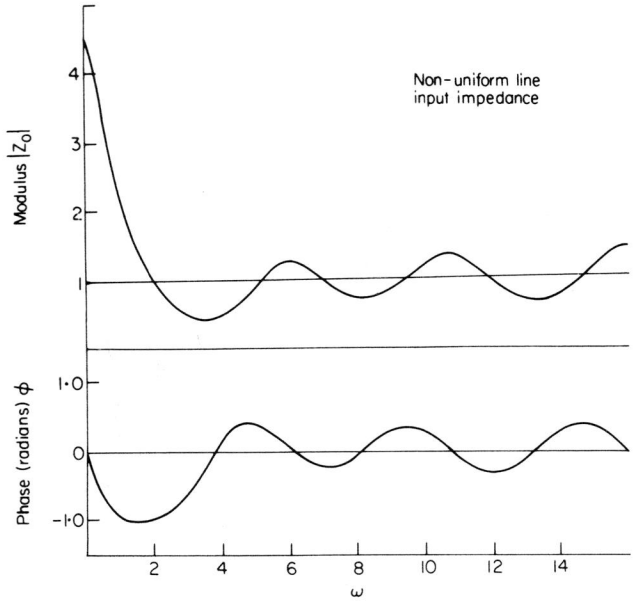

FIG. 9.11.   Input impedance of Taylors non-uniform line. Note greater similarity to aortic input impedance (Fig. 7.10) than shown by the simpler tube model (Fig. 7.12). From Taylor (1964).

tic impedance increase with distance. The most important effect of this is on the reflection coefficient. For the uniform system this is given by:

$$R = \frac{Z_T - Z_0}{Z_T + Z_0}$$

(Z_t = terminal impedance, Z_0 = characteristic impedance), i.e. the amount of reflection depends on the mismatch between the two impedances. In the non-uniform system, Z_T is modified by a term including rate of change of the log of the impedance with distance and frequency so that for high frequencies the impedances become nominally matched and very few high frequency reflections occur; only low frequency reflections occur. At high frequency, the input impedance of the arterial bed decreases as one tracks towards the heart.

Taylor has summarised the advantages of such a system as follows:

(1) High wave velocity and characteristic impedance in peripheral arteries leads to
  (a) low overall distensibility of the system
  (b) approximate matching with the peripheral terminations
  (c) small reflections leading to small fluctuations of input impedance with frequency.

(2) Low wave velocity at the origin of the system so that the heart only 'sees' the terminal impedance at low frequencies. At high frequencies the heart does not see the terminal impedance but the low characteristic impedance of the aorta.

Taylor checked his theoretical predictions in a simple computer model of such a system. The input impedance (Fig. 9.11) has much smaller oscillations with frequency

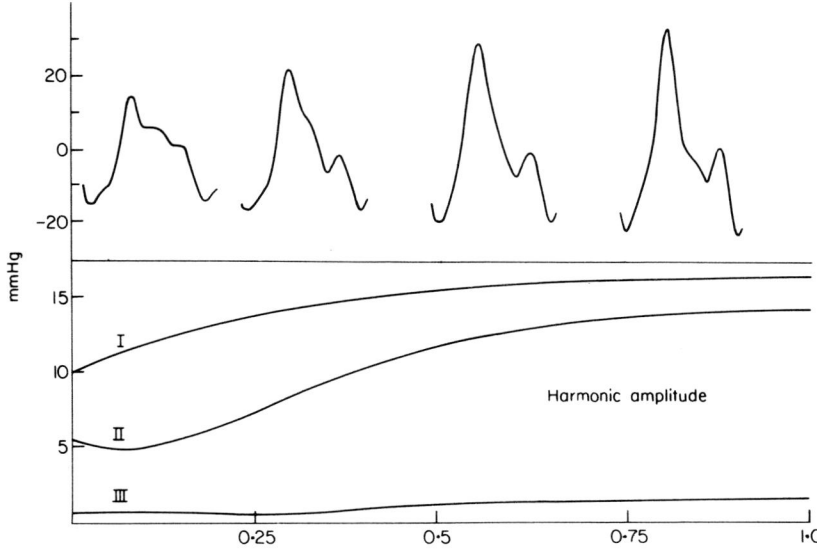

FIG. 9.12. Increase in pulse pressure (above) and pressure harmonics (below) with distance down. Taylor's non-uniform line. Compare with Fig. 9.9b. Note greater increase in second than in first harmonic. From Taylor (1964).

than the uniform tube (Fig. 7.10). A striking characteristic of this model and of a hydraulic model (Barnard *et al.* 1966) was amplification of pressure oscillation with distance (Fig. 9.12).

To this type of system, in which the presence of reflections is minimised, we must add the features outlined in the previous section which minimise backward travel of reflected waves, i.e. the branching pattern and the asymmetric design of the upper half/lower half main arteries. Thus both of these features help to ensure that the input impedance of the system (and therefore cardiac work) is minimised and fluctuates little with frequency. This ensures optimal matching of the left ventricle to the system. The matching of the periphery of the system to the peripheral resistance results from the non-uniformity as does the low overall distensibility.

If the design results from natural selection it is interesting to speculate on the different results of natural selection in birds. In the turkey for instance, the arterial system has been shown to be like a simple Windkessel, the thoracic aorta being the distensible damper and the distributive arteries being stiff conduits. Increase in pulse pressure with increasing distance from the heart is not found. The aortic input impedance, like that of the Windkessel model, is similar to that of mammals. Are these different end results the effect of chance or does the Windkessel design have some superior survival advantage for birds, while the non-uniform transmission system confers comparable advantage in the mode of life of mammals ?

REFERENCES

ANLIKER M., HISTAND M.B. & OGDEN E. (1968) Dispersion and attenuation of small artificial pressure waves in the canine aorta. *Circulation Res.*, **23**, 539–551.

BARNARD A.C.L., HUNT W.A., TIMLAKE W.P. & VARLEY E. (1966) Peaking of the pressure pulse in fluid-filled tubes of spatially varying compliance. *Biophys. J.*, **6**, 735–746.

BERGEL D.H. (1961a) The static elastic properties of the arterial wall. *J. Physiol.*, **156**, 445–457.

BERGEL D.H. (1961b) The dynamic elastic properties of the arterial wall. *J. Physiol.*, **156**, 458–469.

COX R.H. (1971) Determination of the true phase velocity of arterial pressure waves *in vivo*. *Circulation Res.*, **29**, 407–418.

HARKNESS M.L.R., HARKNESS R.D. & MCDONALD D.A. (1957) The collagen and elastin content of the arterial wall in the dog. *Proc. Roy. Soc. B.*, **146**, 541–51.

KORTEWEG D.G. (1878) Uber die Fortpflanzungsgeschwindigkeit des Schalles in elastischen Rohren. *Ann. Phys. Chem.*, Ser. *3*, **5**, 525.

LEAROYD B.M. & TAYLOR M.G. (1966) Alterations with age in the viscoelastic properties of human arterial walls. *Circulation Res.*, **18**, 278–292.

MCDONALD D.A. (1968) Regional pulse-wave velocity in the arterial tree. *J. Appl. Physiol.*, **24**, 73–78.

MCDONALD D.A. (1974) *Blood Flow in Arteries*. Edward Arnold, London.

MOENS A.I. (1878) *Die Pulskurve*. Brill, Leiden.

NEWMAN D.L. & BOWDEN N.L.R. (1973). Effect of reflection from an unmatched junction on the abdominal aortic impedance. *Cardiovasc. Res.*, **7**, 165–172.

NICHOLS W.W. & MCDONALD D.A. (1972) Wave velocity in the proximal aorta *Med. Biol. Engng.*, **10**, 327–35.

PORJÉ I.G. (1946) Studies of the arterial pulse wave, particularly in the aorta. *Acta. Physiol., Scand.*, **13** (suppl) 42, 1–68.

ROY C.S. (1880) The elastic properties of the arterial wall. *J. Physiol.*, **3**, 125.

TAYLOR M.G. (1959) An experimental determination of the fluid oscillations in a tube with a viscoelastic wall, together with an analysis of the characteristics in an electrical analogue. *Phys. Med. Biol.*, **4**, 63–81.

TAYLOR M.G. (1964) Wave travel in arteries and the design of the cardiovascular system. In *Pulsatile Blood Flow*. E.O. Attinger, Ed. McGraw-Hill, New York.

TAYLOR M.G. (1965) Wave travel in a non-uniform transmission line in relation to pulses in arteries. *Phys. Med. Biol.*, **10**, 539–550.

TAYLOR M.G. (1966) Wave transmission through an assembly of randomly branching elastic tubes. *Biophys. J.*, **6**, 697–716.

WESTERHOF N. (1968) *Analog studies of human systemic arterial hemodynamics*. Ph.D. Thesis, University of Pennsylvania. University Microfilm, Ann Arbor, Mich. 69–5676.

WESTERHOF N., ELZINGA G., SIPKEMA P. & VAN DEN BOS G.C. (1977) Quantitative analysis of the arterial system and heart by means of pressure-flow relations. In *Cardiovascular Flow Dynamics and Measurements*. N.H.C. Hwang and N.A. Normann, Eds. University Park Press, Baltimore.

WESTERHOF N. & NOORDERGRAAF A. (1970) Arterial viscoelasticity: A generalized model. Effect on input impedance and wave travel in the systemic tree. *J. Biomech.*, **3**, 357–379.

WOMERSLEY J.R. (1957) An elastic tube theory of pulse transmission and oscillatory flow in mammalian arteries. *Wright Air Development Tech. Rept.* WADC-TR, 56–614.

INDEX